THE CANADIAN PAEDIATRIC SOCIETY

Guide to

Caring

for Your

Child from

Birth to Age

Five

THE CANADIAN PAEDIATRIC SOCIETY

Guide to
Caring
for Your
Child from
Birth to Age
Five

Collins

Canadian
Paediatric
Society

Diane Sacks, MD, FRCPC, Editor-in-Chief

The Canadian Paediactric Society Guide to Caring for Your Child from Birth to Age Five
Copyright © 2009 by the Canadian Paediatric Society
All rights reserved.

Published by Collins, an imprint of HarperCollins Publishers Ltd.

Originally published by John Wiley & Sons Canada, Ltd.: 2012
First published by HarperCollins Publishers Ltd in this Collins trade paperback edition: 2014

This publication contains the opinions and ideas of its author(s) and is designed to provide useful information in regard to the subject matter covered. The author(s) and publisher are not engaged in rendering
medical, therapeutic, or other services in this publication. This publication is not intended to provide
a basis for action in particular circumstances without consideration by a competent professional. The
author(s) and publisher expressly disclaim any responsibility for any liability, loss, or risk, personal or
otherwise, which is incurred as a consequence, directly or indirectly, of the use and application of any of
the contents of this book.

HarperCollins books may be purchased for educational, business, or sales promotional use through our
Special Markets Department.

HarperCollins Publishers Ltd
2 Bloor Street East, 20th Floor
Toronto, Ontario, Canada
M4W 1A8

www.harpercollins.ca

Library and Archives Canada Cataloguing in Publication Data is available upon request.

ISBN 978-1-44342-788-3

Printed and bound in the United States
RRD 9 8 7 6 5 4 3 2 1

Table of Contents

273 CHAPTER 5: Off to School: Ages Four and Five

373 CHAPTER 7: Keeping Your Child Safe

459 APPENDIX

LIST OF QUICK REFERENCE TABLES

About the Canadian Paediatric Society

OUR MISSION

The Canadian Paediatric Society is the national association of paediatricians, committed to working together to advance the health of children and youth by nurturing excellence in health care, advocacy, education, research, and support of its membership.

WHO WE ARE

As a voluntary professional association, the CPS represents more than 2,500 paediatricians, paediatric subspecialists, paediatric residents, and other people who work with and care for children and youth.

WHAT WE DO

- **Advocacy.** The CPS works to improve public policy that affects the health of children and youth.

- **Public education.** The CPS helps parents and caregivers make informed decisions about their children's health by producing reliable and accessible health information.

- **Professional education.** The CPS supports the continuing learning needs of paediatricians and other child and youth health professionals through position statements, a peer-reviewed journal, and educational events.

- **Surveillance and research.** The CPS monitors rare diseases and conditions, and ensures continued research into vaccine-associated adverse reactions and vaccine-preventable diseases.

Because the needs are so great, the CPS also works with many other organizations to promote the health of children and youth.

ON THE INTERNET

www.cps.ca This is the primary online home of the Canadian Paediatric Society. Visit this site to access position statements—written by the country's leading paediatricians—on a range of child health topics, and to learn more about the organization.

www.caringforkids.cps.ca Caring for Kids is the CPS website for parents and caregivers. On Caring for Kids, you'll find more than 150 documents with practical, easy-to-use information on pregnancy and babies, healthy bodies, immunization, safety and injury prevention, growing and learning, behaviour and development, childhood illnesses, teen health, and much more. You can also sign up for a monthly electronic newsletter dedicated to child health and well-being. To access the French version of the site, Soins de nos enfants, visit www.soinsdenosenfants.cps.ca.

Editorial Advisory Board

The Canadian Paediatric Society Guide to Caring for Your Child from Birth to Age Five reflects the collective wisdom and experience of some of Canada's most respected paediatricians. Led by Dr. Diane Sacks, the Editorial Advisory Board reviewed all the content in this book, providing insight and expertise from years of caring for Canadian children and youth. We also enlisted the help of a number of experts for specific topics.

We are indebted to the Canadian Paediatric Society's many committees who, over the years, have produced guidelines and information on a vast range of topics affecting the health and well-being of children and youth. Their work forms the backbone for many of the recommendations and guidance on these pages. The CPS is grateful to committee members past and present for their dedication and commitment.

Editor-in-Chief

Dr. Diane Sacks, a paediatrician for more than 30 years, has a practice in Toronto and is an assistant professor at the University of Toronto. She is a past president of the Canadian Paediatric Society, and currently chairs the CPS Mental Health Task Force. With a special interest in both mental health and adolescent medicine, Dr. Sacks has been involved with organizations such as the Canadian Attention Deficit Hyperactivity

Disorder Resource Alliance (CADDRA), the Canadian Association of Adolescent Health, and the American Academy of Pediatrics. She was involved in the development of guidelines for diagnosing depression in primary care. Dr. Sacks appears regularly in newspapers, magazines and on television, speaking about a range of issues affecting the health and well-being of children and youth.

Members

Dr. Krista Baerg is a consultant paediatrician in the Division of General Pediatrics at the Royal University Hospital in Saskatoon, Saskatchewan. She is also an assistant professor of paediatrics at the University of Saskatchewan, where she completed her medical degree and speciality training in paediatrics as well as a bachelor of science in nursing prior to entering medicine.

Dr. Shirley Blaichman has practised paediatrics at the Montreal Children's Hospital and in her community practice since 1980. The parent of four young adults, Dr. Blaichman says, "I understand how parenting is one of life's greatest challenges and joys. I hope that this book will help guide parents through the early childhood years."

Dr. Leona Fishman-Shapiro practises consultant paediatrics in the community and is on staff part-time at Toronto's Hospital for Sick Children in the division of clinical and metabolic genetics, and at North York (Ontario) General Hospital. Married with two grown children, Dr. Fishman is originally from Montreal, where she trained in genetics at McGill University. She later went to the University of Toronto to study paediatrics and paediatric endocrinology.

Dr. Fabian Gorodzinsky has practised paediatrics in London, Ontario, for nearly 30 years and also serves the nearby communities of Goderich and Clinton. He is an associate professor of paediatrics at the University of Western Ontario, with a special interest in learning disabilities and attention deficit disorder. Dr. Gorodzinsky is a former member of the CPS Community Paediatrics Committee and serves on the Public Education Subcommittee. He has been organizing medical relief missions to Honduras for the last 10 years. Dr. Gorodzinsky has three grown children and three grandchildren.

Dr. Bob Issenman is a professor of paediatrics at McMaster University and Chief of Pediatric Gastroenterology and Nutrition at McMaster Children's Hospital in Hamilton, Ontario. A long-time active member of the Canadian Paediatric Society, Dr. Issenman is a past president of the Board of Directors. He is currently president of the CPS charitable foundation Healthy Generations. Dr. Issenman was educated at Harvard, McGill, and McMaster universities. His interests include advocacy for children and youth, health promotion through encouragement of early literacy, and appropriate paediatric nutrition and physical activity.

Dr. Ken Schelberg, a community paediatrician in North York, Ontario, is on staff at North York General Hospital and the Hospital for Sick Children. He is an assistant professor at the University of Toronto, where he received his medical degree and training in paediatrics. Dr. Schelberg, who also specializes in adolescent medicine, is married with three children.

Dr. Alyson Shaw is the mother of two young children who are a humbling reminder of the delights and challenges of parenting. She is a consultant paediatrician in the Division of Paediatric Medicine at the Children's Hospital of Eastern Ontario, and an assistant professor of paediatrics at the University of Ottawa. Dr. Shaw's advocacy interest is in early literacy and health promotion, and she is a consultant for the Canadian Paediatric Society's *Read, Speak, Sing* program.

Dr. Henry Ukpeh is a consulting paediatrician at the Kootenay Boundary Regional Hospital in Trail, B.C., and a clinical associate professor of paediatrics at the University of British Columbia. He is the founding president of Kootenay Friends for Children Foundation and author of a 485-page personal-development book, *Only Be Afraid of Standing Still: Practical Lessons from the Lives of Children*, which he uses to conduct seminars on maximizing human potential. He was awarded a Certificate of Merit by the Canadian Paediatric Society for outstanding commitment to the welfare of children and youth in his community in 2005.

Dr. Glen Ward is a community paediatrician practising in White Rock and Langley, B.C. He is also a member of the clinical faculty at the University of British Columbia's Department of Pediatrics. Dr. Ward completed his medical training at McGill University, and did his paediatric residency at Montreal Children's Hospital and the Hospital for Sick Children in Toronto. He notes that his formal paediatric education was supplemented by the birth of twins in 1992, requiring a great deal of retraining! A former member of the Canadian Paediatric Society Board of Directors, Dr. Ward is Chair of the CPS Public Education Subcommittee.

Dr. David Wong is a community paediatrician in Summerside, P.E.I. In addition to his clinical work, he actively advocates for the well-being of children through a monthly column in a local newspaper as well as through his involvement with the Premier's Council on Healthy Child Development. He is also involved in teaching medical students and passing on his knowledge to the next generation. He and his wife have two grown children, both of whom are physicians.

Other Expert Reviewers

The Canadian Paediatric Society is grateful to the following members for their careful review of portions of this book.

Dr. Anne-Claude Bernard-Bonnin
CHU Sainte-Justine
Montreal, Quebec

Dr. Clare Gray
Children's Hospital of Eastern Ontario
Ottawa, Ontario

Dr. John C. LeBlanc
IWK Health Centre
Halifax, Nova Scotia

Dr. Jorge L. Pinzon
Alberta Children's Hospital
Calgary, Alberta

Dr. Ted Prince
Alberta Children's Hospital
Calgary, Alberta

Dr. Michelle Ward
Children's Hospital of Eastern Ontario
Ottawa, Ontario

How to Use This Book

Raising your child is a journey that spans many years. This book covers the years from birth (and before) to age five. Many of the age-related chapters start with the developmental milestones your child will meet during each stage, but don't be afraid to flip back or skip ahead. Children develop at their own rate, so you may want to recall information from the last few months or find out what's in store for the next year.

The age-related chapters are followed by chapters that deal with issues that are relevant at every age: common illnesses, your child's safety, and emotional health and well-being. Although age-specific aspects of these issues are dealt with in the first five chapters, the final three chapters provide comprehensive information.

This book is meant to be used as a reference you can turn back to any time you have a question, as well as read chapter by chapter. Many of the unique tools will enable you to quickly access answers to specific questions.

FIVE QUESTIONS FOR THE FIRST WEEK

When you're poised over your newborn with one hand holding him steady and the other hand holding a perplexing diaper mess, you probably won't want to casually search through the index to find out what on earth it is. That's what "Five Questions for the First Week" is for. In one convenient spot (pages 40-41), you can find the answers to the questions you're bound to have in the first week: how many diapers he'll go through, and what they'll look like; how often he'll sleep and eat; how much he'll cry, and what you can do about it; and what will affect his skin, and how you should care for it.

QUICK REFERENCE TABLES

Quick, how much should your two-year-old be sleeping? What should you do if you think she has pinkeye? The answers are all in here somewhere, but sometimes a table is more convenient when you need to find the information again. Quick reference tables appear throughout the book (see page xiv for a list of the tables we have included and their page numbers), summarizing the information in the text so you can easily find out when your newborn should get her first vaccinations and what they should be, or how many wet and dirty diapers she should have at different stages. As we stress, however, the range of normal and healthy in a child's physical and emotional development is wide, so be sure to read more about the topic if you have any concerns.

MAKE A NOTE, MAKE AN APPOINTMENT, OR GO TO THE HOSPITAL?

A doctor's waiting room or emergency room can be a lifeline when you're worried about your child's health, but they can also be unhealthy, unpleasant places to hang out. If your child doesn't really need to be there, you could be giving him lots of care and attention comfortably at home. To save yourself time and stress, look for the "Make a Note, Make an Appointment, or Go to the Hospital?" boxes in this book. These will let you know when your child's symptoms warrant an appointment with his doctor or a trip to the emergency room, and when you can wait to mention them at his next well-child visit.

DR. SACKS SAYS

Dr. Diane Sacks has helped a lot of parents raise healthy children, and she's seen it all. Look for the boxes offering her no-nonsense words of wisdom that will help you put your priorities in order. For instance, keeping your child strapped into her car seat is imperative; keeping up with the Joneses' bizarrely talented kids is not worth the effort.

MYTH BUSTERS

Whether it's on the Internet or courtesy of your ever-helpful neighbour, new parents are inundated with a lot of advice and information. Highlighted in boxes throughout the book, our Myth Busters help you sort out the truth from the rumours and folklore.

YOUR CHILD'S DEVELOPMENT

Throughout the text you'll find many references to when children are expected to meet certain developmental milestones. These milestones are also provided in a chart in the Appendix so that you can easily check how your child is doing and what you should be prepared for next. Remember, though, that these are just guidelines, and your child probably won't meet all of them at exactly the times noted. Your doctor will be able to tell you whether your child is developing at a healthy rate.

RESOURCES

This book covers a lot of ground, but it can't cover everything—nor should it, given that some information changes regularly. Also, there are specific professionals who can give you much more information on some subjects than we can. So when you need to find the most up-to-date children's product recalls or if you suspect your child has asthma and want to know more, we'll direct you to the Resources section in the Appendix, where you'll find relevant websites and books that the Canadian Paediatric Society considers reliable.

Introduction

Your child's health and safety will be your priority for years to come and, as a mother of three grown-up children, I can tell you that never changes. In my 35 years as a paediatrician, I have been very fortunate to have been asked by families to accompany them on their child's journey to adulthood. What a privilege! I could never have done this without the parents who were willing to work hand in hand with me and share their wishes and concerns for their children. We walked together; sometimes they led, sometimes I took the lead, but the goal of a healthy, happy child always guided the way.

However, in recent years I have noted that with the thousands of experts, TV shows, books, and websites claiming to "teach" people how to parent their children, parents have become less confident, and they have less fun raising their kids. It is more important than ever for parents to join with their child's healthcare providers to sort through this information and distill the knowledge that's really relevant to their child's health and development.

This book is designed to help parents participate fully in this endeavour. It will give you current, basic knowledge of the wide, wide range of normal that we see in children. It will provide you with comprehensive information on every aspect of your child's health, for every stage of his life from birth to the age of five. It will guide you on when and where to seek help. It will help you formulate the questions you may want to ask your child's doctor about growth and development, health, nutrition, and injury prevention, and will help you get the most out of your visits to the doctor. It is never appropriate to leave a medical appointment with your questions unanswered. Sometimes it may mean scheduling another visit for when the doctor has more time, but you should always leave the office with the answers you need or a plan for action.

Did you know that one of the original meanings of the word doctor is "teacher"? The doctor you choose to care for your children should be a resource you can draw upon to help you with the health issues that come up during your child's early years. One of the main reasons the Canadian Paediatric Society decided to write this book was to help ensure parents make the most of this relationship. Family health care is more than a one- or two-person job. It's a team effort: parents, caregivers, physicians, and other healthcare providers, all working together to keep your child healthy. The role of the physician includes

- seeing that your child's growth and development are occurring as expected;
- picking up early signs of potential health problems;
- educating you about your child's nutritional, emotional, and physical needs;
- being knowledgeable about current health innovations that could be important for your child;
- having a network of professionals to call upon when and if your child has other needs; and
- preventing problems and promoting healthy development by

    · providing up-to-date information on childhood immunizations;
    · providing nutritional information;

· providing up-to-date information on safety and injury prevention; and

· identifying possible emotional health issues that may affect your child.

The role of the parent includes

- becoming knowledgeable on issues that affect your child, and staying up-to-date through reliable sources;
- knowing yourself and your limits;
- becoming your child's advocate;
- joining with trusted healthcare professionals to keep your child healthy;
- knowing and appreciating your child; and
- having appropriate expectations of your child (and forgetting about the neighbour's genius kids).

One of a parent's most important duties is to become informed about children's health in general, and their child in particular. We want to give parents the essential knowledge they need to feel confident when it comes to the health and safety of their children. No one knows your child as well as you do, and your instincts are almost always right. With the information provided here, you'll have the confidence to know when to trust your instincts.

I hope this book gives you a good foundation in children's health. The information on growth and development, health, nutrition, and injury prevention in Chapters Two through Five, as well as the development chart in the Appendix, applies to all young children, but remember that every child is unique. Just ask any parent with more than one child, or look to your own siblings. Active children often need a different approach than those who are very quiet, for instance. Children with specific conditions and disabilities will need a more customized approach. By giving you a foundation on which to learn about your own child's needs, this book can become a very personalized resource.

Even the most informed parent still needs to rely on medical experts. Medical science changes as rapidly as your child grows. (Even during the writing of this book, new immunizations were brought to the public.) This book is a great starting point to help you ask the right questions and give you an idea of where to turn for the answers. Because it's based largely on information developed by the Canadian Paediatric Society, which I had the honour of leading in 2003, and has been written and reviewed in collaboration with a team of paediatricians from across Canada, this book provides you with guidance you can trust. You'll also find additional information on many topics in Resources, located at the end of the book, as well as on the Canadian Paediatric Society website for parents, Caring for Kids: www.caringforkids.cps.ca.

Chapters One through Five deal with the different stages of your child's life up to age five, but because many health issues are common to children of all ages, we have included additional information on illnesses and safety in Chapters Six and Seven. Finally, because your child's emotional and mental health is just as important as her physical health, we have included a chapter on emotional health and well-being. This chapter is intended to help parents feel comfortable talking about these issues. If stigma surrounding mental health issues still exists, we hope to eradicate it. Knowledge should empower parents to seek the care their children need. The more confident parents are, the more likely they will be to give their children space to thrive and become the happy and healthy people we all want them to be.

—*Diane Sacks, MD, FRCPC, FAAP*

Preparing for Your Baby

Pregnancy is an exciting time, full of anticipation and amazement, whether you're pregnant for the first time or the fourth. It's also a time of planning. Having everything you need in place before the big day definitely makes the first few days of parenthood easier, but it's just as important to be emotionally prepared. The more you can do to prepare your home and your head before the due date, the easier it will be to make the transition into a completely new routine. Part of your preparation will be to assemble your team of eager assistants: healthcare providers, friends, and family who can offer you and your baby expert advice, emotional support, and a little help around the home when you need it. Luckily, the Canadian medical system offers a network of experts who are ready to help you prepare for your birth and advise you as you raise a healthy, happy child.

INCLUDED IN THIS CHAPTER

BUILDING YOUR TEAM OF EXPERTS

In the months and years ahead, you will receive a lot of support and encouragement from your healthcare providers. An obstetrician, family doctor, or midwife can see you through pregnancy; a paediatrician or that same family doctor can help care for your child. If you are considering a midwife for the delivery, you'll still want a doctor to monitor your pregnancy. (In British Columbia, midwives are independent providers, so they will not involve a family doctor unless there are concerns about a birth.) Your doctor can answer any questions you might have about your own health during your pregnancy, and can treat your child after she is born.

If you don't already have one, you should start looking for a paediatrician or family doctor early on in pregnancy so you can talk to her about any questions or concerns you have before your baby comes. Word-of-mouth is one of the most effective ways to find a doctor, so ask friends who have children about their doctors. If your local hospital has a family practice unit, they may be able to help you find a doctor. You can also look in the Yellow Pages under "physicians and surgeons." If you're having a difficult time finding a doctor, contact your province's college of physicians and surgeons or your territory's government. The provincial colleges grant licences to doctors, and many have referral services that help people find doctors who are accepting new patients. Good communication is essential for good medical care, so if English is not your first language, ask your local community centre or immigrant assistance agency for a list of doctors who speak your language.

Once you find a doctor, schedule an appointment so you can meet her. Some things you'll want to know are listed below.

- What are the office hours?
- How many other doctors are in the practice?
- What hospital does she send patients to?

- How long will it usually take to get an appointment?
- Is there a medical lab or X-ray facilities in the building or nearby where tests can be done?
- Whom do you call after hours and for emergencies?
- How does she provide on-call service, and who is likely to attend the labour and delivery?

Also ask yourself if you feel comfortable talking to the doctor. Did she answer all your questions? Remember, it takes time to build a relationship with your doctor.

Schedule of well-child visits

Age	Visit Details
1 week	Sometime in the first week after you and your baby have gone home from the hospital, your baby will have his first doctor's visit. The doctor will ask how feeding is going, how your family is adjusting, and if you have any concerns. He will also complete any tests that weren't done while you were in the hospital, examine your baby to check his general health, weigh him, and check him for jaundice.
2 months	
4 months	
6 months	
9 months (optional)	When you take your child to a well-child visit, the appointment will last 10 to 20 minutes. The doctor will ask about your child's eating habits, developmental milestones, language milestones, and social and emotional issues; do a physical examination; check his weight, height, and head circumference; give him his vaccines; and answer any questions you have.
12 to 13 months	
15 months (optional)	
18 months	
2 years	
3 years	
4 years	
5 years	

Once your child is 5 years old, he will see the doctor every 1 or 2 years until he is 18 years old.

Source: Adapted from the Rourke Baby Record (www.rourkebabyrecord.ca).

What Is a Paediatrician?

Paediatricians are doctors who have at least four years of additional training after medical school in the care of infants, children, and adolescents. They are certified by the Royal College of Physicians and Surgeons of Canada, and most belong to the Canadian Paediatric Society. Many paediatricians are subspecialists, such as paediatric cardiologists, paediatric surgeons, paediatric allergists, neonatologists, and developmental paediatricians. You can find a paediatrician through your province's college of physicians and surgeons or your territory's government, but in some areas of the country you'll need a referral from a family doctor, usually for a specific problem.

What do paediatricians do?

Paediatricians provide a wide variety of services for children, youth, and their families. Their work with patients runs the gamut from taking care of a seriously ill newborn baby, to helping families make decisions about immunization, to treating a teenager who's been involved in a car accident. Most perform one or more of the duties discussed below.

- **Provide primary health care.** Paediatricians provide day-to-day care to help sick children get better and to prevent healthy children from getting sick. They conduct physical exams, diagnose and treat problems, provide education and advice, and administer immunizations. Paediatricians check that children are reaching their milestones, and can determine whether a child needs to be seen by another health professional for more specialized service.

- **Investigate, diagnose, and manage acute or chronic illness.** Many paediatricians take care of children with complex medical needs, including long-term disabilities or conditions such as asthma, ADHD, Crohn's disease, cystic fibrosis, diabetes, heart disease, and mental health problems. They also support the families of children with chronic illnesses.

- **Promote health.** Paediatricians provide guidance on issues such as injury prevention, nutrition, physical activity, and behaviour. They do this with patients and parents, through the media, and by working with other healthcare professionals, the public, and government.

- **Research new treatments.** Paediatricians conduct research that contributes to new treatments and approaches for disorders in children.

- **Evaluate treatment measures.** Paediatricians assess current therapies and approaches for paediatric disorders to check that they are appropriate.

- **Collaborate with other professionals.** Paediatricians work with other professionals who care for children, including child protection workers, teachers, and psychologists.

- **Advocate for children and youth.** Paediatricians give presentations to community and parent groups, and talk to politicians about improving services for children.

THE BIG DECISIONS

Before your due date, you're going to have to make some big decisions: whether to breastfeed, whether you'll use cloth or disposable diapers, and, if you're expecting a boy, whether to have him circumcised. The busy days following childbirth are not the best time to make these decisions. If you discuss these things with your partner well ahead of time and are comfortable with your decisions, you'll be able to focus only on your baby in his first days.

Breastfeeding

Perhaps the most important decision you'll make before your baby is born is whether you are going to breastfeed. The Canadian Paediatric Society, Health Canada, and the World Health Organization all recommend that new mothers breastfeed exclusively for a baby's first six months of life. After that, your baby will begin to eat a variety of foods, but you can continue to breastfeed until the age of two years or older. The benefits of nursing are many: breast milk is nutritionally balanced, it contains antibodies that help babies fight off sickness and infection, and it's easy on their digestive systems, which means there's less chance of constipation and diarrhea. Once your breastfeeding routine is established, it's an easy and convenient way to feed your baby.

As a mother, you'll also benefit from breastfeeding. Nursing right after birth causes your pituitary gland to release the hormone oxytocin, which then causes your uterus to contract. These contractions reduce the likelihood of postpartum haemorrhaging and encourage the uterus to go back to its pre-pregnancy state. Perhaps most importantly, the skin-to-skin contact during breastfeeding creates a powerful bond between you and your baby.

Breastfeeding doesn't come easily to every new mom. It can take a while for both you and your baby to figure things out. Before you leave the hospital, ask the nurses or your midwife for guidance. They can introduce you to a lactation consultant, a specialist who can show you how to breastfeed and help if you have problems.

Having supplies and information ready before you bring your baby home will also make the early days of breastfeeding easier. A breastfeeding pillow, a curved pillow designed especially for nursing, can make you and your baby more comfortable during feeding. Lanolin cream helps if your nipples become sore, a very common problem in the early days of breastfeeding. For peace of mind, ask your doctor for the number of a good breastfeeding clinic or lactation consultant so you can call an expert if you have questions.

Naturally, mom will be doing most of the feeding for the first few months, but there may be times when you won't be able to breastfeed. Your partner will also want to spend time feeding your baby. A breast pump, either manual or electric, can help you express milk so you can maintain your milk supply. It lets your partner participate in feedings, as well as giving you time to take a shower (you'll be surprised at how much of a challenge it can be to find the time!). It also means that you can confidently leave your baby with someone else for more than a couple of hours if you need to. (For information on breastfeeding for the working mother, see page 161 in Chapter Three.) Pumps can be expensive, but you can rent them, or you may know someone who can lend you her pump. You'll also need some bottles to hold the extra milk.

Diapers

The choice between cloth and disposable diapers is really just a matter of preference. Both have many benefits and drawbacks, and the question of which one is better for the environment and for your baby is still the subject of much debate. Disposable diapers are more convenient than cloth, are good at moving moisture away from the skin to prevent diaper rash, and are less likely to leak. You'll have to buy thousands of diapers for your baby, however, adding to municipal solid waste.

Cloth diapers can be more affordable if you wash them yourself, and they can be more environmentally friendly because they don't go in the garbage. But if the thought of washing them is enough to convince you to opt for disposables, you may be able to use a diaper service. Diaper services are a great solution for those who want to use cloth but don't want to deal with the laundry, and the cost is about the same as buying disposables. Despite their eco-friendly reputation, it takes a lot of energy and water to wash and dry cloth diapers properly.

From your baby's point of view, cloth does a good job as long as you change her shortly after the diaper is soiled. Babies who use disposables may get diaper rash less often. Diaper rash is caused by wet skin and prolonged contact with urine and stool, so regardless of the type of diaper you choose, the key is to change them often.

Baby wipes are a popular product for cleaning up at diapering time, but along with the excess waste they produce, they're also unnecessary. A warm, damp washcloth is efficient, environmentally sound, and almost always non-irritating.

Circumcision

If you're having a boy (or if you don't know yet, but want to be prepared), it's a good idea to decide before the birth whether you want to have him circumcised. Circumcision is a surgical procedure to remove the layer of skin (called the foreskin or prepuce) that covers the head (glans) of the penis and part of the shaft. It is usually done during the first few days after birth. Circumcision is a non-therapeutic procedure, which means it is not medically necessary. It also means the cost of circumcision is not covered by provincial/territorial health care.

The Canadian Paediatric Society has reviewed the evidence for and against circumcision, and does not recommend it for newborn boys. (For the CPS's position statement on circumcision, see "Publications & Resources" at www.cps.ca.) However, parents who decide to circumcise their newborns often do so for religious or cultural reasons, rather than health reasons. You should know about the benefits of circumcision and the problems that can occur from the procedure before making your decision.

Risks and benefits of circumcision

Problems from the surgery are usually minor. Although serious complications are rare, they do occur. Of every 1,000 boys who are circumcised, 20 to 30 will have a surgical complication, such as an infection or too much bleeding; two or three will have a more serious complication, such as having too much skin removed or serious bleeding; and about 10 babies will need to have the circumcision done again because of a poor result.

The benefits of circumcision are also minor. Of every 1,000 boys who are not circumcised, seven will be admitted to hospital for a urinary tract infection before they are one year of age (compared with two circumcised boys), and 10 will have a circumcision later in life for medical reasons, such as a condition called phimosis (a narrowness of the opening of the foreskin). When older children are circumcised, they may need a general anaesthetic, and they may have more complications than newborns. Circumcision slightly lowers the risk of developing cancer of the penis in later life, but this form of cancer is very rare: one of every one million men who are circumcised will develop penile cancer each year, while three men who are not circumcised will develop it. There is also some recent evidence that circumcision may lower the risk of HIV.

If you decide to have your baby boy circumcised

Newborn babies do feel pain, and studies have shown that the amount of pain they experience depends on the circumcision method used (the Mogen clamp seems to cause less pain than the Plastibell or Gomco technique). Talk to your baby's doctor about the different methods before deciding. Your baby will also need pain relief—without pain relief, circumcision is very traumatic for babies (and probably for you too). Your baby will need a local anaesthetic given by a needle, and he should receive acetaminophen, such as Tempra or Tylenol, to relieve discomfort when the local anaesthetic wears off. The needle can cause bruising or swelling, and anaesthetics can carry risks, so talk to your doctor first so you know what to expect. Giving your baby a pacifier or gauze soaked with a sugar solution may also help reduce his pain.

After the circumcision, the penis will take a few days to heal. The area may be red for a few days and you may see some yellow discharge, but that should decrease as it heals. Keep the area as clean as possible, washing gently with mild soap and water, and be sure to clean away any bits of stool. If there is a bandage, change it each time you change your baby's diaper, and use petroleum jelly to keep the bandage from sticking. The best comfort you can give your baby is to hold him and nurse him often.

> ## MAKE A NOTE, MAKE AN APPOINTMENT, OR GO TO THE HOSPITAL?
>
> **Make an appointment** with your baby's doctor if you see more than a few drops of blood at any time during the healing process, the redness and swelling around the circumcision doesn't start to go down within 48 hours, your baby develops a fever (rectal temperature of 38.0°C/100.4°F or higher), or he seems to be sick.

DATE OF DELIVERY

When the day of your baby's arrival finally comes, be ready for it by having your bag packed in advance. (You might want to do it well in advance—some babies do arrive early!) Don't forget the diapers: some hospitals do not provide diapers, so bring some newborn diapers with you. Pack a receiving blanket, a couple of newborn sleepers, a hat, and booties for your new baby. You should also bring sanitary pads, a nursing bra, and comfortable clothing for yourself. And, of course, the camera.

The Apgar Test

One minute after your baby is born, and again at five minutes after birth, she will receive her first test: the Apgar test. Developed by anaesthesiologist Virginia Apgar in 1952, the test's name is also an acronym: Activity, Pulse, Grimace, Appearance, Respiration. Your baby will be given a score between 0 and 2 in each area, for a total score out of 10. The test quickly evaluates her physical condition right after delivery so that doctors can identify if she requires emergency care.

The Apgar scores are determined as follows:

Activity (muscle tone)

0 — Limp and floppy; no movement

1 — Some flexing of arms and legs

2 — Active, spontaneous movement

Pulse (heart rate)

0 — No heart rate

1 — Fewer than 100 beats per minute

2 — At least 100 beats per minute

Grimace (reflex response)

0 — No response to stimulation

1 — Facial movement only with stimulation

2 — Grimace and pull away, cough, or sneeze with stimulation

Appearance (colour)

0 — The baby's whole body is bluish-grey or pale

1 — Good colour in body, but bluish hands or feet

2 — Good colour all over, including hands and feet

Respiration (breathing)

0 — Not breathing

1 — Weak cry, like whimpering; slow or irregular breathing

2 — Strong cry; normal rate and effort of breathing

A score between 7 and 10 means a baby is in good health and doesn't need additional intervention beyond routine post-delivery care. A baby who scores between 4 and 6 might need some special immediate care, such as some oxygen or suctioning of the nose to help her breathe. A score of 3 or lower requires immediate lifesaving measures, such as resuscitation. Some babies—those born by Caesarean section, or those who are premature or who have a heart or lung condition—will have lower-than-normal Apgar scores.

The Apgar test does not predict long-term health, intellectual capacity, or behaviour in any way. Even the healthiest babies rarely achieve a perfect 10, and most babies who score lower than 7 on the Apgar test do just fine.

BRINGING HOME BABY

Preparing Your Home

One thing you'll quickly realize about having a baby is that you need a lot of stuff just to feed, clothe, protect, and amuse him. (Why does a 7-pound infant require 300 pounds of equipment, anyway?) Setting up your home for your new child is a significant task that requires lots of research, so start early. To help you get started, we've included a shopping list of the essentials at the end of this chapter.

What to consider when you're looking for the most important equipment—the car seat, the crib, and the first-aid kit—is described below. Safety standards are constantly changing and improving, so if you plan to use second-hand equipment, make sure it meets current standards. Visit Health Canada's website regularly to ensure that the furniture, toys, and equipment you have meet current safety standards and to check for advisories and recalls. For directions to Health Canada's website and other sites that offer guidance on safe toys and equipment, see "Product Safety" in Resources.

Car seat safety

The first safety issue you'll encounter is making sure your baby is safe in the car for his ride home from the hospital. For at least the first year, your baby must be in a rear-facing infant car seat every time he travels in the car, from the moment you get in to the moment you're ready to leave the vehicle. It may be tempting to save money by getting a used seat, but many seats now have expiry dates because the plastic can become brittle after just a few years. Never re-use a car seat that has been in a car crash, however minor.

The way to correctly install and use car seats has changed a lot in recent years and will probably continue to change. If you have any doubts about installing and using yours, your local public health unit, police department, or fire department can help you figure it out. In some communities, local fire or police departments hold clinics to make sure car seats are properly installed and correctly used. Try to attend these clinics every time you install a new car seat.

Before using your car seat, check that the label indicates that the car seat is appropriate for infants. Car seats don't fit the same in every vehicle, so also make sure it fits well in the rear seat. Read and follow the manufacturer's and your vehicle's instruction manuals carefully, and install it according to the instructions. Install the seat in the "kid zone"—the middle of the back seat. A child should never be in the front of a vehicle or near a front passenger air bag. Once it's installed, you shouldn't be able to move the seat more than 2.5 centimetres (1 inch) forward or from side to side.

Your baby's position in the car seat is important too. Harness straps must be snug and threaded at or just below his shoulders, and the chest clip must be at armpit level. If you can put more than one finger between the shoulder harness and your baby's collarbone, the harness is too loose. A bunting bag keeps the harness too loose and prevents it from being properly secured between a baby's legs, so take the bunting bag off before putting your baby in the car seat. If it's cold, tuck a blanket over him after he is secured with the harness, not before.

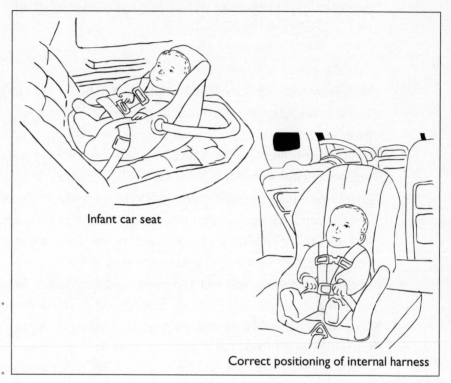

Infant car seat

Correct positioning of internal harness

**Figure 1.1:
Rear-facing
seats**

Source: *Well Beings: A Guide to Health in Child Care*, 3rd Edition. Canadian Paediatric Society, 2008.

SAFETY DOESN'T STOP WITH THE SEAT

Once your baby is secure, you'll still need to watch out for him. Don't put the car seat on the trunk or roof of the car when your baby is in it, don't leave him in the car seat to sleep, and never leave him alone in the car. In hot weather, children can get heatstroke in a closed car; in cold weather, they can get hypothermia, or if the car's exhaust pipe is blocked by snow or the car is left idling in the garage, they can die from carbon monoxide poisoning.

Car seat safety will be an ongoing concern until your child is at least eight years of age, so check Transport Canada's website regularly for age-specific guidelines, as well as travel-related product advisories and recalls (see "Travel" in Resources).

A safe place to sleep

Your baby's crib is his most important piece of furniture. For his first six months, the safest place for him to sleep is on his back in a crib in his parents' room—as long as the crib meets all current safety standards and you take some precautions. Any crib made before 1986, when government safety regulations changed, is not safe. Whether your crib is new or used, check that it has a permanent label with the manufacturer's name, model number or model name, date of manufacture, instructions for assembly, and a warning statement about mattress size and proper crib use. If you have a used crib, buy a lead test kit at a paint, hardware, or home improvement store, and test the paint on the crib. Babies will mouth anything in reach, including the crib rails, so they can be poisoned by lead-based paint. If it does contain lead, strip the old paint and repaint with high-quality enamel paint.

When you're shopping for a crib, look for a few important safety features. Make sure the crib bars are no more than 6 centimetres (2⅜ inches) apart, are securely fastened, and are all present. Corner posts should be either no higher than 3 millimetres (⅛ inches) above the top of the end panels or, with four-poster–style cribs, should be too high to catch on clothing. Simple is safe: there should be no cut-out designs in the head or footboards, or openings between the corner post and top rail—anywhere a baby could get his head stuck.

Dr. Sacks Says

There is no compromise with a crib: first comes safety and security, then comes style.

The drop-side latches should lock securely in place when the side is raised. The mattress support hangers should be secured with bolts or closed hooks—don't use a crib where these hooks are Z- or S-shaped. These fixtures should all be tight and strong. The mattress should fit tightly within the crib frame. If there is more than 3 centimetres (1¾₆ inches) between the mattress and crib side when you push it toward a corner, the mattress is too small. A baby can get his head caught in that space and suffocate.

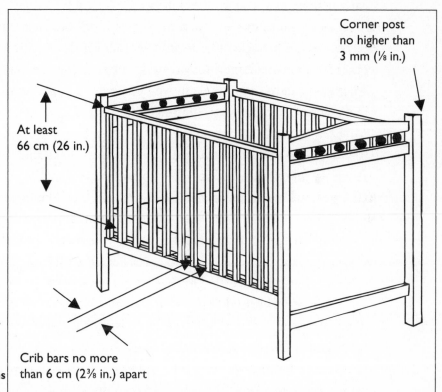

Figure 1.2: Crib safety specifications

Corner post no higher than 3 mm (⅛ in.)

At least 66 cm (26 in.)

Crib bars no more than 6 cm (2⅜ in.) apart

Source: *Crib Safety*. Health Canada, 2003. © Adapted and reproduced with the permission of the Minister of Public Works and Government Services Canada, 2008.

Take a good look around your baby's room before deciding where to place the crib. You might feel like giving your baby a great view, but window coverings and blind cords are hazards. Place the crib away from windows, and don't let any strings or cords dangle in or near the crib. The mattress should be firm and flat with well-fitting crib sheets. Don't use bumper pads, and keep pillows, lambskins, quilts, and comforters out of the crib as they could cause overheating, suffocation, and sudden infant death syndrome (SIDS). (For information on SIDS, see page 66 in Chapter Two.) For the same reason, even stuffed toys should be kept out of the crib. Hang mobiles out of reach, fastened solidly on both sides of the crib, and remove them as soon as your baby is four months old or can push up on his hands and knees.

Bassinets and cradles used to be common, but now they are not recommended because there are no safety standards for them, and infants outgrow them quickly. At only three months old, your baby's increasing weight, strength, and active movement make it possible to fall or tip in a cradle.

Stocking your first-aid kit

A well-stocked first-aid kit will help you calmly handle any illness or emergency. Pre-packaged children's first-aid kits contain many of the essential items, but no store-bought kit will contain everything you need, so start with a pre-packaged kit and add to it as necessary. Put together a first-aid kit for your diaper bag too, and keep the kits in securely locked boxes so that curious little hands can't get into them.

You may never need to use some of these things (and you probably won't use some of them until your child is a little older), but you should have them on hand. Familiarize yourself with how to use everything—how to take your baby's temperature and how to administer pain relief, for instance—so you'll feel calm and confident if a situation arises.

Your first-aid kit should include everything on this list.

- An assortment of adhesive bandages
- Cotton gauze with non-allergic gauze tape
- Hydrogen peroxide to clean cuts and scrapes

- Antibiotic ointment for burns, cuts, and scrapes
- Tweezers
- Sharp scissors
- A couple of pairs of non-latex or vinyl gloves
- Pain medication (acetaminophen or ibuprofen—**not** aspirin). Carefully check dosage and age requirements, and do not use on a baby younger than three months unless instructed to by a physician.
- Antihistamine for allergic reactions
- Saline drops to loosen mucus in a stuffy nose
- Thermometer
- Petroleum jelly (for use with a rectal thermometer)
- Liquid soap or gel hand sanitizer
- If your baby is allergic to peanuts or shellfish, or has any other life-threatening allergy, keep a dose of his emergency medicine in here. Also send a dose with your baby wherever he goes, and keep one on yourself.
- A small, easy-to-read first-aid manual
- A list of names and phone numbers of emergency contacts. This may be the most important thing in your first-aid kit. It should be clearly printed or typed, and attached to the inside lid or other visible area of the kit, as well as beside all telephones. Include the following people:

  - Your family doctor or paediatrician
  - Your local hospital
  - Alternate caregivers, such as grandparents or aunts and uncles
  - The local or provincial poison control hotline
  - Your local police and fire squads
  - Two close neighbours (in case you need emergency assistance such as a ride to the hospital or child care for a sibling)
  - Your contact information (all numbers) in case of emergency

Don't rely on your excellent memory to remember these numbers in an emergency. Post them in a central area of your home and program them into your cell phone too, as you'll often forget them in a panic.

Dr. Sacks Says

Taking a first-aid course before your baby is born is truly one of the most important things you can do to prepare for parenthood.

Babyproofing your home

Your baby won't really be mobile for the first several months of her life, but it doesn't hurt to put some of these measures in place well before you need them. She may roll over or crawl for the first time when you're not looking, and stairs, wall sockets, and loose wires are all potential hazards for a baby on the move. Taking these precautions before there is a baby in your home will give you peace of mind. Look at your home from a baby's perspective: get down on your hands and knees to find potential hazards your adult eyes might not normally see.

The suggestions below are for the first 12 months, but childproofing is an ongoing process. Start with the basic precautions and continue to modify and add to them according to your baby's development. At times, she will develop new skills overnight, so try to keep one step ahead of her curiosity and ability level. Injury and poisoning are two of the leading causes of death in infants and toddlers, so it is vitally important that you take these suggestions seriously.

Kitchen and dining area

Install cabinet latches on all lower cabinetry and drawers so your baby can't open them. Keep plastic bags stored in a latched cupboard. You might want to make one cabinet accessible with safe playthings like wooden spoons, plastic dishes, and pots and pans. If your baby wants to explore, this might be enough to satisfy her curiosity. As a further precaution, store all cleaning products, including dishwashing liquid, in a locked upper cabinet. That way, even if your baby does manage to invade a cabinet or two, these potentially lethal products are out of reach. Glassware should also be placed in high cupboards. Keep garbage and recycling bins locked or firmly latched so your baby can't get into them, and keep all alcoholic beverages locked away and out of reach.

You can keep stoves and dishwashers from becoming tipping hazards by installing anti-tip brackets that screw into the floor and attach to the bottom of these appliances. Install corner cushions on sharp table and countertop corners. Tablecloths should be secured to the table or replaced with placemats so your baby can't pull them—and whatever is on top of them—onto the ground.

Baby's room and other bedrooms

Once again, the crib is your baby's most important piece of furniture, so make sure it meets government guidelines. Soft fabrics can be dangerous, so limit her bedding to a fitted crib sheet and a light blanket for the first six months of her life. Never allow her to sleep wearing a bib, jewellery, or clothes with strings, and don't fall for those adorable crib pads—they're unnecessary, and they can be dangerous. Avoid using curtain or blind cords, or keep them far away from your baby. Check that knobs on dressers and armoires are securely fastened, and keep drawers closed at all times. In your bedroom, keep small jewellery, perfumes and colognes, shoe polishing materials, belts, scarves, and ties out of reach. And never lock your baby alone in a room.

Bathroom

What seems hot to you can burn your baby's sensitive skin, so install anti-scald devices on your hot water faucets and change the temperature on your hot water heater (Safe Kids Canada recommends 49°C/120°F).

If you have difficulty adjusting the temperature, contact your landlord or local utility company for help.

Put toilet latches on all toilet seats, and keep all medicines, cosmetics, perfumes, and razor blades in a latched cabinet well out of reach of your baby.

Dr. Sacks Says

Don't answer the phone when your baby is not in a secure spot—and never when bathing her. That is why you have voicemail. The real meaning of call waiting? Calls can wait; my baby cannot.

Living room and family room

Securely anchor bookcases, TV cabinets, and other top-heavy furniture to the wall to prevent them from tipping over if your baby hangs or climbs on them once she's mobile. Keep fans and space heaters out of your baby's reach, as she could be severely cut or burned if she comes into contact with them. If you have a fireplace, set up a fireplace guard—even cold ashes can be harmful to your baby's eyes. Move fireplace tools out of your baby's reach, and if you have a stone or brick hearth, it's a good idea to pad the edges.

General whole-home safety

There are lots of little hazards scattered throughout your home. Some are as obvious as staircases and electrical outlets; others you might not even be able to imagine. For instance, paint used in older homes could be lead-based, and there is a chance your baby will eat chipped or peeled paint. Make sure paint on all surfaces is lead-free by using a paint test kit, available at hardware, home improvement, and paint stores. Older homes may also have radiators, which can cause severe burns when touched, so if you have them, consider installing radiator covers. Install electrical outlet plugs over all outlets in your home, including ones on extension cords and powerbars, and wrap and tie all appliance cords.

Use carbon monoxide detectors and smoke detectors on every level of your home. There should be one near each sleeping area. Test them monthly, changing the batteries every six months, or use a long-life battery, which may last up to 10 years. Replace alarms that are more than 10 years old. In some newer homes, smoke alarms may be connected to your home's wiring.

Secure all vent covers to the floor so your baby can't pull them up. Use non-slip carpet tape or non-slip mesh underneath rugs so they don't slide. Try to keep floors clean; given the opportunity, babies will eagerly put small objects in their mouths, which can cause them to choke.

Install safety gates at the top and the bottom of all staircases. Those on the top should be secured into the wall; those at the bottom can be pressure-type gates. Bars on stairway railings should be no more than 10 centimetres (4 inches) apart so your baby can't get her head through them. If they're further apart, replace them, or consider putting in a clear wall made of Plexiglas.

Keep plants out of any area that your baby will be in; even if a plant isn't poisonous, she could choke on leaves and dirt. (For a list of poisonous plants, see page 423 in Chapter Seven.) Put away any fragile or breakable items and knick-knacks or put them up high, well out of your baby's reach. While you might feel like leaving out a couple of these types of items to teach her about being gentle and not touching, it's a lot safer and less frustrating to just remove them until she is older. In the meantime, replacing your crystal vase with a sturdy plastic version will keep baby safe and parents sane.

Windows can be dangerous for two reasons: the risk of your baby falling out, and the risk of strangulation from cords used on drapes and blinds. Install window guards that allow the window to open only a few inches, or opt for double-hung windows and open them from the top down. Keep windows latched at all times when they're not open. Purchase cord winders for blinds and make sure cords are kept well out of reach of your baby.

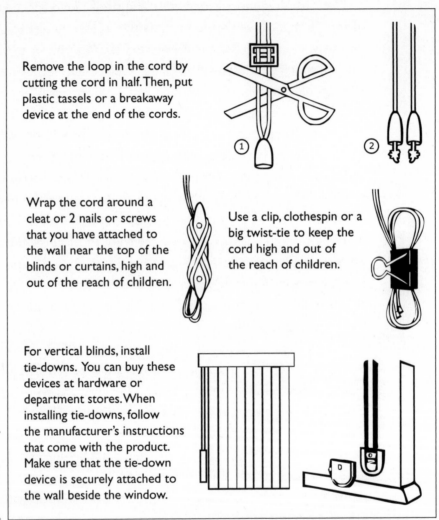

Remove the loop in the cord by cutting the cord in half. Then, put plastic tassels or a breakaway device at the end of the cords.

Wrap the cord around a cleat or 2 nails or screws that you have attached to the wall near the top of the blinds or curtains, high and out of the reach of children.

Use a clip, clothespin or a big twist-tie to keep the cord high and out of the reach of children.

For vertical blinds, install tie-downs. You can buy these devices at hardware or department stores. When installing tie-downs, follow the manufacturer's instructions that come with the product. Make sure that the tie-down device is securely attached to the wall beside the window.

Figure 1.3: Dealing with hanging cords

Source: *Danger! Children Can Strangle on Blind and Curtain Cords*. Health Canada, 2005. © Adapted and reproduced with the permission of the Minister of Public Works and Government Services Canada, 2008.

On doors, avoid metal coil doorstops; the end cap can be a choking hazard, and if you remove the cap, the metal coil can be sharp. Instead, use one-piece plastic or wooden doorstops. Keep exterior doors locked at all times, and make sure screens are locked and have no holes or gaps. Interior doors can be latched with a simple hook and eye mounted high up on the door, to secure any rooms that you don't want your baby getting in once she's mobile, like the bathroom or laundry room. Child-resistant doorknob covers can also prevent children (and some frustrated adults) from opening doors.

Install safety latches on washing machine and dryer lids if they are in an area where your baby has access to them. Keep laundry room supplies, gardening supplies, and pet food in a latched cupboard, and litter boxes in an area entirely out of your baby's reach. To her, that nasty litter box might look like a sandbox at the park. Also, keep purses and briefcases closed and out of reach. Children have an insatiable urge to explore, and these bags are treasure chests to them, but they contain countless hazards, including coins, pens, paper clips, medications, cosmetics, and keys. Pick a specific, secure place for both yours and your guests' purses, knapsacks, and briefcases.

FORMULATING YOUR FIRE ESCAPE PLAN

While you're taking a careful look at your home, it's a good time to create a fire escape plan. Try to plan a main escape route and an alternate route out of every room, if you can. Pick a safe place to meet after exiting your home. Be sure that everyone in your family knows the plan, and that they know to yell "fire!" and leave your home immediately if the alarm goes off or if they hear someone yell. Practise your fire escape plan once every season. (See "Injury Prevention" in Resources for tips from the Canadian government on preparing for emergencies.)

Preparing Your Family

Being the parent of a new baby is a huge responsibility, but you'll be amazed at how quickly the nuts-and-bolts aspects of baby care—feeding, bathing, changing diapers—will become second nature. But who's taking care of you? In the early days after childbirth, the focus is so squarely on the newborn that new parents can often feel neglected and ignored.

Dr. Sacks Says

Having a baby may make you tired, but it should not weaken or diminish you. It should teach you about yourself and help you grow into a stronger person.

When a new baby comes into the home, parents can feel a whole range of emotions, many of which they were not expecting. In addition to euphoria and wonderment, there may be fatigue and anxiety. Sometimes the sadness caused by hormonal changes lingers, and can be troubling or embarrassing, but it's completely normal. Try to recognize and accept the challenges you're facing, and take time to take care of yourself and your partner. If you do, you'll have more to give your baby and everyone in your family will be happier. Here are some tips that may help you remember to occasionally put yourself first.

• **Help each other out.** Make sure the division of labour between parents is clear, defined, and flexible so resentment doesn't build. Try not to focus on how tasks are done: your partner may not clean, cook, or change diapers the way you do, but their way is probably fine. Remember that you're both doing the best you can.

- **Take time off.** Don't be afraid to ask for help, or accept it if it's offered. Ask family or friends to help with shopping, cleaning, cooking, or babysitting your older children. You and your partner should take time for yourselves without your baby, both together as a couple and separately. Even an hour or two of alone time or adult conversation can make a world of difference.

- **Know when to draw the line.** For a while after your baby is born, you may be inundated with calls and requests by people to come and visit. While some company is nice, it's perfectly okay to let people know you're just not up for a visit yet. Most people will understand completely. Plus, it's important to surround yourself with people who are supportive and don't place demands on you when you're learning how to manage being a new parent. If some of your guests don't fit that bill, delay the visit until you've established your own routines.

EVERYONE'S AN EXPERT

During your pregnancy you likely received all sorts of unsolicited advice from family, friends, and complete strangers. Some of it probably helped you; some of it may have been way out in left field; much of it you probably learned to ignore. That won't stop with the arrival of your baby; if anything, it will only increase.

Your parents will probably be your number one source of child-raising advice, often accompanied by the familiar refrain "That's how I raised you, and you turned out all right." But keep in mind that many things have changed since your mother-in-law raised her kids. For instance, immunizations, car seats, and sleep recommendations have all evolved over the last couple of decades, but older friends and family members probably won't be aware of those changes. When they give advice, they (usually) don't mean to be critical. They care about your child, and they just want to be involved. Help them be supportive by suggesting websites and books that will bring them into the twenty-first century.

No matter what you do, you're going to do something wrong in someone's opinion. There is no one right way for you to raise your child—if there were, most of us would be the same, and how dull would that be? So listen to the advice of others, but don't take it personally; instead, decide with your partner how the two of you want to raise your child.

In the first few weeks, quiet time with just your immediate family is essential for successful breastfeeding. Screen your calls and return them when you want. Turn off the ringer and your cell phones—but tell the grandparents you're doing this so you don't find the fire department breaking down your door. When you do go out, set a limit on social occasions. It's okay to drop in somewhere for just a few minutes or to leave early—especially when you will probably be up several times that night feeding your baby.

- **Take care of yourselves.** Get some rest; you need sleep to restore your energy. If and when your baby decides to sleep, that's your cue to put your feet up. Try to resist the temptation to do laundry or housework when your baby is sleeping. (Don't worry, it will still be there tomorrow...and the day after that.) Eating well, drinking plenty of fluids, and getting as much rest as you can are essential for a good milk supply. When you're feeling ready physically, try to get outside every day, even for a walk. Fresh air and exercise are great stress relievers, and your baby will love it too. (But don't take your newborn to the mall or supermarket yet; a well-meaning admirer may pass on a cold.)

Let your partner take the baby out for a walk while you do something you enjoy. As time passes, you should become more comfortable leaving your baby with another trusted adult, even if it's just for a short time. It will be refreshing to know he is well cared for and that you don't need to respond to every cry. Most importantly, don't try to be a super-parent; there's no such thing. The days of daily to-do lists are over for now, so just set your priorities and stick to them. Some days, caring for your baby is all that you'll be able to get done.

- **Seek support.** Other new parents can be a great source of camaraderie and conversation. Try joining a parenting support group or playgroup so you can meet other families. Seek out friends who also have children so you can reconnect with them. Consider joining a moms-and-tots group or planning a reunion with the other couples from your childbirth preparation class.

  If you do feel overwhelmed, anxious, or blue—and many new parents do at one time or another—talk to people about it. Friends, family, and religious leaders can lend an ear and offer support if you are having trouble coping. If the feeling lasts more than a few days, talk to your doctor about it. You don't have to go through it alone, and there's no need to be embarrassed by your feelings. Just make sure you don't ignore them.

WHEN THE BABY BLUES WON'T GO AWAY

Childbirth is an emotional experience, so, understandably, women are at increased risk of depression while they are pregnant and during the weeks and months after having a baby. Often this depression is confused with the symptoms of pregnancy or with the "baby blues," which many experience right after birth.

Depression can cause mothers to be inconsistent in how they care for their baby. They may be loving one minute and withdrawn the next; they may respond negatively to their baby's behaviour or not respond at all. Forming a secure attachment is one of your most important jobs in the early days of your baby's life, but a depressed mother's response can lead to an insecure attachment. A baby who doesn't develop a secure attachment may not be comfortable with her mother, she may be withdrawn or passive, and she may develop skills later than other babies. (For more on attachment, see page 437 in Chapter Eight.)

What's the difference between baby blues and postpartum depression?

Many new moms experience the baby blues, which is a mild form of postpartum depression that is very common and starts a couple days after birth. With baby blues, many women have mood swings—they're happy one minute and crying the next—and they may feel anxious or confused, or have trouble eating or sleeping. The baby blues will go away on its own in a few weeks.

About 13 per cent of new mothers experience postpartum depression, which is more serious and lasts longer. Mothers who have suffered from depression before or have a family history of depression have a higher risk of developing postpartum depression. It can start up to a few months after childbirth. Symptoms include sadness, hopelessness, and extreme anxiety or panic. A mother with postpartum depression will have difficulty making decisions, will feel out of control, and will feel inadequate, thinking she is not able to care for her baby. No one knows exactly what causes postpartum depression.

Treating postpartum depression

Fortunately, postpartum depression can be treated. Treatment often includes medication; individual therapy with a psychologist, psychiatrist, or other professional; family therapy involving your partner or older children; and social support such as community services and parenting education.

MAKE A NOTE, MAKE AN APPOINTMENT, OR GO TO THE HOSPITAL?

Make an appointment with your doctor if you think you have postpartum depression. If left untreated, depression can lead to problems for you and your child. If you are breastfeeding, remind your doctor in case he prescribes medication.

Sibling rivalry: Preparing your older children for the new baby's arrival

If you're an older child yourself, you probably remember how the arrival of a younger brother or sister turned your world upside down. The arrival of a new baby means a major life change for everyone in the family, including siblings. Some children just naturally adapt to being the big sister or brother and take on the role with ease. Others may resent all the attention the baby is getting; they may become angry or aggressive, withdraw, become highly needy or emotional, or regress in their development. A toddler who has long been toilet trained may suddenly start having "accidents" again, for example.

You can make the transition a little easier for the entire family by taking steps to prepare your older child for all this change. Start telling her about the new baby as early as you feel comfortable. Explain your pregnancy in terms that make sense to her. Start by saying, "When you were born…" and answer any questions she has, but keep discussion to a minimum. There is no right or wrong way to tell your child about the new baby; let her comfort and maturity level guide you. A two-year-old may understand there's a baby in mommy's tummy and want to kiss and hug it; a four-year-old may want to know how the baby got there and how it's going to come out. If you're stuck for an answer, it's a good idea to err on the side of providing less detail. If your child wants to know more, she'll ask. And don't be surprised if she isn't as excited by the prospect of a new baby as you are. Most children quickly tire of hearing all the "new baby" talk.

There are lots of activities you can do to prepare your child for a new baby's arrival. Do things together that are baby-related, like looking at her own baby pictures, visiting friends who have infants, and thinking of names for the new sibling. Check your local library or bookstore for age-appropriate books about being a big sister or brother. Read them together several times before the new baby is born. Some hospitals offer sibling birth classes to provide orientation for soon-to-be siblings, with lessons on how babies are born and how to hold them, and opportunities to discuss their feelings about having a new brother or sister. You can also bring your child to a prenatal appointment so she can listen to your baby's heartbeat.

Consider getting a special gift for the baby to give to the older sibling. Buy or make small cards and treats from mom for each day you'll be in the hospital to remind your child that even though you're not home, you haven't forgotten her and still care as much for her as for the new baby.

As your due date draws near, keep your older child's routine as regular as possible. If you are making any room or furniture shifts (for example, if you're moving her out of the nursery to make room for Number Two), do so several weeks before your due date. If your child is old enough, let her know what is going to happen when you go into labour. Tell her she'll be going to her grandparents' or a friend's home for a couple of days, but her parents will be home again soon. It can be very upsetting for a child of any age to leave a parent behind at the hospital, so don't bring older children to the hospital until you're ready to be discharged. However, if you're hospitalized for more than the usual one or two days, a visit will let your child see that you're okay.

After your baby comes home

Once your baby is home from the hospital, there are some things you can do to help your older child adjust to all the changes. If you're breast-feeding, keep him occupied with toys or other activities so he doesn't feel left out. Include him as much as he seems to want in the care of the new baby. If he is old enough, he can bring you a fresh diaper during a diaper change, hold the baby for a few minutes while sitting on the floor, and sing to the baby or even push the stroller. This means that it will take longer to do simple tasks, but be patient. It's important to let older siblings feel needed and to allow them a chance to interact with the baby in a positive way.

If your older child wants to hold the baby, sit the two of them on the floor with a blanket and stay close by. If all he hears is "no" or "don't touch" whenever he is near the baby, he'll start to feel negatively about his new sibling. Tell him that just as you wouldn't let anyone hurt him, you won't let anyone hurt the new baby either.

Most importantly, make opportunities for one-on-one time with your older child. Ask someone to take your baby for an hour or two so you and your child can do something special together. Or alternate special alone time with each parent; one parent can take him to the zoo one day, the other can take him to the park the next. Special time doesn't have to be a new experience. It's important to maintain routines, so it can be everyday experiences like reading alone together. Having this exclusive time, however short, may help reduce any anger or resentment he has about the new baby.

If he's old enough, encourage him to talk about his feelings where the new baby is concerned. Let him know that his feelings are important and that they're okay. If your older child doesn't express any interest in his new brother or sister, don't be alarmed, and don't force it. Listen to and respect his cues. He will eventually come around; it may just take some time.

READY OR NOT . . .

The nursery is set up and your home suitably babyproofed, the car seat is purchased and strapped in, and you're ready for your baby's arrival. You've also got an idea of the range of emotions you will have—and how you can manage them. One way to deal with any less-than-positive moments is to remember to put the experiences of your baby's first days into perspective. Moms waiting for their children at the end of the first day of school have only the slightest memory of anything negative from those early days. People are blessed with the ability to forget a lot of the stress of these first few days, weeks, and months—that's why Number Two comes along.

It also helps to talk to your partner about how you plan to support each other during the early days and months of parenthood. If you're on your own, make sure you've arranged a strong support network from among your family and friends. Having a team of healthcare experts and people who care about you in place will help you be a wonderful parent to this baby you're about to bring into the world.

One last thing to do before your baby arrives is to sit down with your partner and make a short list of hopes and wishes for your child. As the months and years go by, when your two-year-old won't go to bed or your three-year-old is still struggling with toilet training, you can refer back to the list to remind yourself of what's really important.

Dr. Sacks Says

Have fun and don't forget to laugh. Think of all those times your mother said she hoped you'd have a child just like yourself!

Shopping list—Just the essentials

Furniture	· crib · dresser · change table
Equipment	· rear-facing infant car seat · carriage stroller and/or front baby carrier · first-aid kit · breast pump (buy, rent, or borrow) · baby tub
Supplies	· fitted crib sheet · baby bottles · infant diapers (cloth or disposable) · petroleum jelly (for diaper rash) · soft washcloths · mild soap · receiving blankets · infant sleepers, hats, and booties · infant mittens (to cover your baby's sharp nails) · pacifier · lots of books
Childproofing Accessories	· cabinet and toilet latches · anti-scald devices for hot water faucets · electrical outlet plugs · safety gates · window guards · padding for sharp furniture edges · child-resistant doorknob covers · paint test kit (if you have an old home)
For Mom	· nursing bras · lanolin cream

Five Questions for the First Week

1 **How much should my baby sleep?** Newborns may sleep as much as 16 hours a day, for three to four hours at a time, with no regular pattern. Your baby's little stomach can hold only enough food to keep her satisfied for three or four hours at a time, so she will often wake up during the night to feed. As she gets older, she will stay awake longer during the day, and she'll sleep for longer periods at night.

2 **How often should my baby eat?** In the early weeks, you'll be doing a lot of feeding on demand—feeding your baby whenever he's hungry, which is usually every two to three hours throughout the day and night. You can expect to breastfeed 8 to 12 times over a 24-hour period, although small babies may need to be fed more frequently.

3 **How many diapers should my baby go through, and what will they look like?** In the first few days of your baby's life, she will typically have one dirty diaper and one wet diaper for each day of her life (one on day one, two on day two, etc.).

Days 1 and 2. Your baby will pass a thick greenish-black substance called meconium. Her urine may be pinkish in colour.

Day 3. After the meconium has passed, your baby's stool will turn to a yellowish-green colour and will be loose.

Day 4. Your baby's urine should be pale yellow or clear.

Day 5. Her stool will usually be yellow, with the consistency of scrambled eggs, and she should have at least three stools a day that are the size of a loonie or larger, as well as five or six wet diapers.

4 **Why is my baby crying?** Healthy newborns usually cry for about two to three hours a day. At this age, you should respond immediately to your baby's cries. When he begins to cry, first check to see if he is hungry, wet, tired, or feverish.

If none of these are the reason, he may be bored, so try singing or talking to him, or offer him a distraction, or just keep him in the same room as you so he can see you. If there's a chance he's over-stimulated, try putting him in a quiet, dimly lit room, taking a warm bath with him, or lying down for a nap together (not in the same bed). If he won't soothe himself, try giving him a pacifier or swaddling him. Some babies are soothed by noise, so create some white noise by turning on some music or even the hair dryer, washing machine, or vacuum cleaner. Some babies are soothed by motion, so you can also try walking with him, rocking or swaying in a gentle, rhythmic motion, or going for a car ride.

Most newborns have a fussy period late in the day that can last for several hours. As long as your baby has been fed and changed and he doesn't have a fever, he's most likely fine. Do your best to soothe him, and take turns with your partner so you don't become frustrated.

5 **Is there something wrong with my baby's skin, and how do I care for it?**
Your baby's skin may have a greasy white film on it during the first week or so. This is vernix, which protected her skin when she was in your uterus. It is harmless and can be wiped off, but as it's being lost during the first week of life, it may cause the skin to peel. It may help to moisturize your baby's skin with petroleum jelly. Vernix will go away on its own.

If your baby's skin and the whites of her eyes are yellow, she has jaundice. Jaundice is common in newborns, and is usually not harmful. It typically becomes noticeable during a baby's first three to five days of life, and disappears as her liver matures. See page 75 for information on when jaundice is serious.

Your baby may develop a splotchy red rash called erythema toxicum. The rash tends to come and go on different parts of the body, and is usually in the form of small white pustules surrounded by a flare of red, like small mosquito bites. It is most common on the second day of life, but can appear at birth or within the first two to four weeks. The individual splotches may stay for only a few hours, or they may linger for several days. There is no treatment, but it will gradually disappear.

To care for your baby's skin, all you need to do is bathe her with soap and comfortably warm water every other day. Between bathings and during diaper changes, clean her with a warm, moist cloth. Use a barrier cream, such as a paste of petroleum jelly and cornstarch, on her diaper area to prevent diaper rash.

CHAPTER

Your New Baby, from Birth to 12 Months

After all those months of anticipation, your baby has arrived! Now the extraordinary task of parenting begins. Your baby's first year will undoubtedly bring a mixture of amazement and perplexity, as well as the most incredible joy you've ever experienced. From dealing with the onslaught of well-wishers, to establishing feeding and sleeping schedules, to learning how to bathe your baby, change his diapers, and use a car seat, the first weeks with a newborn can feel like a crash-course in parenthood. The most important thing you can do is learn to trust your instincts and your ability to learn. In a very short time, the tasks that were once daunting will be routine, and you'll quickly learn to interpret the curious behaviour—the squirms, sounds, and facial expressions— of the new little person in your life.

Babies need physical and intellectual stimulation, proper nutrition, and attentive health care. But what they need most of all is love. Holding your baby and responding to his cries is essential to building a strong, healthy bond. This is the easy part of your job, but it's also the most important, so cuddle, sing, and talk to your baby as much as you can. It's impossible to spoil a newborn baby with too much affection.

INCLUDED IN THIS CHAPTER

GROWTH AND DEVELOPMENT

During this year, your newborn will go from a sleepy little bundle to a distinct presence in your home. With her ever-increasing muscle control, she will learn to hold her head up, roll onto her back and stomach, sit, and stand up. She'll smile and laugh, play peekaboo, and say her first words. And by her first birthday, she may even be taking her first steps.

Developmental Milestones

Every baby is different, and yours will develop at his own pace. Most babies will achieve certain milestones by a particular age, but don't worry if he doesn't reach all these milestones at exactly the times shown in the list below. It's much more important that he continues to gain new skills.

One month
- Turns his head from side to side while lying on his back
- Responds to sound
- Looks at faces

Two months
- Smiles in response to your smile when you play with him
- Raises his head while lying on his back
- Makes sounds, and starts to gurgle and coo
- Holds his head steady for short periods of time
- Focuses his eyes to see objects about a foot away, like mom's face while breastfeeding
- Tries to mimic facial expressions
- Sees complex designs and a variety of colours
- Starts to follow moving objects with his eyes

Three months
- Holds his head steady
- Raises his head, shoulders, and chest up while lying on his stomach
- Recognizes his parents' faces and smells
- Bats at things with his hands
- Tightly grasps a ring or rattle placed in his hands

Four months
- Rolls over from his stomach to his back
- Reaches for things and brings his fingers to his mouth
- Laughs
- Holds his head up steadily
- Coos when talked to
- Picks up large objects like blocks, and rakes things toward himself
- Knows the difference between night and day, and sleeps in a pattern—maybe even for nine hours at a time!

Five months
- Distinguishes between bold colours
- Amuses himself by playing with his hands and feet
- Pushes things away when he's no longer interested
- Repeats sounds back to you ("ooh" and "aah")
- Rolls from his back to his stomach and onto his back again

Six months
- Passes things from one hand to another
- Turns his head toward sounds and voices
- Blows bubbles
- Makes new baby sounds such as "bababababa"
- Bears his weight when he's held upright

Seven months

- Imitates speech sounds
- Reaches for things with a sweeping motion

Eight months

- Says "dada" and "mama," but not to a specific parent
- Starts to crawl

Nine months

- Combines syllables into word-like sounds
- Stands while holding on to something
- Waves goodbye
- Constantly puts things into his mouth
- Sits upright without support

Ten months

- Picks things up with a pincer grasp (between finger and thumb)
- May be crawling well
- Cruises along furniture
- Expresses himself with gestures and sounds instead of cries
- Starts to babble in a conversational way

Eleven months

- Says "dada" and "mama" to the right person
- Plays pat-a-cake
- Stands up alone for a couple of seconds

Twelve months

- Imitates others' activities
- Jabbers word-like sounds
- Indicates wants with gestures

- Picks up almost anything
- Takes a few unassisted steps
- Says a few one-syllable words
- May be triple his birth weight
- Plays side by side with other children
- Understands the word "no"
- Is aware of what others are doing

Feeding milestones

Birth to four months
- Opens his mouth when a nipple touches his lips
- Has a strong rooting reflex (turns and opens his mouth when his cheeks or mouth are touched)
- Sucks and swallows

Four to six months
- Has increased sucking strength
- Brings his fingers to his mouth
- Socializes during feeding

Six to nine months
- Drinks from a cup held by an adult
- Eats soft food from a spoon
- Enjoys holding food and feeding himself with his fingers
- Loves to be included at the table for meals
- Begins to show likes and dislikes for certain foods

Nine to twelve months
- Tries to use a spoon
- Starts to finger-feed with a more advanced grasp
- Feeds at regular times

Literacy milestones

(Adapted with permission from the Reach Out and Read National Center in Somerville, Massachusetts.)

Birth to six months

- Vocalizes while you read to him
- Looks at the pictures in a book
- Shows a preference for pictures of faces

Six to twelve months

- Reaches for books
- Puts books in his mouth
- Sits on the reader's lap
- Turns the pages, with help
- Pats pictures

MAKE A NOTE, MAKE AN APPOINTMENT, OR GO TO THE HOSPITAL?

Not all babies will be able to do these things according to the timeline provided above. Premature babies in particular will reach these milestones at a different rate. It's usually not a cause for concern if your baby develops a bit slower, but **make a note** to talk to her doctor at your next scheduled appointment if she doesn't reach the following milestones:

Two months

- Your baby doesn't respond when you put a toy in front of her.
- She still feels very stiff or floppy.

Three months

▷ She stiffens or crosses her legs when you have her bear weight on them, or scissors her legs when you pick her up under the armpits.

▷ She has trouble lifting her head up even slightly.

Four months

▷ She doesn't grasp or reach for toys, or bring objects to her mouth.

▷ She doesn't try to stand when her feet are placed on a firm surface.

▷ She doesn't try to hold her head up.

▷ She isn't imitating the sounds her parents make.

▷ She doesn't focus on someone's face.

▷ She doesn't turn toward a sound.

Six months

▷ She isn't laughing or squealing.

▷ She can't sit, even with help.

▷ She makes little attempt or no attempt to turn over.

▷ Either of her hands is still constantly in a fist.

Seven months

▷ She has poor head control when pulled to a sitting position.

▷ She refuses to bear weight on her legs.

Eight months

▷ She can't sit by herself without lots of support.

▷ She isn't using sounds to get your attention.

Nine months

▷ She hasn't begun babbling.

Ten months

▹ She doesn't respond to her name.

▹ She doesn't look at you when you talk to her.

Your Baby's Growth

Just like adults, children come in a wide range of shapes and sizes. Your child may be taller or shorter and heavier or lighter than other children of the same age. Yet changes in height and weight follow a regular pattern determined mostly by genetics. The way a child grows indicates a great deal about his health. His growth could be affected if he's having problems with health or nutrition. Since growth and weight gain are very sensitive indicators of how your baby is doing, it's important that his doctor measures and weighs him regularly at his well-baby visits. The doctor will take his undressed weight and measure his length and head circumference, then compare him with other babies of the same age and sex, and with his measurements at previous checkups. These measurements help your doctor make sure your baby is growing in a healthy and consistent way.

Interpreting the growth chart

The growth charts used in Canada to measure length, weight, and head circumference in babies were developed by the Centers for Disease Control and Prevention in the United States in 1977 (see "Growth" in Resources). They were revised in 2000 because the original growth charts were based mainly on a sample of white, middle-class infants who were nearly all bottle fed. The data used to construct the new charts is more reflective of the U.S. population.

The growth chart is a good way to get a general picture of your baby's general health. After taking his measurements, the doctor will tell you into which percentile he falls. For example, if your baby is in the 45th percentile for weight and the 65th percentile for height, it means that 55 per cent of boys his age weigh more than him and 45 per cent weigh less, and 35 per cent of boys his age are taller and 65 per cent are shorter.

More important than these numbers is whether your baby is growing at a steady rate. If he's always around the same percentile in both height and weight, his growth pattern is fine. Small peaks and valleys aren't a cause for concern. Babies have growth spurts, and their weight gain ebbs and flows. However, if he has a very sudden and rapid weight gain or loss or change in head circumference, or if he falls into the extreme areas of the growth chart (the top or bottom 5 per cent), your doctor may want to investigate further.

MYTH BUSTERS

Myth: A fat baby is a healthy baby.

Fact: Looking at a baby's pattern of growth is the best way to determine if her growth is healthy. Excessive weight gain may be due to a physical or emotional illness, or it may just reflect poor eating and drinking habits.

—*Dr. Glen Ward, MD, FRCPC*

Dealing with Diapers

Inspecting the contents of your baby's diaper will soon become your new habit. Believe it or not, you will quickly become an expert on variations in your baby's stools. The variety you find may not seem normal, but it usually is, and it will change dramatically as she ages and as her diet changes.

In the first couple of days of her life, your baby will pass a thick greenish-black substance called meconium, which is made up of amniotic fluid and other cells that have built up in her intestines while in the womb. After the meconium has passed, your baby's stool will turn to a yellowish-green colour. In the first few days, she will typically have one dirty diaper and one wet diaper for each day of her life (one on day one, two on day two, etc.). Her stool should be loose, not formed. Her urine may be pinkish in colour, but that's normal too, and is due to uric acid crystals in her urine. After day three, your baby's urine should be pale yellow or clear. After day four, her stool is usually yellow, with the consistency of scrambled eggs. Your baby should have at least three stools a day that are the size of a loonie or larger, as well as five or six wet diapers in 24 hours.

After she is a few weeks old, the range of normal for wet and dirty diapers varies greatly. Breastfed babies tend to have frequent bowel movements for the first month or two because they easily digest breast milk. Their stool is softer, fairly odourless (it may smell faintly like buttermilk), and may look seedy due to undigested breast milk proteins. Formula-fed babies, on the other hand, may have slightly firmer and smellier stool. They are more likely to become constipated, so watch for straining and hard, pellet-like stool, which are signs of constipation.

The frequency of bowel movements also varies from baby to baby. Some pass a stool after each feeding; others may have only one or two dirty diapers a week. From two to three months of age, many breastfed babies have infrequent bowel movements because they digest almost every bit of nutrition they can get out of breast milk, leaving very little waste. Their bowel movements may be a bit uncomfortable, but as long as your baby's stool is soft and she's gaining weight at a steady rate, everything is normal.

How many diapers will my baby go through?

Time	Number of Wet Diapers	Number of Dirty Diapers
Day 1	1/day	1/day
Day 2	2/day	2/day
Day 3	3/day	3/day
Day 4 to 1 month	5 or 6/day	3 or 4/day

After a month or so, the frequency of wet and dirty diapers may change dramatically, and almost any amount is normal. Your baby may have several dirty diapers a day, or she may go several days without a dirty diaper. The number of dirty diapers will go down a bit for breastfed babies after a couple of months. Keep a diary so you know what is normal for your baby and can tell when there has been a significant change.

MAKE A NOTE, MAKE AN APPOINTMENT, OR GO TO THE HOSPITAL?

Make an appointment to see your baby's doctor if

▷ your baby's urine is dark in colour or has a pinkish discolouration after day three;
▷ her stool is still very dark in colour after day four;
▷ she suddenly has far fewer wet or dirty diapers than she has been having;
▷ she passes hard or pellet-like stool, appears to be straining, or there is blood in her diaper; or
▷ she has diarrhea.

Diarrhea is often difficult to judge in newborns, but **make an appointment** with her doctor if she starts having much more frequent bowel movements with a high liquid content.

　　Take her to the hospital immediately if she has no wet or dirty diapers within a 24-hour period, especially if she is feeding poorly.

Diaper changing

You don't have to love changing diapers, but you can make it easier on yourself. Before you start, make sure your supplies are all within reach. Don't ever leave your baby unattended—even newborns can wiggle, so you must keep a hand on your baby or be right by her side at all times. A clean washcloth and water is all you need for cleaning her. Wipes can dry out a baby's tender skin, so if you do use them, be sure they are alcohol-free and unscented.

Wipe your baby clean from front to back. This is especially important for girls, since wiping from back to front can transfer harmful bacteria from the rectum into the vulva area and cause urinary tract infections. If you have a boy, you'll probably want to keep a clean diaper or washcloth over his penis during changing to prevent an unexpected soaking of both him and you. Point his penis downward before you fold up the diaper to minimize leakage at the waistline. If you see creases or red marks around your baby's legs or waist, it means her diaper is too tight—just fasten it a little more loosely next time. When you're done diapering, remember to wash your hands well with soap and water to prevent the spread of germs.

Baby powder has been associated with lung problems in babies, so skip it. If your baby has a diaper rash, protect and lubricate her skin by applying unscented petroleum jelly or a cream that contains zinc oxide. Babies can be sensitive to certain brands of diapers, particularly some that include a moisturizer designed to act like a barrier cream, so if a rash develops around her legs or waist, try changing the brand of diaper.

If you're using cloth diapers, your biggest fear (besides washing them) will be diaper pins. Use safety pins with a sliding lock head, and always keep your hand between the point of the pin and your baby's skin when fastening her diaper. Sticking the point of the pin in some soap will help it glide through the fabric more easily. If pins make you nervous—just take a deep breath and relax. Or use diaper tape instead, or buy cotton diapers with Velcro straps.

Whenever possible, put solid waste in the toilet before putting a soiled cloth diaper in the laundry. You can buy handy flushable liners that make this part relatively painless. If you're washing the diapers yourself, wash them in lots of hot water, and separate them from your other laundry. Use a mild detergent recommended for infant clothing, and don't use fabric softener or dryer sheets as they can irritate your baby's skin.

Crying

Here's the shocking truth: all babies cry. In fact, healthy newborns usually cry for about two to three hours a day. Crying is their way of communicating: they cry because of hunger, discomfort, frustration, fatigue, and even loneliness. As you get to know your baby better, you'll get to know his different cries, and you'll be able to figure out what he needs, whether it's food, a diaper change, or just a cuddle. During the first few months, you should respond immediately to your baby's cries. Don't worry about spoiling him at this stage. He'll feel reassured and comforted, and your attention will help him bond to you.

Most of the time, your crying baby will be easily consoled, but sometimes newborns cry for no apparent reason. Most have a fussy period, often during the late afternoon or early evening, when they're tired but unable to relax. This fussiness can last several hours, but is completely normal. When your baby begins to cry, check for all the usual reasons. Is he hungry, wet, tired, or feverish? If none of these are the problem, there are a whole host of other things you can try.

Babies are often soothed by motion, so try walking with him, rocking or swaying in a gentle, rhythmic motion, or going for a car ride. Some babies like noise, so turn on some background music or white noise—even the washing machine or vacuum cleaner. He might be bored and in need of some stimulation, so try singing or talking to him, or offer him a toy. On the other hand, he may be over-stimulated. (Isn't this game fun?) Try putting him in a quiet, dimly lit room, taking a warm bath with him, or lying down for a nap together (but never in the same bed). Or he may just want to be in the same room as you so he can see you.

Swaddling

Swaddling is the age-old technique of wrapping a baby snugly in a sheet or blanket to make him feel secure, and it just might help your fussy baby calm down. It creates a slight pressure around the body that gives most newborns a sense of security because it is similar to the pressure they felt in the womb. Newborns have a startle-like reflex, called the Moro Reflex, that causes them to arch their backs and extend their arms and legs unexpectedly, waking them up. This will go away after a few months, but in the meantime, keeping his limbs snugly at his sides minimizes this reflex, allowing him to sleep longer and more soundly. When he's bundled up, he'll know there's a long sleep ahead.

Most maternity ward nurses are proficient in the art of baby swaddling, so you'll probably receive a lesson in swaddling technique before you bring your baby home. After a month or so, it's a good idea to stop swaddling your baby during his waking hours as it could interfere with his development and mobility. It's fine to keep swaddling him at night as long as he seems to enjoy it and it helps him to sleep soundly.

Pacifiers

Once you've ruled everything else out, it's okay to give your baby a pacifier to help him stop crying. See if other solutions satisfy him first, and check if he is hungry, tired, or bored before giving him the pacifier. Babies are born wanting to suck, and some even suck their thumb or fingers before they are born. It's a natural behaviour that allows them to feed and grow, but it also comforts them. A pacifier can satisfy your baby's need to suck between feedings, but it should never be used instead of feeding, and never without the extra comfort and cuddling a parent provides.

Sucking on a pacifier is better than a thumb or finger because it causes fewer problems with future tooth development. You can control the use of a pacifier, but it's hard to control thumb-sucking. And when it's time to stop using a pacifier, you can throw it away. (You can't throw away a thumb!) Also, the latest medical research finds that there is some early evidence that using a pacifier may decrease the risk of sudden infant death syndrome (SIDS) or crib death. However, not using a pacifier properly can lead to problems with breastfeeding, dental problems such as cavities and overbite, and possibly ear infections. Homemade pacifiers, sweetened pacifiers, or pacifiers tied around a baby's neck are not safe. Pacifiers made out of bottle nipples, caps, or other materials can cause choking if they break. Dipping a pacifier in sugar or honey will damage new teeth, and in rare cases honey can lead to botulism, a type of food poisoning. Instead of tying a pacifier around your baby's neck, which can cause strangulation, buy pacifier clips with short ribbons that attach to his clothes.

Never start using a pacifier until breastfeeding is fully established. Talk to your doctor or lactation consultant if you feel your baby needs to use one earlier. An exception is often made for premature or sick babies in the hospital because it may comfort them when they can't be fed. As some medicines can cause the material in pacifiers to break down, don't give your baby a pacifier right after giving him medicines such as a pain reliever, antibiotics, or vitamins.

Before its first use, sterilize a pacifier by putting it in boiling water for five minutes. Make sure it has cooled down completely before giving it to your baby. Then, keep it clean by washing it with hot, soapy water after each use. Don't try to clean it by sucking on it yourself; you're more likely to spread germs to your baby. Always check for cracks or tears before giving it to him, and throw it out if you find any. Don't let your baby chew on a pacifier as it could break down and cause him to choke. Replace the pacifier every two months, before damage occurs.

Pacifiers are a fantastic invention, but you shouldn't rely on them completely. In the second half of your baby's first year, a pacifier can interfere with speech development, and may cause dental problems if you let him use it all day. Pacifier use should be stopped between 9 and 12 months.

Colic

There may be times when you try everything to get your baby to stop crying, but nothing works. When a baby cries long and hard without a break, even though he's been fed, changed, and cuddled, he is said to be colicky. For a long time, people thought that colic was a condition afflicting some babies. New information suggests that it's actually a normal part of a baby's development. All babies go through a period early in life when they cry more than at any other time. During this peak period—which is usually sometime between three and eight weeks— some babies may cry much more than others. Their crying may seem stronger, and it may be harder (and sometimes impossible) to soothe them.

Some experts believe that babies who cry more than others have a more sensitive temperament and have difficulty controlling their crying. They may have more trouble self-soothing and settling into their natural body rhythms when they are very young. It was once thought that colic was caused by bowel problems, gas, or food allergies, but there's no strong evidence for that argument. In fact, crying actually causes infants to swallow air, which they then burp up or pass as wind when they strain and tighten their stomach muscles.

THE COLIC HOLD

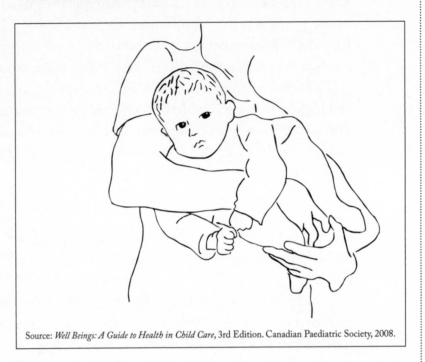

Source: *Well Beings: A Guide to Health in Child Care*, 3rd Edition. Canadian Paediatric Society, 2008.

Try calming a colicky baby by holding him face-down along your arm and rocking him. Place your arm down his front with your hand between his legs so that your elbow cradles his head. Hold him in place by steadying his feet with your other hand.

Although some over-the-counter and natural remedies claim to help colic, talk to your baby's doctor before using them. The good news is that colic is normal, there's no lasting effect on your baby, and it won't go on forever. This period of strong, intense, and unexplained crying can end as quickly as it started, or it may gradually decrease over time. It's usually over by the time your baby is three to four months old.

MAKE A NOTE, MAKE AN APPOINTMENT, OR GO TO THE HOSPITAL?

If your baby's crying is accompanied by fever, vomiting, diarrhea, or a significant change in his behaviour, or you think it could be due to an injury, **make an appointment** with his doctor.

If your baby cries intensely after many of his feedings, he could have gastroesophageal reflux disease (GERD). See "When spitting up is serious" on page 88. **Make a note** to mention it to his doctor at his next appointment if you suspect your baby has GERD.

The early days of taking care of a new baby aren't always easy. You're probably not sleeping much, and you might be trying to meet your baby's needs around the clock. As the days pass, you'll start to find what works for your baby when he cries for long periods. Although these crying jags are completely normal, they can be very stressful, especially when you're tired. The most important thing to know is that it is not your fault, and it will get better. No matter how frustrated you become, *never shake your baby.* You and your partner should take turns holding your baby during his fussy period. If you're alone and you become angry or frustrated, put him down in his crib, close the door, and go to another room for a few minutes. There is nothing wrong with taking a short break to collect yourself. It may be all you need to find the strength to return to your baby and try another soothing tactic. If you identify a pattern in his fussiness, plan for extra help during that period. Have a friend or relative come over for an hour or two to relieve you and your partner.

Be sure to take care of yourself. It sounds simple, but eating and sleeping well can make a big difference in how well you can cope. Try to get at least three hours of sleep in a row, twice a day. If your baby's crying is very bad, consider scheduling an appointment with his doctor more frequently than usual, perhaps every two weeks, just to reassure yourself that nothing is wrong. Your peace of mind will help your baby feel secure and will help him to settle easier.

SHAKEN BABY SYNDROME

If a baby is shaken with force in a moment of anger, it can lead to a lifetime of disabilities. Shaking can injure a baby's brain, it can cause permanent brain damage and developmental disabilities, and can even be fatal. Babies younger than one year of age are particularly at risk if shaken violently, but older children can also be seriously injured. Protect your child by talking to your babysitter, daycare workers, friends, and relatives so that they're aware of the dangers of shaking a child.

What parents should do

Plan ahead so that you're not tempted to shake your baby. If he cries a lot, arrange for regular childcare relief so that you can get some rest. Form a back-up plan so that you can call on reliable help when your baby's crying seems impossible to deal with. Reliability is key—pick a reliable friend or family member, or a babysitter with good references. Never leave your child with someone you don't trust, or who tends to react intensely or violently to everyday situations. Pay attention to your instincts and get references directly from other parents.

Shaking is not first aid

If a baby is not breathing, shaking will not help. The appropriate treatment is artificial breathing, or CPR. Many community organizations, such as St. John Ambulance or the Red Cross, offer affordable courses for these first-aid skills, and a first-aid course is great preparation for parenthood. See "Injury Prevention" in Resources for information on first-aid courses.

Where parents can go for help

There are many resources and professionals who can help you if you have concerns or questions. (See "Newborns" in Resources for some helpful organizations.) Talk to your paediatrician, family doctor, or public health nurse, and look for local community resources that support parents and caregivers. Check the first pages of your local phone book for the emergency numbers in your area.

If your baby won't stop crying and you've exhausted all the possible causes, stay calm and check your own state of mind. Are you upset? Are you frustrated? If you feel like you might lose control, place him safely in the crib and leave the room for a few minutes. If the problem continues, talk to a friend or family member you trust, and get some support. And if you really feel that you might hurt your baby, call for help: a local crisis line, your child welfare agency, or the police. Remember, no matter how upset you feel, don't shake your baby.

Sleep? What Sleep?

Newborns may sleep as much as 16 hours a day, for three to four hours at a time, with no regular pattern. They don't know the difference between day and night, and their little tummies can only hold enough food to keep them satisfied for three or four hours at a time, so your baby will often wake up during the night to feed. In the early weeks she needs to be fed every few hours. As your baby gets older, she will stay awake longer during the day, and she'll sleep for longer periods at night. After about eight weeks, some babies may even sleep through the night. (Of course, your idea of "sleeping through the night" will have changed drastically. A five-hour stretch—from midnight to 5 a.m., for instance—will seem decadent.) Other babies won't make it that long until they're a year old, or even older. Your baby will sleep through the night when she is ready.

Some time after three months, your baby's sleep habits will become more predictable and you can start to develop a regular nap schedule. Keeping a sleep diary might help you recognize a regular sleeping pattern, but it's also important to trust your baby's cues—she will let you know when she is tired. Try to develop a naptime routine, such as a quiet cuddle time in a darkened room before it is time to nap. By four months, most babies need three naps a day: one in the morning, the afternoon, and the early evening.

Dr. Sacks Says

If you want your baby to sleep through the night before she starts high school, teach her to fall asleep by herself in her own crib by five months of age.

Babies, just like adults, need the right cues to learn when it is time to sleep. If you always put your baby in her crib to sleep, she'll learn that this is the place where she sleeps, and eventually she'll learn to go to sleep when you put her to bed. Put her in her crib when she is drowsy but still awake, as an over-tired baby will have more trouble sleeping. Napping actually helps her sleep better at night, so keeping her awake during the day will probably have the opposite effect of what you were hoping for. Occasionally she will wake up during the night, but give her a few minutes to settle back to sleep on her own. When you feed her or change her diapers during the night, keep the lights dim to avoid stimulating her.

After six months, babies will sleep an average of 14 hours in a day, but anything less or more is also normal. By this time you should have a regular routine of naptimes, bedtime, and wake times. Your baby will probably go from three naps a day to two longer naps—one each in the morning and afternoon. Every baby's napping needs are different; some will nap for as little as 20 minutes at a time, while others nap for three hours or more.

How much should my baby sleep?

Time	Hours of Sleep per Day	Details
Newborn	16 hours	3 to 4 hours at a time
4 months	16 hours	will probably take 3 naps during the day
6 months	14 hours	2 naps during the day
12 months	14 hours	probably sleeps through the night

To promote your baby's healthy sleep, try to maintain regular daytime and bedtime sleep schedules. Set up a consistent bedtime routine, such as the three Bs—take a warm bath, read a book, and settle into bed. If your baby wakes at night and cries, make sure nothing is wrong, such as being too cold or too warm, but don't take her out of the crib. Comfort her by stroking her forehead or talking softly to reassure her that you are there. Never put her to bed with a bottle.

MYTH BUSTERS

Myth: Infant cereal helps newborns sleep.

Fact: Sleep is a neurobiologic process that differs from child to child. Unfortunately, cereal doesn't change this sleep clock.

—*Dr. Krista Baerg, MD, FRCPC*

Creating a safe sleep environment

Starting from birth and for the first year of life, place your baby to sleep on her back at nighttime and for naps. When she can turn over on her own, you no longer need to force her onto her back. Check that her crib meets Health Canada's most current safety standards (see page 20 in Chapter One). Use a firm, flat surface for sleep. Waterbeds, air mattresses, pillows, sofas, and other soft materials like quilts and comforters are not safe sleep surfaces for babies. Bumper pads and stuffed animals should also be kept out of her sleep environment. She could turn onto her stomach and bury her face and not get enough air to breathe. Keep her warm, but not too warm, with a light blanket or sleepers.

Having her in your room will make nighttime breastfeeding easier and may help protect against SIDS. Keep a chair in the room for cuddling and breastfeeding, though. When you bring your baby into bed with you to breastfeed, it's too easy for both of you to fall asleep, especially when you're lying down.

PREVENTING SIDS

Babies need a safe sleeping environment to reduce the risk of injury and sudden infant death syndrome. SIDS occurs when a baby dies unexpectedly while sleeping and no cause is identified after a thorough investigation and full autopsy. Not a lot is known about the exact cause of SIDS, but we do know that babies whose heads become covered while they sleep or who are exposed to cigarette smoke in the womb or after birth have an increased risk of dying from SIDS. The Canadian Paediatric Society recommends that for the first six months, your baby should sleep lying on her back in a crib in your room. All she needs in her crib is a light blanket; stuffed toys, cushions, and bumper pads could suffocate or overheat her and cause SIDS. Recent medical research suggests that using a pacifier may decrease the risk of SIDS.

Bedsharing

Some parents decide to bedshare, which means sleeping on the same surface with your baby. Adult beds are not designed with infant safety in mind, though, so they're not a safe place for babies to sleep. Not only can an adult roll over and suffocate a baby, but a baby can become trapped in a space between the mattress and the wall or the mattress and the bed frame, she can fall off the bed, or she can become overheated if soft bedding covers her head.

If you fall asleep with your baby, you may not be able to wake up easily and respond to her. This is more likely to happen if you've had alcohol, taken drugs that could make you sleepy, or are just really tired. Never lie down or sleep with your baby or let her sleep alone on a sofa or armchair. She can become trapped down the sides or in the cushions and suffocate. The safest place for your baby to sleep is in a crib close to your bed.

MAKE A NOTE, MAKE AN APPOINTMENT, OR GO TO THE HOSPITAL?

If you have any concerns about how much or how little your baby sleeps, **make a note** to mention it to her doctor at her next appointment.

Make an appointment if your baby seems overly irritable and cannot be adequately soothed, or if she is difficult to rouse from sleep and generally seems uninterested in feeding.

Preventing flat head

Babies who always sleep with their head to the same side can develop flat spots. The medical term for this is positional plagiocephaly. Babies' skulls are very soft, and the bones can be affected by pressure. Although they have strong vocal cords (you've probably noticed that by now), their neck muscles are weak, so they tend to turn their heads to one side when placed on their backs.

A little bit of flattening will go away on its own. More serious flattening may be permanent, but it will not affect a baby's brain or development. Flat spots can be prevented simply by changing the position of her head each day. Because babies like to have something interesting to look at, they tend to turn their head to look out into their room, rather than toward the wall, so they can see you come and go. Alternate between placing her head at the head and the foot of the crib so she can always look out into the room. You could also put a mobile on the side of the crib facing the room to encourage her to look that way.

Another way to prevent flat head is to give her supervised tummy time several times a day when she's awake. Not only will time on her front help prevent a flat spot on her head, but it is important for helping your baby develop her neck muscles.

MAKE A NOTE, MAKE AN APPOINTMENT, OR GO TO THE HOSPITAL?

If your baby still develops flat spots, **make a note** to mention it to her doctor at her next appointment.

Time to Play: The Importance of Reading, Music, and Games

From the moment you baby is born, your voice, your touch, and your face are the best tools for developing his physical and social skills. But the whole world is filled with fascinating objects, sounds, colours, and textures for him to discover, from a plastic ring, to a bowl of squishy oatmeal, to a set of building blocks. You can encourage this development simply by playing with him. Playtime is fundamental for your baby's ability to interact, learn, and express himself. It encourages self-esteem and confidence. And the right toys and activities for each stage of the first year can make playtime an even richer experience for both of you. Remember, toys don't have to be expensive, and you don't need hundreds of them. In fact, some of the best toys for babies this age are simple things you probably have around your home. Remember, too, that you are your baby's favourite toy, teacher, and friend.

For the first three months of life, your baby is developing his hand-eye coordination. Things like a set of plastic measuring spoons, pieces of bright cloth with different textures, wooden or plastic bracelets that don't have loose parts, and anything with a face on it—dolls, pictures, or stuffed animals—are great toys for this age. Just touching these things and figuring out how to close his hand around them provides wonderful stimulation for your baby.

Between three and six months, his fine and gross motor skills are really getting a workout. His hands have become a source of endless fascination, and he is learning to associate the feeling of his arm and hand movement with his own intention. Great toys for this stage include things like sturdy, well-constructed rattles; doughnut-shaped objects made from plastic or fabric that are large enough to grasp; pieces of textured fabric like terry cloth, silk, and fake fur; and smooth-surfaced toys that light up or make sounds when they are shaken or kicked.

By the second half of your baby's first year, he is sitting up, dropping and throwing things, and happily leaning over and picking them up. Or making you pick them up—his favourite game of all! Things like wooden spoons, plastic cookie cutters and napkin rings, paper-towel rolls, and tennis balls make great toys for this age. Also great are nesting and stacking toys, even if they're household objects like cups, rings, or pots. He will get so much more out of these toys if you are there on the floor playing with him, helping him to discover each new sensation, and encouraging him to explore.

OBJECT PERMANENCE

Sometime around six months of age, your baby will begin to understand the concept of object permanence: the idea that objects and people still exist even when he can't see them. It's this mental skill that puts the fun in peekaboo. Your baby will look for you (or a toy or other object) hidden under a blanket because he knows you still exist and is expecting you to reappear. Toys like jack-in-the-boxes provide hours of fun now, as your baby waits for "jack" to reappear and squeals with glee every time it does. He will continue to learn about object permanence for the next several months.

Unfortunately, an understanding of object permanence also coincides with separation anxiety, as your baby now begins to remember you and call up mental images of you when you're not there. Before this point, when you left the room, he assumed you vanished, and when you returned, you were a new and exciting person. As he begins to understand that there is only one of you, and that when you leave you are somewhere else (and not with him), he may start to get agitated and cry for you. As he begins to understand the signs that you are getting ready to leave, like putting on your coat, he may cry and cling to you. The good news is that this behaviour usually means he has formed an attachment to you. Fortunately for everyone, this phase doesn't last forever, but at this age it's only beginning. Normal separation anxiety peaks somewhere between the ages of 12 and 18 months and tapers off until the end of the second year.

General tips for baby play

Newborn babies learn how to read signals all around them by listening to voices, watching faces, and reading body language. Hearing and using sounds, sound patterns, and spoken language helps prepare them to eventually read printed words. There are some things you can do to provide these opportunities from the moment your baby is born.

- **Use rhymes, games, and songs.** Babies respond to them almost from birth, and they don't need to understand the words for these moments to be learning experiences, especially when they're sharing them with a parent. For newborns and very young babies, try rhymes that involve gentle touch, such as patting his feet or giving him a little bounce while you're talking.

- **Talk about what's going on.** Whether you're changing a diaper, bathing your baby, or taking a walk, use words that describe the actions and the things around him. You'll help him develop vocabulary before he can even talk.

- **Encourage your baby to babble.** It's how he learns to make sounds with his own voice. Repeat these sounds and turn them into real words. You'll help him recognize which sounds form language, and he'll eventually make the connection between the sounds and an object or person, like "dada."

- **Reward your baby's first attempts at making sounds with smiles and hugs.** This early communication is exciting for him, and your approval will encourage him to keep trying.

- **Ask questions.** When you say, "What's that?" and name the picture in a book, your baby learns that things have names.

- **Encourage your baby's involvement.** Babies like to put books in their mouths, so be sure he has access to sturdy and clean board books. At first, he'll need your help to turn the pages, but as he gets older, you can let him turn the pages on his own.

- **Once your baby starts talking,** help him find the words for the things around him. By repeating words, you'll help him remember them.

- **Read to your baby.** Making books, stories, and storytelling a part of his daily routine will help nurture his love of reading. Even very young babies love picture books, and it's a great idea to make storytime a part of your bedtime routine. You don't even have to read the story all the way through. Just talking about some of the pictures is enjoyable for young babies.

- **Sing songs.** Music makes the words easier to remember, and is a fun way to make language come alive.

Reading

When should you start reading books to your baby? Although babies may be six months or older before they can really concentrate for any length of time on a book and turn its pages, there are wonderful benefits to reading together long before that. The soft cadence of your voice and the bonding that happens when you hold him close and spend quiet time together are wonderful for your baby. Reading helps to develop his language skills, creating a natural foundation for later learning. It's also a great way to help him wind down before sleep if you incorporate reading into your bedtime routine.

For babies under six months, books with simple patterns in black and white or strong primary colours are best. One or two large illustrations per page are more appealing than pages cluttered with visuals. At this stage, your baby enjoys hearing repetitive sounds and language, so nursery rhymes, poems, and lullabies are also wonderful.

At six months and older, when your baby's attention span and physical coordination are a little more developed, textured books with realistic photographs (particularly of objects he recognizes, and especially of other babies) are a big hit. Interactive features like pop-ups and flaps may start to hold real appeal by the end of this year. Sturdy board books will take your baby's rough handling best now, instead of easily ripped paper pages.

Dr. Sacks Says

Babies this age love to digest books . . . literally, so cloth or safe plastic books that can be mouthed and then washed are particularly good.

There's no right or wrong way to read to your baby. Try to read together every day. You can achieve enormous benefits even from reading for only a few minutes a day together. A story before bedtime is a great routine, but it shouldn't be the only time you read to your baby. If he only associates reading with going to bed, he might balk at reading together when he doesn't want to go to bed.

Be interactive when you're reading. Tell your baby what's happening, and point out and name objects in the book. Your best vantage point may not be his, so hold your baby close while you read to ensure he can see the pages clearly. Change your voice and facial expressions to dramatize the story. Don't worry if you feel silly—he will love your funny voices.

Some children don't get the most out of a book by reading it from front to back, so let your baby set the pace. Sometimes he'll want to read slowly, sometimes fast; sometimes he'll want to look at a favourite page for several minutes. Focusing on his favourite parts is the best way to foster a love of reading. Get used to a lot of repetition, too. You'll end up reading some books again and again as your baby lets you know which are his favourites. While this may become boring to you, it's not to him. You're developing his long-term-memory skills, so be enthusiastic while you're reading it, even if it's for the hundredth time.

The most important thing is that you both enjoy it, so don't push him if he seems uninterested or starts to fuss. Follow his cues, and stop reading when he seems tired or loses interest. For some variety, visit the public library often—even babies can get a library card! There are lots of resources to encourage your baby's love of reading. Many libraries have free programs for parents and babies or young children that use books, rhymes, and songs. Ask a librarian for more ideas.

Music to your baby's ears

There's no doubt about the impact music can have on babies' lives. Just think about how music affects you; how some songs can relax you while others make you want to get up and dance. Babies are no different. They feel and respond to music as soon as they're born, and maybe even before. While the jury is still out on whether exposure to music can actually make your baby smarter, there's no doubt that it will enrich his life.

Try incorporating music into your baby's life in a number of ways. Instead of having the television on for background noise, turn on the stereo. Play soft music at bedtime to get him in the mood for sleep, although you may want to avoid putting a CD on and letting him fall asleep to it, as this might create a sleep association that could be difficult to break. Sing to him, and while you're at it, dance together as well. Encourage him to make his own music by banging pots and pans, singing through toilet paper tubes, and pounding on a plastic toy piano.

HEALTH

Once you're home from the hospital, your new family will soon settle into a whole new routine. As you'll discover, parenting is a full-time job, especially in these early days. Even the simplest tasks, like bathing and diapering, can be a bit complicated with such a little body. Every little rash and sneeze may seem like a cause for concern. Although instincts are a parent's best tool, being armed with some basic information will help you feel confident in your baby's health, and will help you know when you should seek medical attention.

Jaundice

Even before you leave the hospital, you may encounter your baby's first health issue. Jaundice is a yellow colouring of the skin and whites of the eyes. Babies become jaundiced when they have too much bilirubin in their blood, a pigment produced as red blood cells break down. It's usually processed by the liver and excreted in a baby's stool. With jaundice, either too much bilirubin is being produced or the liver isn't getting rid of it quickly enough. Because a newborn baby's liver is not fully matured, jaundice is common during the first few days of life.

There are two kinds of jaundice. The first is known as physiological jaundice, and is the most common for newborns. It usually becomes noticeable during a baby's first three to five days of life, and disappears as her liver matures. This type of jaundice is not harmful, but in some situations, there is so much bilirubin in a baby's blood that it can be dangerous. This condition is called pathological jaundice. If the level of bilirubin becomes very high, it may affect some of the baby's brain cells. In rare cases, a baby may have seizures, and it may also lead to deafness, cerebral palsy, and mental retardation.

When jaundice is dangerous

For babies with certain risk factors, jaundice is even more common, and it can cause serious problems. Babies who are at risk are those who are born before 38 weeks' gestation, weigh less than 2500 grams (5½ pounds) at birth, needed resuscitation at birth, or have jaundice within the first 24 hours of life. They may also be at risk if they are large infants of diabetic mothers, their blood group is incompatible with their mother's blood group, they are being exclusively breastfed, or their breastfeeding is not going well. If your family has a strong family history of newborn jaundice (associated with red blood cell conditions) or your older children had jaundice, your baby will be at risk. Other risk factors include infections, significant bruising, and cephalohematoma (collection of blood under the scalp, usually due to birth trauma).

Treatment

When a newborn baby shows signs of jaundice, the doctor will do a physical examination and blood tests to help determine its cause, and whether it is serious enough to be treated. One way to reduce bilirubin levels in a baby's body is to expose her skin to light, a process called phototherapy. Her eyes are protected from the light by eye patches, and she may be fed more frequently so she gets more fluids. Phototherapy can cause skin rashes and loose bowel movements, but it is a safe procedure. It's only used when needed, and usually for two to three days, after which the baby's liver takes over. In severe cases, she may need to have new blood transfused and old blood removed.

Once a jaundiced baby leaves the hospital, she will need to be checked again within the following 24 to 48 hours. The doctor will do a physical examination and often blood tests to see how severe her jaundice is, and will determine how it should be treated.

MAKE A NOTE, MAKE AN APPOINTMENT, OR GO TO THE HOSPITAL?

Make an appointment to see your baby's doctor if your baby

- refuses two or three feedings in a row;
- is sleepy all the time;
- has lost a significant amount of weight (more than 10 per cent of her birth weight);
- is extremely jaundiced (her arms, legs, and the whites of her eyes are yellow); or
- still has jaundice by the time she is three weeks old.

Skin Care

When it comes to baby skin products, all you really need to do is stick to the basics—soap and water. As many as there are on the market, baby lotions aren't necessary unless your baby has dry skin, and powders aren't recommended because they can cause respiratory problems. You don't even need to use very much soap on your baby. To keep his skin in good shape you can use a barrier cream, as simple as petroleum jelly mixed with some cornstarch to create a paste, on the diaper area. To clear up a minor diaper rash, creams containing zinc oxide can be used sparingly. Prevent skin problems by taking care when you do your baby's laundry. Some everyday laundry detergents and fabric softeners may cause irritation to his delicate skin, and even if you use a detergent marketed for baby laundry, it's a good idea to rinse an extra time to remove residues.

Bathing your baby

Although the traditional advice has been to give babies a sponge bath until the area around the umbilical cord heals, today many doctors say a full bath is okay once you bring your baby home. You don't need to bathe him every day, as it may be too drying for his skin. A warm, moist cloth will help to keep him clean between bathings. Wash his face and hands and clean the genital area gently after each diaper change. You don't need to use soap, but if you do, make sure it is mild and unscented. Rinse well to prevent irritation.

Keep your baby's safety and comfort in mind when you are bathing him. Bathe him in a warm room, with water that feels comfortable to the touch. You should already have set your water heater temperature to 49°C (120°F). Remove any jewellery that might scratch your baby, and have all of your supplies within reach. Never leave your baby unattended while bathing him, even for a moment, and never answer your phone, even your cell phone, while you're bathing him.

Hold your baby securely, and use a washcloth and clean water to wash his eyes, ears, mouth, and face. If you have a girl, wipe her genitals from front to back, and don't separate the vaginal lips. Keep your baby boy's penis clean by gently washing the area; don't try to pull back the foreskin. Don't use cotton swabs to clean inside your baby's nose and ears; instead, use a clean washcloth wrapped around your little finger to clean the outer areas. Mucus or earwax will work itself out in time. When you're done, pat him completely dry with a towel.

MYTH BUSTERS

Myth: If you get water in your baby's ears, it will cause an ear infection.

Fact: It's okay if you get water in your baby's ears during bathing. Water does not cause ear infections.

—Dr. Shirley Blaichman, MD, FRCPC

Caring for the umbilical cord

By the time you go home from the hospital, the umbilical cord will have started to dry. Until it falls off—and that can take days, weeks, or, in very rare cases, even longer—you should keep it clean and dry. Water is all you need to clean it. It will fall off on its own, so don't pull on the stump, even when it starts to come off. Prevent your baby's diaper from rubbing the area by folding it over so it's under the belly button. For a day or two, you may find a few spots of blood on his sleeper, but that's perfectly normal.

MAKE A NOTE, MAKE AN APPOINTMENT, OR GO TO THE HOSPITAL?

Make an appointment to see your baby's doctor if your baby has a fever (rectal temperature of 38.0°C/100.4°F or higher), or if his umbilical area

▷ bleeds more than a bit;

▷ oozes yellow pus;

▷ produces a foul-smelling discharge; or

▷ appears red and swollen.

Caring for an uncircumcised penis

If you have had your son's penis circumcised, information on caring for him during the healing process can be found on page 14 in Chapter One. An uncircumcised penis is easy to keep clean and requires no special care. Keep your baby's penis clean by gently washing the area during his bath. When your son is old enough, teach him to clean it as you are teaching him how to keep the rest of his body clean.

The foreskin covers the glans and part of the shaft of a boy's penis. At some time during the early years of a boy's life, the foreskin separates from the glans and can be pulled back. It usually becomes retractable by the time a boy is between three and five years old, but sometimes it isn't fully retractable until after puberty. The separation is a natural process that occurs over time, so don't try to force it. You don't need to do anything to make it happen. When the foreskin is fully retractable, teach your son to wash underneath it each day.

When the foreskin separates, skin cells will be shed and new ones will develop to replace them. These dead skin cells will work their way down the penis through the tip of the foreskin and may look like white lumps (called smegma). If you see smegma under the skin, you don't need to force it out. Just wipe it away once it comes out.

Skin Conditions

No matter how well you take care of your newborn's skin, some skin conditions are unavoidable. Most are fairly common and do not need to be treated. One of the first things you may encounter is vernix, a greasy white substance that coats and protects a baby's skin in the mother's uterus. Some babies are born with lots of vernix still on their skin. It is harmless and can be wiped off, but as it's being lost during the first week of life, it may cause the skin to peel. This is normal and will go away on its own, as will most skin conditions, including acne. That's right—your newborn may seem as far as possible from her teen years, but babies can get acne. Baby acne is a red, pimply rash on the face caused by hormonal changes. Babies also often get milia, which look like tiny whiteheads.

Erythema toxicum is a splotchy red rash that commonly affects newborns. The rash tends to come and go on different parts of the body, and is usually in the form of small white pustules surrounded by a flare of red. It is most common on the second day of life, but can appear at birth or within the first two to four weeks. The individual splotches may stay for only a few hours, or they may linger for several days. There is no treatment, but it will gradually disappear. Another common condition is cutis marmorata, which makes the skin look like pinkish-blue marble when it's exposed to cold temperatures. It is not serious and will improve as your baby gets older.

Birthmarks

Birthmarks abound in newborns—hence the name. Mongolian spots are flat birthmarks that can be slate gray or blue-black in colour. They sometimes look like bruises and are often found on the lower back and buttocks. Mongolian spots are present at birth, and most of them fade (at least a bit) by age two, and usually completely by age five. They are very common in babies of African, Asian, Hispanic, and biracial descent.

Another form of birthmark, hemangiomas aren't always present at birth, but like many birthmarks they may appear during the first few weeks. These "strawberries" are a benign overgrowth of blood vessels. After some initial growth over the first six or seven months, they typically shrink after two years or so. A very small proportion of hemangiomas will occur in places that may disturb function, such as around the eyes, and may need treatment.

Storkbites are vascular lesions that occur in almost 50 per cent of babies. They occur over the upper eyelids, on the forehead, or on the nape of the neck. Those over the eyes almost always disappear, those on the forehead usually disappear by age two, while those on the nape of the neck may persist without causing problems.

MAKE A NOTE, MAKE AN APPOINTMENT, OR GO TO THE HOSPITAL?

Make a note to mention it to your baby's doctor if your baby has flat red birthmarks on her skin, particularly if they're on her face.

Diaper rash

Diaper rash, also called diaper dermatitis, is caused by rubbing and moisture. It occurs when urine or stool in the diaper remains in contact with the skin for too long and irritates it, making it tender and red. When it rubs against the diaper, your baby's sensitive skin becomes weakened and is vulnerable to infection and inflammation. Diarrhea only adds to the problem. Acid in the stool burns the skin, and the area around the anus becomes red and sore, causing your baby to fuss even more when you clean the area. Diaper rash can also be caused by snug-fitting, airtight plastic pants or plastic-covered diapers that prevent water from evaporating, increasing the likelihood of skin irritation. Your baby's age also makes a difference. Babies are most likely to have diaper rash around 8 to 10 months, which may coincide with when they start eating more solid foods.

Once a rash develops, your baby's skin must be kept clean and protected. Her diaper should be changed after every bowel movement, and her skin should be washed with warm water, then thoroughly dried. Don't try to get her completely clean, as this will just cause more irritation. Barrier creams, such as a paste made from petroleum jelly and cornstarch, should be applied to her skin before you put on a fresh diaper.

MAKE A NOTE, MAKE AN APPOINTMENT, OR GO TO THE HOSPITAL?

Make an appointment to see your baby's doctor if your baby has a severe case of diaper rash. The doctor may need to prescribe a specific cream.

Candida

If you're taking antibiotics and breastfeeding, or if your baby is taking antibiotics, she may be more susceptible to a rash caused by yeast. Candida is a type of yeast that causes an infection on the skin or in the mouth. Yeast from the stool can affect the skin, causing a bright red rash with small pimples. When it's in the mouth, it's called thrush.

Candida diaper rash tends to be in the deepest part of the creases in the groin and buttocks. The rash is usually very red, with a clearly defined border and small red spots close to the large patches. Candida infections can be cured with a medication that your doctor prescribes and that is applied to the skin. An oral treatment is often used to treat thrush. To help avoid candida, wash your baby's diaper area with mild soap and warm water during diaper changes, rinse her off, and dry. Wash your own and your baby's hands carefully after the diaper change.

MAKE A NOTE, MAKE AN APPOINTMENT, OR GO TO THE HOSPITAL?

Make an appointment to see your baby's doctor if you suspect your baby has a candida infection. If the doctor prescribes medication, follow the directions and recommendations.

To prevent diaper rash and candida, change your baby's diaper often, wash the area well with just a washcloth and warm water, rinse and let dry completely, and apply unscented petroleum jelly to the skin of the diaper area to protect and lubricate it. Avoid using baby powder or talc, and avoid baby wipes unless they are alcohol-free and unscented.

MAKE A NOTE, MAKE AN APPOINTMENT, OR GO TO THE HOSPITAL?

Make an appointment to see your baby's doctor if

> your baby has patches of bright red skin that peels off in sheets;
> the rash is a large, red area;
> the rash is very raw or bleeding; or
> the rash has spread beyond the diaper area.

You should also see a doctor if your baby is a newborn (less than one month old) and has a rash with tiny water blisters or pimples in a cluster, or her rash includes pimples, blisters, open weeping sores, boils, yellow crusts, or red streaks. If she's being treated for candida but the rash has not improved after three days of treatment, **make another appointment.**

Thrush is a common infection that may occur after a baby is treated with antibiotics for some other infection. Babies may develop a rash in their mouths or on the skin if large numbers of candida are present or if the skin is damaged. Thrush appears as a whitish-grey coating on the tongue and the insides of the cheeks and gums. Unlike milk in your baby's mouth, the coating is hard to wipe off. Vigorous attempts to wipe it off may leave a raw, bleeding surface. In severe cases, your baby's mouth may be sore and she may find it painful to suck, but most babies have no pain or complications with thrush. To help avoid thrush, regularly sanitize bottle nipples and soothers by boiling them for 10 minutes. If breastfeeding, wash your breasts before and after feeding. Thrush is treated with a prescribed anti-fungal liquid.

MAKE A NOTE, MAKE AN APPOINTMENT, OR GO TO THE HOSPITAL?

If your baby refuses to suck, **make an appointment** to see her doctor.

Cradle cap

Cradle cap, also called seborrheic dermatitis, appears as scaly patches on a baby's scalp. There may be some redness around the scaly skin. You may also notice redness on other parts of your baby's body, including the creases of her neck, armpits, behind the ears, on the face, and in the diaper area. It's not as common as it once was because so many parents shampoo their babies' hair daily.

Cradle cap will usually go away on its own, so it doesn't need to be treated. If you want to help control the condition, you can apply oil and wash your baby's hair with a medicated shampoo that is approved for babies. Baby oil or mineral oil may help soften the scaly bits. When applying the oil, rub only small amounts into the skin. About an hour later, shampoo and brush out the oil to avoid more build-up.

If your baby's cradle cap is itchy and irritating, or if it looks red and angry, it should be treated. If baby oil doesn't help, a mild hydrocortisone cream (0.5 per cent) is safe and usually effective.

MAKE A NOTE, MAKE AN APPOINTMENT, OR GO TO THE HOSPITAL?

Make an appointment to see your baby's doctor if your baby's cradle cap persists even after you've treated it with hydrocortisone cream.

Eczema

Eczema is a common, chronic skin rash that shows up as dry, thickened, scaly skin, or tiny red bumps that can blister, ooze, or become infected if scratched. It usually appears on a baby's forehead, cheeks, or scalp, though it can spread to her arms, legs, chest, or other parts of her body. The affected skin will usually be extremely dry and itchy.

Eczema is chronic and may be present for years. Although there's no cure, it can usually be controlled and often will go away after several months or years. Do your best to try to control the discomfort of the itching and inflammation by moisturizing your baby's skin frequently; avoiding frequent baths, but using therapeutic oil products when you do bathe your baby; leaving your baby wet and applying petroleum jelly or other non-perfumed moisturizer before she is completely dry; and dressing her in loose cotton fabrics. Only use medicated creams if your baby's doctor has prescribed them, and follow the instructions carefully. As eczema may last for years, you and your baby's doctor should set out a plan for how to treat outbreaks. If the rash persists and your baby is not comfortable, her doctor may prescribe medication.

Contact dermatitis

Contact dermatitis can develop after your baby's skin comes into contact with something irritating or that she's allergic to, such as metallic snaps on undershirts or dyes in clothing. This contact may cause rashes in areas where the clothing rubs or where there is sweat. Contact dermatitis rash is usually only found on the part of the skin that came in contact with the item your baby is allergic to. The treatment is the same as for eczema, but your doctor will also want to find the cause of the rash by taking a careful history.

Heat rash

Heat rash causes little bumps on the skin that can show up when your baby overheats. The bumps may appear red, especially in babies with light skin colour. You can usually see the rash in the folds of your baby's skin and on parts of her body where clothing fits snugly, including the chest, stomach, neck, crotch, and buttocks. Hot, humid weather is prime time for heat rash, but you might see it in winter if your baby is wearing too many layers of clothing. Treat it by removing excess clothing. Keep your baby comfortably cool by dressing her in loose-fitting, light cotton clothing, especially in warm, humid weather.

Spitting Up

It's normal for babies to spit up a little—or even a lot—from time to time, with absolutely no cause for concern. When they take in air along with breast milk or formula, the air becomes trapped in bubbles between the liquid. When they burp, the air forces out the liquid that's sitting on top of it. Sometimes babies will just take in too much liquid in one sitting for their stomachs to digest. If your baby is generally happy and gaining weight at a normal rate, occasional or even frequent spitting up is not harmful, and it will have no long-term effects. Most babies outgrow this rather unpleasant habit by about six to nine months of age.

There are a few things you can do to help your baby avoid spitting up. Feed him in a quiet, calm atmosphere. Noise or other distractions can make him agitated or upset, increasing the air he swallows during feeding. To keep pressure off his stomach, hold your baby upright during feedings, check that his diaper and clothing waistbands aren't too tight, don't lay him over your shoulder while burping, and don't put him into his car seat immediately after eating. Burp your baby frequently during feedings to eliminate any trapped air. If you use a bottle, make sure the hole in the nipple isn't too small (which will frustrate him and increase his air intake) or too large (which can cause him to gag and ingest more air). You can tell it's the right size if liquid comes out in a steady flow of about a drop per second when the bottle is held at feeding angle.

Try not to overfeed your baby; feed him a little each time, but feed him frequently. Don't stimulate or jostle him too much after he's eaten—and remember to keep a towel handy.

MAKE A NOTE, MAKE AN APPOINTMENT, OR GO TO THE HOSPITAL?

Make an appointment to see your baby's doctor if your baby is spitting up frequently and you suspect he's not gaining weight, or he vomits forcefully or frequently, with almost each feed.

Take him to the hospital immediately if he projectile vomits—spits up forcefully a few times and in larger quantities than normal. It could be the result of a number of problems, such as a condition called pyloric stenosis, in which the muscles at the bottom of the stomach thicken and don't allow food to pass into the small intestine, or a blockage in his intestines, which could require surgery. If projectile vomiting starts suddenly (especially if it contains green bile, a sign of a potential blockage), **call 911.**

When spitting up is serious

It's perfectly normal for babies to spit up from time to time, and they may vomit as a result of a general infection. If your baby is vomiting, keep him hydrated with breast milk or oral rehydration fluids. If he is also listless, it could be serious, and he needs to be checked quickly.

Dr. Sacks Says

If you need to change your shirt, he's spitting up. If you need to mop the floor halfway across the room, it's projectile vomiting.

If the spitting up is severe and persistent (more often than twice a day), your baby could be suffering from gastroesophageal reflux disease (GERD). Reflux is most often the result of a weak esophageal sphincter, the valve connecting the esophagus to the stomach. It allows acidic stomach fluids to flow backward into the esophagus and sometimes up into the mouth (and out—hence the frequent spitting up). Severe cases are relatively uncommon—about 3 per cent of infants get it. Most babies outgrow it in their first year as their esophageal sphincter gets stronger, and there is usually no need for medication. If your doctor determines that your baby has GERD, he may prescribe medication to help ease your baby's suffering. Some doctors feel that waiting and carefully checking weight gain is all that is needed.

Other than that, you can employ the same techniques as used to help control spitting up: holding your baby in a vertical position while feeding, burping frequently, and feeding him small portions frequently. You may also want to try adding a little rice cereal to his bottle, but you should talk to his doctor first.

> ## MAKE A NOTE, MAKE AN APPOINTMENT, OR GO TO THE HOSPITAL?
>
> **Make an appointment** to see your baby's doctor if your baby is not gaining weight, or if you suspect he has GERD.

Eyes and Eye Care

Neonatal opthalmia

Your newborn's eyes are very delicate, and an infection could easily damage them. Fortunately, Canadian hospitals are one step ahead. Neonatal opthalmia is any infection that occurs in the eye of a newborn within the first 30 days of life. Babies get opthalmia from bacteria, usually from a maternal infection or STD, that are passed to them during vaginal delivery. Since the potential for serious eye damage from infection is so great, and since the mother may not have symptoms with some infections, it is standard treatment in Canadian hospitals to give infants antibiotic eye drops or ointment, called an eye prophylaxis, within an hour of delivery.

Blocked tear ducts

Blocked tear ducts are a common problem in infants. As many as one-third may be born with this condition. Fortunately, more than 90 per cent of all cases resolve themselves with little or no treatment by the time a baby is one year old.

The most common cause of blocked tear ducts is that a baby is born with a duct that is more narrow than usual, so it becomes blocked easily or does not drain properly. Less often, a baby has a web of tissue over the end of the duct that did not dissolve during fetal development. This condition is more likely to require surgical probing.

Babies with blocked tear ducts usually develop symptoms of the condition between birth and 12 weeks of age. The most common sign of blocked tear ducts is excessive tearing, even when a baby is not crying. You also may notice pus in the corner of your baby's eye, or he may wake up with a crust over his eyelid or in his eyelashes.

Most discomfort from a blocked tear duct can be relieved by gently massaging the eye several times a day for a few months. If your baby develops an infection as a result of the blockage, his doctor will prescribe antibiotic eye drops or ointment to treat the infection. If he still has excess tearing after nine months, develops a serious infection, or has repeated infections, his tear duct may need to be surgically probed. His doctor will recommend a consultation with an opthamologist.

MAKE A NOTE, MAKE AN APPOINTMENT, OR GO TO THE HOSPITAL?

Make an appointment to see your baby's doctor if his eyes tear excessively but show no sign of infection. Early treatment can prevent the need for surgery.

If your baby shows signs of infection such as redness, pus, or swelling, **make an appointment with his doctor for that day** *or* **take him to the hospital.** An infected tear duct can lead to a serious infection if not treated.

Your Baby's First Teeth

Caring for your baby's teeth begins when that first tooth peeks through her gums. Proper mouth care includes cleaning the tongue, gums, and new teeth as they erupt. Such early practices as giving your baby water, gently cleaning her mouth after feeding, and not leaving her in bed with a bottle will lay the groundwork for healthy teeth for life.

Primary teeth start forming during the first three months of pregnancy, so some antibiotics taken during pregnancy can affect them. The first tooth usually arrives at about 6 months of age, but it's normal for some children's teeth to appear as early as 3 months or as late as 12 months. Most children will have all 20 primary teeth by the time they are three years old.

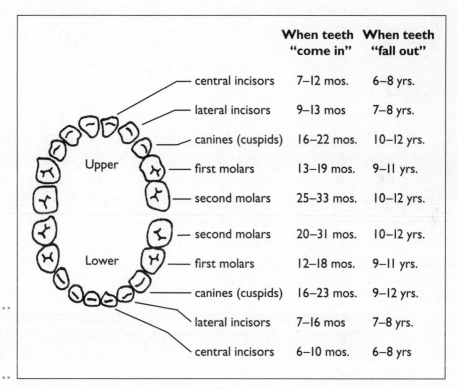

	When teeth "come in"	When teeth "fall out"
central incisors	7–12 mos.	6–8 yrs.
lateral incisors	9–13 mos	7–8 yrs.
canines (cuspids)	16–22 mos.	10–12 yrs.
first molars	13–19 mos.	9–11 yrs.
second molars	25–33 mos.	10–12 yrs.
second molars	20–31 mos.	10–12 yrs.
first molars	12–18 mos.	9–11 yrs.
canines (cuspids)	16–23 mos.	9–12 yrs.
lateral incisors	7–16 mos	7–8 yrs.
central incisors	6–10 mos.	6–8 yrs

Figure 2.1: Primary teeth

In the past, the care of primary or "baby" teeth was not considered important because they eventually fall out, to be replaced by permanent teeth. However, healthy primary teeth are an essential component of normal overall growth. Primary teeth give shape to your baby's face, help guide permanent teeth into the right position in her mouth, and help her learn to eat and speak. Unhealthy teeth and gums may lead to poor nutrition if your baby's mouth hurts too much when she feeds, and may even lead to serious infections.

MYTH BUSTERS

Myth: Teething causes fever and diarrhea.

Fact: Teething rarely causes a significant fever or diarrhea. Look for other causes.

—*Dr. Ken Schelberg, MD, FRCPC*

Teething

When your baby's primary teeth are coming in, her gums may be swollen and tender. To help ease her discomfort, rub her gums with a clean finger, and give her something to chew on, such as a teething ring made of firm rubber or a wet facecloth that has been in the freezer for half an hour. Never rub gel on her gums, as she may swallow it, or give her teething biscuits, which contain a lot of sugar and aren't the best treatment for sore gums.

MAKE A NOTE, MAKE AN APPOINTMENT, OR GO TO THE HOSPITAL?

Teething causes mild discomfort, but it does not make babies sick or give them a fever. If your baby is younger than six months and has a fever, **make an appointment** with her doctor.

Make a note to talk to her doctor at her next appointment if she seems very distressed by teething.

Decay

Tooth enamel is a thin, hard, white substance that covers the tooth. Primary teeth have a thinner enamel than permanent teeth, which puts them at risk of early childhood tooth decay. This used to be called baby bottle tooth decay, and is defined as decay that occurs before a child is six years old. However, it can begin as soon as the first tooth arrives. It can be caused by repeated and prolonged exposure to sweet liquids, which include breast milk, formula, milk, juice, and soft drinks. One sure way to fend off early childhood tooth decay is to prevent any liquid but water from remaining in your baby's mouth for a long time. This means limiting the amount of juice she drinks, not putting her to bed with a bottle, and not sweetening her pacifier.

Plaque, which is a thick, whitish bacterial film, forms on primary teeth immediately after they appear. Bacteria in plaque can cause inflammation of the gums (gingivitis). Carbohydrates in a child's normal diet can stimulate bacterial growth, and bacteria produce the acids that cause cavities. Check your baby's mouth for signs of decay every month. Lift her upper lip and look for chalky white or brown spots on her teeth or along the gum line, and take her to the dentist if you see any of these.

Early childhood tooth decay can cause pain that makes it difficult for her to sleep, eat, speak, or concentrate and learn. Children who have tooth decay at an early age are more likely to suffer decay throughout their childhood.

Guidelines for good dental care

After your baby is born, and up to 12 months, wipe her mouth with a soft, clean, damp cloth twice a day. As soon as her first tooth appears, clean it with a soft-bristled toothbrush designed for babies. To clean her teeth, cradle her head in your lap or on a flat surface.

After six months, try giving her a sippy cup for water and formula, and give her water between meals. After 12 months she can switch to a regular cup. If you give her juice, avoid sugared juices (and definitely avoid other sugary drinks), and only give it to her as part of a meal. Give her no more than 125 to 175 millilitres (4 to 6 ounces) per day in a regular cup rather than a bottle, and encourage her to hold the cup by herself. If she needs a bottle before a nap or bedtime, give water as the before-bed drink, but don't put her to bed with a bottle.

Always wash your hands before and after brushing your own teeth and your baby's teeth. Rinse toothbrushes thoroughly after brushing and ensure that each one can dry without touching others. Replace toothbrushes every few months, when the bristles become flattened with use. Take your baby for regular dental visits about every six months, starting at 12 months old, unless otherwise suggested by your dentist.

KNOW YOUR FLUORIDE NUMBERS

Fluoride is a natural compound that protects teeth from cavities. Natural water sources, such as wells and springs, may contain fluoride, but it is also added to the local water supply in many communities. Fluoride is added to toothpastes, and dentists sometimes apply it to teeth as part of your child's normal checkup.

In Canada, the optimum amount of fluoride in drinking water is 0.7 parts per million (ppm). This is the amount that prevents tooth decay but does not cause a condition called fluorosis. Fluorosis happens when a child ingests too much fluoride when teeth are forming—from birth to about three years of age. Although fluorosis is not a health problem, it can cause chalky-white or even brownish spots or blotches on the teeth.

Check with your municipality to find out how much fluoride is in your water, or have your water tested. In municipalities where the level of fluoride is 0.3 ppm or less, ask your dentist or doctor whether your child needs a fluoride supplement.

Immunizing Your Child

Vaccination is the best way to protect your child against many diseases that caused serious illness and death in the past. Children in Canada no longer have to get dangerous illnesses like measles, mumps, chickenpox, or whooping cough thanks to vaccines. Vaccination becomes even more important as old diseases develop new complications. For instance, chickenpox has long been considered an inevitable inconvenience of childhood, but with the prevalence of antibiotic-resistant bacteria, or superbugs, it can actually lead to deadly flesh-eating disease.

To be thoroughly protected, your child needs to receive his shots at the right times. The schedule may vary slightly in different parts of Canada, so if you're moving to another province or territory, talk to your child's doctor first to ensure he won't miss any vaccines. Keep a complete copy of his vaccinations, and make more than one copy to avoid losing track. This record is a very important health document and it is essential that it is kept up to date.

Immunization schedule

Vaccine	2 mos.	4 mos.	6 mos.	12 mos.	18 mos.	4–6 yrs
5-in-1	★	★	★		★	see below*
MMR				★	★ or	★
Chickenpox				★		
Pneumococcal	★	★	★	★		
Meningococcal	★	★	★			
			or			
		between 4–11 mos., 2 shots 4 wks. apart				
			or			
				★		
Hep B	3 doses in infancy			or	from 9–13 years	
Flu				once a year after 6 mos.		

*Children receive a booster shot of 4-in-1 (Diphtheria, Tetanus, Pertussis, and Polio) at 4–6 years.

Immunization schedules may vary depending on the province or territory in which you live. In particular, the hepatitis B vaccine may be given to infants in a series of three shots, or it may be given when children are in their pre-teens, depending on where you live. See the Canadian Paediatric Society's Caring for Kids website (www.caringforkids.cps.ca) for a detailed immunization schedule, and "Immunization" in Resources for more sources of information on immunization.

Vaccines that are covered by health plans

Certain vaccines are covered by provincial or territorial health plans, which means that parents don't have to pay for them. These vaccines are described below.

The 5-in-1 vaccine

As the name suggests, you can protect your child from five diseases with one shot. The 5-in-1 shot (also called DPTP-Hib) protects children against diphtheria, tetanus, pertussis, polio, and hib. In Canada, most children get the 5-in-1 shot when they are 2 months old, 4 months old, 6 months old, and 18 months old. A booster is also given at around four years of age. Premature babies get their shots at the same ages as their full-term friends. The only children who should not get the 5-in-1 shot are those who had trouble breathing or had severe swelling of the skin or mouth as a result of receiving the previous shot.

Diphtheria is an illness caused by germs that infect the nose, throat, or skin. It causes serious breathing problems, and can also cause heart failure and nerve damage for a person's entire life. It can be fatal, especially in babies.

Tetanus is also known as lockjaw. Tetanus germs live in dirt, and when they get into an open cut, poison from the germs spreads to nerves and then muscles. Muscles may lock or go into painful spasms. The first muscles affected are the ones in the jaw. A person with tetanus can die very quickly if it reaches the muscles that control breathing.

Children who survive tetanus may have long-lasting problems with speech, memory, and thinking.

Pertussis is also called whooping cough, and is caused by germs that get into the throat and lungs. Whooping cough may cause babies to have seizures or go into a coma, and some babies under a year old can end up with brain damage. Very young infants or those with lung disease may die. Older children who get whooping cough will have two to three weeks of severe coughing spells, and they may cough so long and so hard that they can't breathe. The disease can last from 6 to 12 weeks.

Polio is caused by three types of the polio virus. It can cause fever, headache, vomiting, strong muscle pain, and paralysis. It can also make children very tired, and cause stiffness in the neck and back. Some people with polio don't feel sick at all, while others are paralysed for the rest of their lives. Polio can also be deadly.

Hib stands for *haemophilus influenzae* type b. In spite of its name, it has nothing to do with the flu. It is a bacteria that can infect the fluid around the brain and spinal cord. Hib can cause meningitis, a very serious disease that infects the brain and spinal cord, and it can also lead to other deadly diseases. Meningitis can cause seizures, deafness, or brain damage. Symptoms include high fever, stiff neck, headache, vomiting, fussiness, and loss of appetite.

The MMR vaccine

The MMR vaccine protects your child from three diseases: measles, mumps, and rubella. In Canada, children get the MMR shot twice, either when they are 12 months old and 18 months old, or when they are 12 months old and just before they start school (between ages 4 and 6). The only children who should not get the MMR shot are those who have had it before and had trouble breathing or had severe swelling on their skin or in their mouth as a result.

Measles is caused by a virus that spreads quickly and easily by sneezing and coughing. Sometimes it is called red measles (or rubeola) so it will not be confused with German measles (or rubella). There is no treatment for it. It begins with a fever, runny nose, cough, and very red eyes. You may think your child has a cold, but in a few days, a rash begins around his face and spreads to his chest, arms, and legs. His eyes may hurt in bright light. Measles can cause an ear infection or pneumonia, and in rare cases can also cause a swelling of the brain called encephalitis, which can lead to seizures, deafness, or mental retardation, or can be fatal. In parts of the world with no vaccination programs, measles is a leading cause of death.

Mumps is caused by a virus that is spread by close contact between people, including by sneezing and coughing. Mumps causes fever, headache, and painful swelling of the saliva glands that makes the cheeks puff out. Sometimes, mumps can cause deafness and even meningitis. In older boys, mumps can cause a testes inflammation that may lead to sterility.

Rubella is also known as German measles. Like red measles, it is caused by a virus that is spread by close contact between people, like through sneezing and coughing, but it is milder than red measles. Children get a low fever and a mild cold, the glands in the neck may swell up, and a rash may follow. The sickness lasts about three days. An infected child can pass rubella on to a susceptible pregnant mother, causing severe damage to the fetus.

The dTap vaccine

The dTap vaccine is a booster shot for teenagers. It protects against diptheria, tetanus, and pertussis (whooping cough), and is given to children once the vaccines for those diseases have worn off.

Hepatitis B vaccine

Hepatitis B is a disease caused by a virus that infects the liver. It is spread through direct contact with body fluids. Some people who have hepatitis B will not feel sick but may be carriers of the disease for the rest of their lives. Others will be very sick for several weeks or even months, with a fever, fatigue, loss of appetite, and jaundice. Children who become infected are more likely to be infected for life, and are at high risk for developing cirrhosis, liver failure, and liver cancer later in life.

Depending on where you live, the hepatitis B vaccine may be given to your child in infancy or when she is in her pre-teens. It is commonly given in a series of three shots over a six-month period: the second shot one month after the first, and the third shot five months after the second. Children older than one year may receive a combination vaccine that also includes the hepatitis A vaccine.

Chickenpox vaccine

Chickenpox is a very common illness caused by the varicella-zoster virus. People with chickenpox get an itchy rash or spots on their skin like small water blisters. It spreads very quickly from person to person through direct contact. You can get chickenpox if you touch a blister, the liquid from a blister, or the saliva of a person who has chickenpox. It can also spread through the air if you are near someone with chickenpox who is coughing or sneezing. A pregnant woman with chickenpox can pass it on to her baby before birth with possible severe consequences, depending on when she has the infection.

Most people get chickenpox by the time they are 15 years old. It's long been considered an inconvenient but normal part of childhood, but chickenpox can cause bigger problems. If the blisters get infected, your child may end up with scars. If open sores get infected, flesh-eating disease, a life-threatening skin infection, may develop. Babies who get chickenpox from their mothers before birth could be born with birth defects, such as scars, eye problems, or arms and legs that are not fully formed. Children with chickenpox may get pneumonia or have problems with other organs, including the brain. Chickenpox can be very severe or even life-threatening for newborn babies and adults, or for anyone who has a weak immune system.

The days of "chickenpox parties" are over. Instead of hoping your child gets chickenpox young so that he doesn't get it as a teenager or adult, when it can be dangerous, you can vaccinate your child and avoid it altogether. Most provinces and territories offer the chickenpox vaccine at one year of age, and children from one to 12 years of age can get the shot once, at the same time as the MMR vaccine. The vaccine is very safe, but some people will get a very mild case of chickenpox (fewer than 50 spots) one or two weeks after they get the shot. If your child is not vaccinated but is exposed to another child who has chickenpox, there's still a chance he can be protected from severe infection if he is vaccinated within 72 hours.

Pneumococcal vaccine

Pneumococcal infections are caused by a germ called *streptococcus pneumoniae*. This germ can cause several different infections, including meningitis (brain infection), bacteremia (bloodstream infection), pneumonia (lung infection), and otitis media (middle ear infection). See page 96 under "The 5-in-1 vaccine" for information on meningitis.

Bacteremia is an illness caused when germs infect the blood. The symptoms are similar to those of meningitis. Sometimes it goes away on its own, but if the germs multiply and travel to other parts of the body, it can cause permanent damage.

Pneumonia is an infection that fills the lungs with fluid, causing breathing problems. Children who get pneumonia will have a fever and cough that may bring up thick mucus, and they will become very ill quickly.

Otitis media (middle ear infection) is caused by many different germs, including the pneumococcal germ. When a person has a middle ear infection, the eardrum turns red and the space behind it fills with fluid or pus. Children under two years old sometimes get middle ear infections when they have a cold. Middle ear infections can cause ear pain, fever, lack of energy, fussiness, and a loss of appetite. For more on middle ear infections, see page 349 in Chapter Six.

All of these infections can also be caused by other germs, so the pneumococcal vaccine will not protect your child from these infections if they are caused by another germ. The pneumococcal vaccine is least effective for otitis media. The germ spreads from the nose and throat of one person to another by close, direct contact like kissing, coughing, or sneezing. It can also be spread through saliva when people share things like food, cups, water bottles, straws, or toothbrushes. However, the germ dies quickly when it is outside of the body.

Children are most at risk of infection if they are under two years old; have weak immune systems; have sickle-cell anemia or HIV (the virus that causes AIDS); have serious problems with their heart, lungs, or kidneys; are missing their spleen or have other spleen problems; or attend daycare.

Two kinds of pneumococcal vaccine are available. One is recommended for all children up to five years of age, and it is best to get it as a newborn. Babies get four doses of the vaccine: when they are 2 months old, 4 months old, 6 months old, and 12 to 15 months old. The other vaccine is for children at high risk of severe disease such as sickle-cell anemia, chronic heart and lung disorders, diabetes, and HIV. They receive it at two years of age, followed by a booster between three and five years. Both forms of vaccine are safe, but some children will have a mild fever after getting the vaccine. Other possible side effects include fussiness, drowsiness, restless sleep, decreased appetite, vomiting, diarrhea, rash, or hives (itchy red bumps). Children who have had a bad allergic reaction to a previous dose of the vaccine should not get it again.

Meningococcal vaccine

Meningococcal diseases are caused by a germ called meningococcus. This germ can cause two serious diseases: meningitis and septicemia, a serious blood infection.

The germs that cause the most infections are known as group B and group C. Since 1989, there have been outbreaks of group C disease among teenagers in many parts of Canada. Without treatment, the majority of children who get meningitis will die or suffer damage that lasts the rest of their lives. Even with treatment, some will die, and some who survive will have brain damage. Septicemia can also kill very quickly. Even with treatment, about half the children who get septicemia will die or have permanent damage.

The germs that cause meningococcal diseases are quite common. They live in the back of the nose and throat of about one in five teenagers and adults without causing any sickness. These people are called healthy carriers. The germs are spread mostly by healthy carriers, and not by people who are clearly sick with the disease. The germs are not very strong, and they die quickly outside the body. For the disease to spread, people must have close, direct contact such as kissing, coughing, or sneezing. The germs can also be spread through saliva when people share things such as cigarettes, lipstick, food or drinks, cups, water bottles, pop and juice cans, drinking straws, toothbrushes, toys, mouth guards, and musical instruments with mouthpieces. Smoking and overcrowding increase the risk that the germs will spread.

Early signs of meningococcal meningitis are fever and a major change in behaviour, including drowsiness, reduced consciousness (your child doesn't seem awake), irritability, fussiness, and agitation. Other symptoms include severe headache, vomiting, stiff neck, pain when moving the head or neck, aches and pains, joint pain, and convulsions. About two-thirds of children with meningococcal meningitis have a skin rash made up of red spots (tiny broken blood vessels, known as petechiae) that don't disappear when pressed. The spots may get quite large over a short period of time.

Early signs of meningococcal septicemia are fever, aches, joint pain, and headaches. Children with this disease get sick very quickly, in only a few hours. They are drowsy, semi-conscious, irritable, or agitated. Almost all children with septicemia have a skin rash that starts as red spots. The spots increase in size and number in just a few hours. Complications include low blood pressure (shock), coma, convulsions, and severe breathing trouble.

When someone has meningococcal disease, doctors will often give specific antibiotics to their family members or the people they live with, as well as close contacts, such as other children and staff at school or daycare. This can stop the germs from spreading and protect exposed individuals from getting the disease.

There are two kinds of meningococcal vaccines available in Canada, and they each protect people from different strains of the germ. One is more effective in babies and young children, but it only protects against one type of the meningococcus germ, group C. The other vaccine only protects children two years of age and older, teenagers, and adults, but it may cover up to four different types of the germ. Your child's doctor can tell you which vaccine is best for your child.

Very young babies get three shots: at 2 months old, 4 months old, and 6 months old. Babies 4 to 11 months old get two shots, at least four weeks apart. Children over 12 months old get one shot. Both forms of the vaccine are very safe, but they often cause redness, swelling, or pain at the place where your child gets the needle, so ask your doctor what you can do to control pain or swelling. Children who have had a bad allergic reaction to a previous dose of the vaccine should not get it again.

Influenza vaccine

If your child is over six months of age, you may want him to get a flu shot to protect him and those around him, especially if he is at high risk for complications from influenza. Children are considered at high risk between 6 and 23 months of age. They are also at high risk if they need to be treated for long periods of time with aspirin, have heart or lung problems (like cystic fibrosis or asthma), have a chronic condition that weakens the immune system (like cancer, HIV, or anemia), have a metabolic disease like diabetes, or have a neurological or neuromuscular disorder that affects their breathing.

The Canadian Paediatric Society recommends that all children over six months old get a flu shot each year. Although the vaccine is not harmful to babies younger than six months old, it doesn't work for them. If there are children younger than two years old in your home, everyone living in your home who is able should get a flu shot. This is especially important if you have a baby under six months old, since he can't get the shot yet and could become infected if a family member gets the flu. Babysitters and others who take care of children younger than two years of age outside of the home should also be immunized. If your baby is around anyone in the high-risk group, including elderly or sick relatives, he should get the shot to prevent the flu spreading to that person.

Dr. Sacks Says

Your child will have about 10 colds a year until he is 10 years old, and most of them will happen between October and March. That's almost two a month. If he gets sick after getting a flu shot, it's likely just a coincidence.

Unless the flu shot is given under close medical supervision, your child should avoid it if he has a severe egg allergy (as the vaccine is made in chicken eggs) or if he has had a severe allergic reaction to a previous flu shot. If he has an allergy to thimerosal (a preservative), ask if a thimerosal-free vaccine is available. Currently, the flu shot is the only vaccine in Canada that contains thimerosal.

MYTH BUSTERS

Myth: If you get a flu shot, you will become dependent on it each year.

Fact: You need a new flu shot each year because influenza viruses change quickly, often from year to year, not because your system becomes dependent on it. The shot helps prepare your system to fight the flu.

—Dr. Krista Baerg, MD, FRCPC

Flu shots are usually given once a year from October to mid-November. Children under the age of nine years who have never had a flu shot will need two doses of the vaccine given at least four weeks apart. The shots provide protection throughout the flu season, from October to March.

The influenza vaccine being used right now is made from killed flu virus, so it cannot cause the flu. Side effects are usually mild, and limited to soreness at the place where the needle goes into the arm, and a slight fever or aching for the first day or two after immunization, especially after the first dose of vaccine. Acetaminophen will help reduce these symptoms. In rare cases, a person may have red or itchy eyes, a cough, and mild swelling of the face within a few hours of vaccination, but this usually goes away within 48 hours.

A new type of influenza vaccine that is given as a nose spray rather than by injection is available in some countries, but not in Canada yet. It contains live influenza virus that has been changed so that it can no longer cause disease. In the United States, it is used only in healthy children who are five years old or over.

Are vaccines safe?

Vaccines are very safe, so there is rarely a reason to not get vaccinated. Immunizations are offered only when the consequences of getting the disease far outweigh any risks of the vaccines. Just ask your grandparents—it wasn't that long ago that deadly diseases like polio, measles, and meningitis were a common threat. However, if your baby is very sick and feverish when it's time for a vaccination, talk to your doctor first.

Much has been made of a possible link between vaccines and autism, but there is no scientific evidence to support this theory. Because signs of autism may appear around the same age that children receive the MMR vaccine, some people believe the vaccine causes the condition. However, just because two things happen at the same time doesn't mean that one causes the other. Many significant studies have confirmed that there is no link between the MMR vaccine and autism. There is also no proven link between thimerosal, a mercury-based preservative used in some vaccines, and autism. However, all routine childhood vaccines in Canada are made without thimerosal. For more information on vaccines and autism, go to www.caringforkids.cps.ca/immunization/MMRMythsFacts.htm.

With any vaccine, there may be some redness, swelling, or pain at the place where the needle went into the arm or leg. If your baby has an allergic reaction to a vaccine, such as breathing problems or severe swelling of the skin or mouth, talk to his doctor before he receives another shot. Some children may have a fever after a vaccination, so ask the doctor what to give your child for fever or pain. If you still have questions about the risks and benefits of vaccinations, talk to the doctor. More sources of information are provided under "Immunization" in Resources and on the Caring for Kids website (www.caringforkids.cps.ca), where the Canadian Paediatric Society statement on vaccine safety is available.

MYTH BUSTERS

Myth: Vaccines can cause autism.

Fact: It has been proven beyond a doubt that vaccines do not cause autism.

—*Dr. Ken Schelberg, MD, FRCPC*

You should also consider vaccines that can protect your child while travelling. Depending on where you are travelling, you may have to consider other vaccines, such as vaccinations against hepatitis A, typhoid fever, and yellow fever; dukoral (ecoli/traveller's diarrhea prevention); and malaria prophylaxis. For more on travel vaccines, see "Immunization for Foreign Travel" in Chapter Three on page 196.

A rotavirus vaccine, which helps prevent acute diarrhea caused by the rotavirus germ, is also now available in Canada.

The Things You Can't Control

Despite your best efforts to keep your baby healthy, there are some conditions you can't prevent. The following are some physical problems that may present themselves during her first year. No one knows your baby better than you do, so trust your instincts, but mention it to her doctor at her next appointment if you see any of them.

- **Tongue tie.** The frenulum, the connective tissue that attaches the tongue to the bottom of the mouth, is connected too tightly. In almost all cases, it will eventually stretch out by itself, but in rare cases it can interfere with breastfeeding.

- **Umbilical hernia.** A bulging around the belly button without discharge or discolouration. In most cases it will close by itself by age two, but if not, a cosmetic procedure can correct it.

- **Inguinal hernia.** A lump in the crease between a baby's thigh and lower abdomen that may appear and disappear. Surgery can easily correct this problem.

- **Diastasis rectii.** A soft-tissue bulge (which may look sort of like a pouch) from the bottom of the sternum along the abdomen. This occurs when the muscles of the abdomen don't completely come together. Generally it will go away on its own.

- **Hemangiomas.** Blood-filled birthmarks that occur during the first six months of life. Most disappear by age two, but some types need attention. Your baby's doctor will determine if attention is necessary.

- **Natal teeth.** Teeth that are present at birth or shortly thereafter. If they are secure in your baby's mouth they will most likely be left alone, but a dentist may need to make that judgment.

- **Metatarsus varus.** A flexible in-turning of the front of the foot that is not so stiff that the leg can't be pushed out. This almost always self-corrects when a child starts walking. If it is stiff and can't be pushed out into a straight position, it may be a club foot, which requires medical attention.

- **Ear tags.** Little flaps of skin that, if cosmetically unappealing, can be removed. They are generally composed of skin, but can also contain cartilage. If an ear tag does contain cartilage, a plastic surgeon can remove it.

- **Mongolian spots, dark spots, or moles.** A Mongolian spot is a darkened area on a baby's lower trunk that can be mistaken for a bruise. They are common in Asian and black babies, and they fade as the child gets older. Any spots or moles on the skin should be checked by a doctor.

- **Undescended testes.** If one or both of a baby boy's testes has not descended into his scrotum, the doctor will monitor the situation and may decide to bring the testes down surgically.

- **Extra digits.** Usually on the hand, extra digits may be associated with other physical issues that need to be addressed. A doctor will make sure there are no associated anomalies, and decide when and if the extra digit needs to be removed surgically.

- **Fused toes.** Toes that are connected together usually pose little or no significant problems. If the situation appears to be interfering with a baby's ability to walk, however, a doctor may need to separate the toes.

NUTRITION

For the first six months of life, all your baby's nutritional needs, with the exception of vitamin D, can be met with milk—preferably breast milk. At six months, your baby will be ready for other foods, and will probably need some extra iron in his diet. You can continue to breastfeed until he is two years of age or older.

Breastfeeding

The Canadian Paediatric Society recommends exclusive breastfeeding for the first six months of life. Breast milk is the best food you can offer your newborn. It has the right amount and quality of nutrients to suit his first food needs. Since it is naturally and uniquely produced by each mother for her own baby, your baby can avoid exposure to foreign allergenic material. It is easy on his digestive system, so there's little chance of constipation or diarrhea. Breast milk also contains antibodies and other immune factors that help your baby prevent and fight off illness. The only addition needed to a breastfed baby's diet is a vitamin D supplement.

MYTH BUSTERS

Myth: Breastfeeding alone provides all the nutrients a baby needs until six months of age.

Fact: Babies also require a vitamin D supplement. Vitamin D is essential to healthy development, and breast milk alone does not provide enough vitamin D to meet your baby's requirements.

—Dr. Leona Fishman-Shapiro, MD, FRCPC

Not long ago, many people in western countries believed that bottle-feeding was better than breastfeeding. Today, we know that breastfeeding offers your baby the best start, and it is the natural way to feed your newborn. Still, it may take a bit of practice. Like all aspects of motherhood, you'll learn through experience, not just through instinct. Your doctor or midwife can counsel you about the principles and practice of breastfeeding. Most hospitals have lactation consultants and breast-feeding clinics, and there are many community-based programs that support breastfeeding families. Before you leave the hospital, ask to see a lactation consultant, who can guide you when you're starting to breastfeed, and keep their phone number handy once you're home.

COLOSTRUM, FOREMILK, AND HINDMILK

In the early days after your baby is born, you will produce colostrum milk. Colostrum milk is usually yellowish in colour and is very rich in protein, vitamins, minerals, and immunity factors that are found only in breast milk. These help protect your baby against infections.

After the first week, colostrum changes into milk that is whitish in colour. The milk at the beginning of each feeding is called foremilk. Foremilk is watery so that it satisfies your baby's fluid needs. As the feed continues, foremilk gains fat content until it becomes hindmilk, which is richer and looks much whiter. Hindmilk gives him a feeling of being full and satisfied.

Time for a feeding

Before you offer your breast to your baby, always wash your hands. Feed your baby from each breast for as long as he wants. Alternate the breast you begin with so that each breast has a chance to produce the proper amount of milk.

Your baby is feeding well when the nursing process doesn't hurt you and he is content after feeding. You should hear short swallowing sounds (like a "K" sound) that gradually lengthen and deepen as your milk is released. Your areola, the area around your nipple, and your baby's jaw muscles should move evenly as he sucks. You'll be able to see the movement of his jaw right up to his ears. If you hear a lot of lip smacking, you notice that there's very little swallowing, the nursing process is painful for you, and your baby is not content after feeding, it's time to call your lactation consultant for help.

At first, you'll be doing a lot of feeding on demand—feeding your baby whenever he's hungry, perhaps every two to three hours throughout the day and night. You can expect to breastfeed 8 to 12 times over a 24-hour period. Small or premature babies need to be fed more frequently. Before you leave the hospital, ask what the appropriate feeding interval is for your baby.

Sometimes babies may want to feed more frequently and for very short periods of time. This is called cluster feeding, and often occurs in the evening. It may mean your baby is going through a growth spurt. These usually happen around the age of two weeks, four-to-six weeks, three months, and six months. Just let your baby set the pace.

If you experience cracked or sore nipples, try exposing them to the air after each feeding, allowing them to dry naturally. You can also apply lanolin or breast milk to them. Avoid using soap on your nipples as it will wash away your breasts' natural lubricants.

MAKE A NOTE, MAKE AN APPOINTMENT, OR GO TO THE HOSPITAL?

Some women get mastitis, a bacterial infection that causes swelling of the breasts along with soreness and fever. If you have these symptoms, **make an appointment** to see your doctor. It can be treated with antibiotics, and will clear up if you continue to breastfeed.

Enough to eat

The easiest way to tell if your baby is getting enough to eat is if he is gaining enough weight, which his doctor will check at each visit. Your baby should also have six to eight wet diapers in a 24-hour period. Today's very absorbent diapers may make this hard to judge, but placing a tissue in the diaper will let you know if he has urinated. He should also have one or more loose, yellowish stools per day during the first month. Early on, these may come after every feeding. After the first month, stools may not be as frequent (one every two to seven days), but they will still be loose and yellowish.

Babies who are breastfed should receive a daily vitamin D supplement, which is available in drops. A deficiency of vitamin D is very serious and can cause rickets, a disease that affects the way bones grow and develop. Your baby needs no other supplements while you are breastfeeding.

But are you getting enough to eat?

Breastfeeding mothers need to eat a variety of nutritious foods, and they should continue to take prenatal vitamins to supplement a healthy diet. You require an extra 500 calories per day to sustain good milk production, so avoid dieting while you are breastfeeding. Just as in pregnancy, breastfeeding mothers shouldn't smoke, and you should also limit your use of alcohol.

Expressing your breast milk

If your breasts are large, sore, and feeling extremely full, your newborn may have difficulty latching on. You can express some milk by gently massaging or pushing by hand or by using a breast pump. Once you've got a breastfeeding routine, you can express your breast milk by hand or with a breast pump if you're away from your baby during feeding time. This will allow him to have breast milk from a bottle or a cup, depending on his age. Expressed breast milk is also a way for your baby to drink breast milk while he is in a childcare facility. Make sure the centre or home has a refrigerator, as milk has to be kept chilled until feeding time.

Storing expressed breast milk

Expressed breast milk should be kept in a sterilized glass bottle or plastic container with the date marked on it. Plastic polyethylene bags, such as commercial bottle liners, are not recommended. Breast milk contains essential immune components that help protect your baby, and using plastic bags to freeze expressed breast milk could cause some of these antibodies to be lost.

Store expressed breast milk in the refrigerator for up to 48 hours. You can also store it for two weeks in your refrigerator freezer (but not in the door), for two to three months in a stand-alone upright freezer, or for up to six months in a chest-type deep freezer with a temperature below −20°C (−4°F). When freezing breast milk, do not add warm expressed milk to milk that has been already chilled or frozen, as this may encourage bacteria to grow.

Preparing expressed breast milk for feeding

To prepare stored milk for feeding, first prepare clean bottles and commercial nipples. Thaw frozen milk in the refrigerator and keep it there until you're ready for it. Do not use a microwave to thaw or warm frozen expressed milk. The milk can contain hot spots that can harm your baby, and the quality of the milk may suffer if it boils.

When it's time for feeding, put the thawed milk into a feeding bottle. You may want to warm up the milk again by placing the bottle of expressed milk into a container of warm water before the actual feeding. Shake the bottle of thawed expressed breast milk well to mix any separated layers, and check the temperature on your inner wrist to make sure it's not too warm. After each feeding, throw away any leftover milk.

Is there ever a reason not to breastfeed?

There very rarely is a reason not to breastfeed. Women who have HIV disease or are receiving long-term chemotherapy may be advised not to breastfeed, so if you are concerned, talk to your doctor. If you are sick and are given prescription drugs, remind your doctor that you are breastfeeding. In most cases, you may continue to feed, as only small amounts will pass through breast milk, and there are usually no problems for your baby. The Motherisk Program at the Toronto Hospital for Sick Children offers information on the safety of drugs and substances while breastfeeding (see "Breastfeeding" in Resources).

What to feed when you can't breastfeed

If breastfeeding is not an option, use a store-bought iron-fortified infant formula for the first 9 to 12 months. The formula should be cow's milk–based. Use soy-based formulas only if your baby can't take dairy products for health reasons. Babies who are fed formula won't need a vitamin D supplement, since it's already added. At six months, you can begin to introduce solid foods to her diet.

If you and your baby have problems breastfeeding, don't be surprised if some people encourage you to give up. Before you do, please ask for help or advice from healthcare professionals or experienced friends and relatives. Contact a lactation consultant, a public health nurse, or a breastfeeding coordinator, all of whom are listed in your phone book. Or call La Leche League (see "Breastfeeding" in Resources) for a referral to a volunteer in your community who is an experienced breastfeeding mother trained to offer support to other mothers.

Vitamin D Needs

Babies who don't get enough vitamin D are at risk of getting rickets, a disease that causes poor growth, limb deformity, bone fractures, and delayed motor milestones. Vitamin D comes from food and sunlight. In Canada, it's added to cow's milk and margarine during production, and some foods—like salmon, tuna, liver, and kidney—are good natural sources. Vitamin D forms naturally when skin is exposed to sunlight, but because we live so far north in Canada, we don't get enough sun at certain times of the year (as you've probably noticed). And sunscreen and clothing, which protect babies from the harmful effects of the sun, won't allow vitamin D to be formed.

Meeting your baby's vitamin D needs starts before birth. If you don't get enough vitamin D while you're pregnant, it will affect how much vitamin D your baby has at birth. A baby born to a mother who is vitamin D deficient is more likely to have a deficiency. If you don't eat foods fortified with vitamin D, if you do not have much exposure to the sun, and if you do not take vitamin D supplements, then you are more likely to be deficient. Ask your doctor about how much supplement you might need.

Getting enough vitamin D

Babies are most at risk of vitamin D deficiency if they are exclusively breastfed, their mothers are vitamin D deficient, they are not exposed to enough sunlight, they have dark skin, or they live in northern communities (north of 55°). These babies should get a daily supplement of vitamin D. The recommended dose is 400 IU per day, and babies in northern communities should get 800 IU per day.

Breast milk has all the other nutrients your baby needs, but it has only small amounts of vitamin D (15 to 40 IU per litre). Breastfed babies should receive a daily supplement of vitamin D from birth until they get enough from their diet. Eating a diet rich in vitamin D isn't enough to enrich your breast milk to the level your baby needs. Since vitamin D is already added to infant formula, babies who are formula-fed don't need a supplement.

Iron Needs

Babies need iron for their brains to develop normally. Our bodies need iron to make hemoglobin, which takes oxygen through the blood to all the cells. Hemoglobin is what gives colour to red blood cells. When you don't have enough iron, red blood cells become small and pale, and can't carry enough oxygen to your body's organs and muscles. This is a condition called anemia.

When babies don't get enough iron, they may gain weight very slowly, have pale skin, have no appetite, be cranky and fussy, or have a condition called pica, where they have the desire to eat dirt and other strange non-food items. Babies with an iron deficiency may be less physically active and may develop more slowly.

Getting enough iron

Babies are born with a reserve of iron, which comes from their mother's blood while they are in the womb. For the first six months of life, breastfed babies will get what they need from their mother's milk. If breastfeeding is not an option, a store-bought iron-fortified infant formula that is cow's milk–based is the next best option for the first 9 to 12 months. Full-term babies who are breastfed or those who get iron-fortified infant formula from birth do not need an iron supplement. Once babies start eating solid foods, the amount of iron they need depends on their age. From 7 to 12 months of age, babies need 11 milligrams of iron a day.

There are two different types of iron: **heme iron,** which is found in meats, and is easily absorbed by the body; and **non-heme iron,** which comes from plant sources like legumes, vegetables, and cereals.

Some foods that are rich in iron are

- meats such as beef, lamb, pork, veal, liver, chicken, and turkey;
- fish, although babies under one year old should not eat shellfish such as lobster, shrimp, or scallops;

- eggs (babies can have yolks, but do not give egg whites to babies under one year old); and
- grains and cereals such as iron-fortified cereals, whole grain breads, enriched bread, pasta, and rice.

Other sources of iron are legumes (chick peas, lentils, dried peas, and beans) and vegetables (spinach, broccoli, Brussels sprouts, green peas, and beans). To help the body absorb even more iron, combine these foods with good sources of vitamin C, such as oranges, tomatoes, and red peppers.

Even though cow's milk has about as much iron as breast milk, it's not a good source of iron as it isn't absorbed well by the body. In fact, cow's milk decreases the absorption of heme iron. Wait until your baby is 9 to 12 months old before introducing whole cow's milk. You need to be sure she is getting other sources of iron and vitamin C, as well as eating a variety of solids, before starting to drink cow's milk.

Introducing Solid Foods

After six months, most babies won't get all the nutrients they need from breast milk or formula alone. Though you can continue to breastfeed until your baby is two years and older, you'll need to introduce her to other foods when she is six months old. Your baby will let you know she is ready to start eating other foods when she shows interest in foods other people are eating. She'll seem hungrier than usual, and she will open her mouth when she sees food coming her way. She's ready for solid food when she can sit up without support, has good control of her neck muscles, will hold food in her mouth without pushing it out on her tongue right away, and can let you know she doesn't want food by leaning back or turning her head away.

There are many ways to introduce solid foods. The first foods usually vary from culture to culture and from family to family. Start with foods that contain iron, which babies need for many different aspects of their development. It's common to start with a single-grain, iron-fortified infant cereal such as rice or barley. Meat, poultry, cooked egg yolk, and well-cooked legumes are also good sources of iron. It's best to limit the variety of foods to just a few grains or a few vegetables to start.

Introduce new foods one at a time, waiting about three to five days before trying another. If your baby develops a reaction to a food, you'll have a better idea of what food might have caused it. Healthy foods that your family eats are good to start with as long as they are plain, with no added salt, sugar, or spices. You can also use commercial baby foods, but check the label to ensure there is no added salt or sugar. Or you can make your own; a list of cookbooks with recipes for babies just starting to eat solid food is provided under "Nutrition" in Resources.

Good solid foods

Trying foods with different textures helps your baby learn how to handle food in her mouth, so be sure to vary both tastes and textures.

- **Grain products.** At 6 to 9 months, offer your baby up to 2 to 4 tablespoons of iron-fortified infant cereal twice a day. Then try other grain products such as small pieces of dry toast or unsalted crackers. At 9 to 12 months, offer other plain cereals, whole grain bread, rice, and pasta.

- **Vegetables.** At 6 to 9 months, offer your baby puréed cooked vegetables that are yellow, green, or orange. At 9 to 12 months, progress to soft, mashed cooked vegetables.

- **Fruits.** At 6 to 9 months, offer puréed cooked fruits and very ripe mashed fruits, such as bananas. At 9 to 12 months, try canned fruit packed in water or juice (not syrup), or try soft fresh fruits that have been washed well, peeled, seeded, and diced.

- **Meat and alternatives.** At 6 to 9 months, offer puréed cooked meat, fish, chicken, tofu, mashed beans, and egg yolks. At 9 to 12 months, mince or dice these foods.

- **Milk and milk products.** At 9 months, you can offer dairy foods like yogurt (3.25 per cent or higher), cottage cheese, or grated hard cheese. Wait until your baby is 9 to 12 months old before introducing whole cow's milk (3.25 per cent). After 12 months of age, she should not take more than 750 millilitres (3 cups or 24 ounces) of milk products per day. Cow's milk alone will not supply all the necessary nutrients, and giving milk exclusively for more than 6 months can lead to iron deficiency anemia.

Dr. Sacks Says

A vegetarian diet is fine as long as your baby gets iron-enriched cereal along with her veggies. She can start to eat tofu at six to eight months of age.

How much?

Your baby will know how much food she needs, so follow her cues. Start by offering a teaspoon or two, and don't rush. Some babies need to try a food many times before accepting it. If she's not hungry, she'll turn her head and close her mouth. If she's hungry, she'll get excited and open up. Never trick or coax her to eat more by playing games or offering sweetened foods—a smart child will soon learn that if she refuses to eat, she can avoid eating healthy food and get treats instead. Babies who are allowed to follow their own hunger cues are much less likely to overeat later in life.

Dr. Sacks Says

Food is for healthy growing, not behaviour management.

What to feed when

Your baby's development	How often to feed	Type of food
Sits with support	2 to 3 times a day*	Puréed, mashed food and semi-solid foods
Sits on own	2 to 3 times a day*	Family foods; small amounts of soft mashed foods without lumps
Crawls	3 to 4 times a day*	Family foods; ground or soft mashed foods with tiny soft lumps; crunchy foods that dissolve, such as whole grain crackers; more flavours
Walks	3 meals and 2 to 3 snacks a day*	Coarsely chopped foods; foods with more texture; toddler foods; bite-sized pieces of food; finger foods.

*Plus breast milk, formula, or whole cow's milk, depending on your child's age.

Source: Adapted from *Well Beings: A Guide to Health in Child Care,* 3rd Edition. Canadian Paediatric Society, 2008.

Water and Juice

If your baby is exclusively breastfed, she doesn't need extra water. When she begins to eat other foods, though, you can start to offer her water occasionally. Babies don't need to drink juice, so offer water in between meals and snacks if she is thirsty. Too much juice can cause early childhood tooth decay, and it can also cause toddler's diarrhea, especially apple juice (for more on toddler's diarrhea, see page 337 in

Chapter Six). It can fill up small stomachs and decrease your baby's appetite for nutritious foods. If you do offer juice, be sure it is 100 per cent fruit juice (with no added sugar), and limit it to 125 to 175 millilitres (4 to 6 ounces) per day. Always offer it in a cup as part of a meal or snack.

Foods to Avoid

Although your baby can eat a wide range of foods once he starts to eat solid foods, there are certain foods you should avoid at this age.

- **Sugary foods or drinks.** Do not give your baby candy, pop, and energy drinks. That goes for you too. Encourage good eating habits from an early age by practising them yourself when you are with your child.

- **Honey.** Babies under one year of age are at risk of infant botulism (food poisoning) from honey.

- **Egg whites.** To reduce the chance of an allergic reaction, avoid giving egg whites until your baby is one year old.

- **Nuts and shellfish.** If you have a family history of allergies, you may want to wait until your baby is three years old before introducing peanuts, tree nuts (such as pecans or walnuts), and shellfish.

  Also, some foods can cause choking in young children. See "Preventing Choking" on page 124 for the foods you should avoid and for tips on preparing certain foods so that they are safe.

> ## MAKE A NOTE, MAKE AN APPOINTMENT, OR GO TO THE HOSPITAL?
>
> **Take your baby to the hospital immediately** if he absolutely refuses two to four feedings in a row and looks listless.

Lactose Intolerance

Your baby should experience different tastes and textures, but he doesn't need a wide variety when he's just starting to eat solid food. So the food intolerance you're most likely to encounter at this age is lactose intolerance, which occurs when the body doesn't produce enough of the enzyme lactase to properly break down the sugar lactose found in most dairy products. A child who has an intolerance may have bloating, loose stools, gas, or other symptoms after eating the food. However, dairy products are an important source of calcium and Vitamin D, which are vital for building strong bones and teeth. There has been a lot of focus on lactose intolerance in recent years, but in some cases the problem might be the quantity of dairy products, not the dairy itself. Most children can tolerate milk in moderate amounts.

> ## MAKE A NOTE, MAKE AN APPOINTMENT, OR GO TO THE HOSPITAL?
>
> If you suspect your baby is lactose intolerant, **make a note** to mention it to his doctor at his next appointment before making substitutions for milk in his diet.

Some cultures have high rates of lactose intolerance. More than 80 per cent of First Nations children, for example, are lactose intolerant. Treatment is easy, as there are lots of lactose-free products available, or your baby can take the lactase enzyme in liquid or tablet form before eating dairy products. Other sources of calcium you can include in his diet are broccoli, figs, soy, canned salmon and sardine with bones, fortified juices, almonds, lactose-free milks, and lentils. Many people use goat's milk as a substitute for cow's milk, but children can be sensitive to it too, so check with your baby's doctor before trying goat's milk. In addition, goat's milk does not provide enough vitamin D, so you will need to give your baby a supplement. Unpasteurized goat's milk is not an acceptable alternative to cow's milk.

Keeping Foods Safe

Food safety is always important, but especially when you have a baby in your home. Foods that are contaminated with germs can cause stomach pains, diarrhea, or vomiting. Ensuring your family's food is safe from harmful germs is simple. Always wash your hands with soapy water before and after preparing food. Keep your kitchen clean, using a mild solution of water and soap to clean counters, cutting boards, and utensils, and a mild bleach solution to clean old or stubborn spills. Washable cloths or paper towels are better than sponges. (For more on cleaning, see page 366 in Chapter Six.)

Read the labels on milk and fruit juices to check that they have been pasteurized to kill germs, and pay attention to expiry dates. (See "Product Safety" in Resources to find out how to stay current on food recalls and advisories.) When preparing raw meats and poultry, keep them away from cooked food and fresh fruits and vegetables. Defrost meat, poultry, and fish in the fridge or microwave, not on the counter.

Use separate cutting boards for raw meats and for vegetables. Foods that are not cooked before they are eaten, such as fresh fruits and vegetables, should be rinsed well under running tap water.

Keep hot foods hot (over 60°C/140°F) and cold foods cold (under 4°C/39°F), and make sure your fridge is set at a temperature of 4°C or less. Cook foods thoroughly, especially red meat, poultry, and eggs, to destroy harmful germs. When serving leftovers, reheat foods all the way through. Eat food soon after it has been cooked so that harmful germs don't have time to grow. And always protect your food from insects and animals.

Preventing Choking

Babies have very good gag reflexes, but they can choke if they're given the wrong foods. So be careful when preparing your baby's food. First of all, don't feed him peanuts or popcorn. You should dice or slice other round foods such as wieners or grapes into small pieces. Chop or scrape stringy meat and add broth to moisten it. Raw vegetables such as carrots can be grated to make them easier to chew, or you can cook hard fruits and vegetables to soften them. Make sure you remove pits and seeds from fruits.

INJURY PREVENTION

Babyproofing for Crawling Babies

Once your baby is on the move, which will happen before you know it, babyproofing your home becomes essential. A newly mobile baby requires special safety precautions around your home. You've probably done most of what you needed to do before your due date, but take another look around before she is mobile so you have enough time to get organized. The best way to spot potential dangers is to get down on your hands and knees and crawl around looking at your home from a baby's-eye view. You may feel a bit silly, but remember that it could save her life.

Down on the floor

At this age, your baby uses a pincer grasp to pick up small things between her thumb and index finger—tiny and potentially dangerous things like a loose pill or staple—and put them in her mouth. To prevent her from choking on small objects, keep the floors vacuumed or swept, and check for splinters, pins, or other sharp objects stuck into floors or carpets.

Within reach

Babies spend a lot of time and energy reaching out to grab objects, so keep dangerous things like hot liquids, loose cords, and breakable, sharp, or pointed objects out of reach or, ideally, out of sight. Check for floor or table lamps that could be pulled over if she grabs the cord. Put grandma's china away, and remove small objects that could be choking hazards from low shelves. To be sure, consider anything that will fit inside a toilet paper roll to be a choking hazard. Cover the controls on your TV with safety panels so curious fingers don't play with the buttons.

On the move

Crawling babies can move more quickly than you might expect, so be prepared. If you cannot babyproof your entire home, use safety gates across doorways to restrict your baby to rooms that are safe. You'll also need to look down all the time when she's on the loose or you may step on little hands. Babies are natural climbers, and once they start crawling, they'll also start climbing whenever they can. Move furniture away from windows, and keep chairs, tables, or other objects away from balcony rails. Keep large toys or stuffed animals out of the crib or playpen, as babies can climb on them and fall out.

Whether your baby is crawling, cruising (walking while holding on to a piece of furniture), or starting to walk, she will want to climb up and down any set of stairs, so safety gates, used properly, are essential at this stage. Always supervise your baby once she learns to climb the stairs, and for everyone's safety, keep stairs free of clutter.

All over your home

Use cupboard and drawer locks, especially on cupboards that contain cleaning products, china and glass, plastic bags, or anything breakable or precious. Install fridge and freezer locks and, where necessary, window locks and devices to prevent doors slamming on tiny fingers. Check that internal glass doors are made from safety glass. If in doubt, add a layer of safety film or consult a glazier, who will be able to identify the type of glass and, if necessary, replace it.

Bathrooms and kitchens pose special dangers, so make sure a responsible adult is with your baby any time she is in one of these rooms. Always leave the bathroom door closed when no one's inside, and never leave your baby alone in the bathroom for any reason. Never leave any electrical appliances plugged in near the tub or sink. While you're cooking, try to keep your baby in a high chair or activity centre. Have a fire extinguisher close by and learn how to use it. Move knives and other utensils away from the edge of the counter so they don't tumble to the floor and into your baby's reach, and keep small-appliance cords away from the counter edge. Turn pot handles inward toward the back of the stove and away from curious little hands. Always point knives and forks down in the dishwasher in case she approaches the dishwasher while it's open.

First-aid kits and medicine cabinets

Store your first-aid kit and all medications in a locked or inaccessible cupboard where children can't get to them. Ask the pharmacist to put child-safe caps on all prescription bottles, including adult medications, that come into your home. Always store medications in their original containers, as dosages and cautions are usually listed on the packaging. If your child takes something accidentally, you'll need to know exactly what she has ingested. You should also check the expiration date on packaging every six months and throw out any medication that has expired.

MAKE A NOTE, MAKE AN APPOINTMENT, OR GO TO THE HOSPITAL?

Keep the number of the poison control centre close by each phone, and **call Poison Control immediately** if you suspect your baby has ingested medication, houseplants, cleaning products, or another toxic substance. If you need to take her to the hospital, take the container and what is left of the contents with you.

Even with the best precautions, the most important thing you can do to assure your crawling baby's safety is to keep an eye on her. For those times when you cannot, put her in a playpen with some interesting toys, and check on her often.

Baby Walkers

In April 2004, Health Canada issued a complete ban on selling, importing, and advertising baby walkers (see "Product Safety" in Resources for more information). Baby walkers do not actually help babies learn to walk. They don't help to strengthen their upper-leg and thigh muscles, and they actually deter babies from walking on their own since walkers make it so easy for them to get around.

More importantly, they are not safe, even in a home with safety gates at the top of stairs. Babies in walkers can move very quickly, and the force of a baby hitting a gate with the walker can cause the gate to release. The Canadian Paediatric Society strongly advises parents not to use baby walkers. Instead, consider getting a stationary activity centre that doesn't have wheels.

ooooo

It's true that your life will never be the same now that you have a baby. Just think of the many ways you and your baby will grow in the first year. During this time, you will gain a lot of confidence, some funny memories, some balance in your life, and a great sense of what is really important. You now have a new individual who is starting to develop his own personality—and distinctive likes and dislikes—and who is becoming a vibrant part of your family. Soon he'll be talking, relating to others (especially his parents), and, best of all, sleeping better. Sleep well and eat well during the first year—you'll need energy for year two.

3

From Baby to Toddler:
12 to 24 Months

An entire year has gone by since that memorable day when you became a parent. And the little person who is crawling up the stairs, babbling and singing, and somehow already pushing your buttons is a million miles away from the tiny, helpless little bundle you brought home from the hospital. The second year of life is full of thrilling milestones like walking and talking. Your toddler will spend most of her waking hours finding out how the world works. By the end of the year, she will probably be running and jumping, speaking two-word sentences, and trying to be increasingly independent in every way possible. Wonderful and challenging, this year will see your little one go from a baby to a toddler.

INCLUDED IN THIS CHAPTER

GROWTH AND DEVELOPMENT

Your toddler's brain is growing dramatically through the second year of life, with the creation of a huge number of synapses, or connections between brain cells, that give him all kinds of new mental and physical capabilities. These new synapses allow him to think in ways that are more complex. He will be able to remember things that happened in the past, and by 24 months he will be able to remember things that occurred several days earlier. He is learning about cause and effect; when he opens the music box, he knows that a song will play. Learning to walk and then run will be his biggest motor accomplishments this year, thanks to greater coordination and muscle control. Continually improving fine motor skills will enable him to start to eat with a spoon, draw with crayons, and manipulate small objects.

Although most children reach milestones like walking and talking by a specific age, it is important to remember that development happens at an individual pace. Also, many toddlers tend to make progress in one area, such as talking, while another skill levels off. If your toddler has a slight delay in a specific area, it doesn't always mean there is a problem. For your own peace of mind, make a note to mention these things to his doctor when you have a concern.

When it comes to language development, there is a wide range of normal. Even if your toddler is lagging behind in verbal skills, his speech will likely develop normally if he communicates effectively though expressions, gestures, and other means. It is of more concern if a toddler shows signs of a general communication problem. It's important that he has the desire to communicate, if not yet the ability, and that he makes attempts to relate his desires and thoughts in some way. A lack of interest in communicating could be an indication of autism. For more information on autism, see page 453 in Chapter Eight.

MYTH BUSTERS

Myth: Boys and younger siblings learn to talk later than girls and older siblings, so there's no need to worry if speech seems delayed.

Fact: There seems to be a one-month lag in speech between girls and boys, but it isn't consistent.

—*Dr. Alyson Shaw, MD, FRCPC*

Developmental Milestones

Language explosion

The rate at which children learn to talk varies widely, but most will experience a huge jump in language skills this year, especially between 18 and 24 months. At 12 months, most toddlers can say a handful of one- and two-syllable words, such as "ball" and "doggie," and can say "mama" and "dada" to the right person. He is beginning to understand that words stand for objects, and knows that the word "dog" and the actual dog go together. Between 18 and 24 months, most can speak at least 50 words and will start using two-word sentences, like "more peas" or "doggy run." Your toddler may also be able to understand two-step commands, like "Please get your shoes and sit down next to me." (Whether he decides to follow these commands is a different story.) Despite his limited vocabulary, your toddler may understand up to 10 times as many words as he can say.

Dr. Sacks Says

Don't talk baby talk to a baby you are hoping will speak a real language soon.

Sense of self

Your toddler is now learning by imitation, and is fascinated by many of the things he sees you do—so be careful what you do when he's around! He doesn't yet know the difference between work and play, so make the most of it and involve him in housework. Let him dump the scoop of detergent into the washer, put dirty spoons into the silverware basket in the dishwasher, or wipe up the table with a rag. He is also starting to play pretend, doing things like giving his teddy bear a drink from a cup, or "talking" to grandma on the telephone. At about 18 months, toddlers start to develop a better understanding of the world around them and their place in it. As they begin to see themselves as individuals, separate from others, they also begin to imagine the threat of being apart from you, and can develop separation issues.

Increasing coordination

After mastering the art of walking, your toddler will start to run, usually about six months after walking is well established. Then he'll start to climb, dance, and kick. He will also gain greater control over the small muscles in his hands, fingers, and wrists. This allows him to do all sorts of things, from picking tiny objects off the floor, to throwing a ball, to using a paintbrush. Your toddler is mastering all kinds of new skills this year, including stacking blocks, pulling off his hat and socks, identifying objects in books, recognizing himself in the mirror or in pictures, walking up the steps, brushing his teeth, and drinking from a straw.

As they develop coordination, most toddlers will perform the tasks below by the ages listed.

Feeding milestones
12 to 18 months
* Grasps and releases food with his fingers
* Holds a spoon, but awkwardly
* Turns a spoon in his mouth

- Uses a cup, but his release is poor
- Wants food that others are eating

18 to 24 months
- Has a decrease in appetite
- Likes eating with his hands
- Likes trying different textures
- Prefers certain foods
- Likes routine
- Prefers to drink, rather than eat

Literacy milestones

(Adapted with permission from the Reach Out and Read National Center in Somerville, Massachusetts.)

12 to 18 months
- Holds a book with help
- Turns board pages, several at a time
- No longer mouths the book right away
- Points at pictures with one finger
- Makes the same sound for a specific picture
- Points when asked "Where's ...?"
- Turns a book right side up
- Gives a book to an adult to read

18 to 24 months
- Turns board book pages easily, one at a time
- Carries a book around
- Uses books as comfort objects, maybe
- Names familiar pictures
- Fills in words of familiar stories
- Reads to dolls or stuffed animals
- Recites parts of well-known stories

MAKE A NOTE, MAKE AN APPOINTMENT, OR GO TO THE HOSPITAL?

Make a note to mention to your toddler's doctor at his next scheduled appointment if he doesn't reach the milestones listed below.

12 months

▷ He doesn't point to an object he wants.

▷ He doesn't look at something when you point to it.

▷ He isn't babbling or starting to use words.

▷ He will not sleep alone.

▷ He can't crawl or pull himself up to stand.

15 months

▷ He has not taken his first steps.

Make an appointment to see his doctor if he doesn't reach the following milestones:

12 months

▷ He doesn't know at least one word in addition to "mama" and "dada."

▷ He doesn't gesture, give, show, or point to get something.

18 months

▷ He doesn't understand simple commands like "Go get your ball."

▷ He doesn't make gestures or ask for "more" or "again."

24 months

▷ He doesn't put two words together, like "more juice."

Your toddler's doctor will likely have his hearing checked and talk about setting up a speech and language assessment. You should also **make an**

appointment if he seems to be regressing on some milestones, such as losing language skills he had already mastered or no longer being able to go up or down stairs, or if some of his mannerisms could be associated with autism. These mannerisms may include:

- poor eye contact;
- not interacting with others;
- relating to others more as objects than people;
- not responding to parental cuddling;
- not looking at an object that is being pointed at; and
- being obsessed with spinning or twirling objects.

Separation and Independence

Your toddler is a wonderful dichotomy of wanting to be independent and still needing you close by. She may waver between these two desires in the same day, or even the same hour. As she starts to realize she's separate from you, it can bring up feelings of anxiety when you leave. It can also mean she's figuring out that she has her own thoughts and desires, and that she can do things on her own and in her own way.

Between 12 and 18 months, she is really beginning to explore on her own, thanks to her ever-improving motor skills. In familiar surroundings, and with familiar people, she will continue to explore, test her limits, and try out her new skills. This can be frustrating for her (like when she goes up stairs and can't figure out how to get down), but it's all part of developing her identity. As long as she's safe, resist the temptation to come running every time she hits a snag. Letting her figure things out on her own is important to her self-esteem.

In the second half of this year, her sense of self will develop even further. If she feels secure, she will increasingly assert herself, wanting the same foods over and over, and only wearing that one red sweater. Impose order by allowing her limited choices rather than saying "no" to everything. Let her pick between two outfits, or two snacks, or two books. That way, she'll have a sense of control, and she'll feel like she can do things by herself.

Separation issues

Around her first birthday, it's not uncommon for a toddler to start to develop separation anxiety—a feeling of great anxiety or panic when you leave the room. Most toddlers will begin this phase sometime between the ages of one and two. It can be very unsettling for parents, especially if you're going back to work and have to deal with a hysterical daycare drop-off every morning. It's only a stage, though, and it's actually a good sign. When your toddler is distressed by your leaving, she's successfully bonded with you, and has reached an important emotional milestone. At the same time, you should trust your instincts. If she refuses to go to a certain caregiver or daycare centre, or she shows other signs of tension, such as trouble sleeping or loss of appetite, there could be a problem with the childcare situation.

Separation issues usually happen after your toddler begins to develop a sense of object permanence—the realization that a person or object still exists even when they're out of sight. She now realizes you've gone away when she can't see you, but she doesn't yet understand the concept of time, so she doesn't know when or if you're coming back. As she grows from a baby into a toddler, she experiences the push and pull of wanting to be increasingly independent and still needing you most of the time. This can create a fear of abandonment, and make separation difficult.

The intensity of separation anxiety varies widely from child to child. Most outgrow the severest part of it somewhere between 18 and 36 months. Certain factors like a new sibling, a new childcare situation, or stress at home can make separation anxiety worse.

MAKE A NOTE, MAKE AN APPOINTMENT, OR GO TO THE HOSPITAL?

If your toddler's separation anxiety gets worse as she gets older, or if it appears unexpectedly, **make a note** to discuss it with her doctor at her next appointment.

There are a number of strategies you can employ to make things easier for both you and your child during this phase. Sneaking away isn't one of them. As tempting as it might be to avoid the crying scene by ducking out when your toddler isn't looking, it may only make things worse. If she thinks you are going to disappear with no notice at any time, she may cling to you even tighter. Instead, say a loving but quick goodbye. Stay calm, no matter how distressed your toddler may be, and tell her where you're going and when you'll be back. Give her an estimate of time that she'll understand. Show her where the hands on the clock will be, tell her what the sky will look like, or explain it in relation to her routine, such as after lunch or after her nap. Even toddlers who aren't talking very much yet understand a lot more than you may think. Once you've explained your departure, be sure to leave. If you let a tantrum influence you, she'll learn that it works, and it will only make things worse the next time.

If your toddler is going to start child care, practise by making a few short visits there before her first day. Ask a new babysitter to come over a bit early so the three of you can spend some time together before you leave. Your toddler will be comfortable with caregivers if she sees that you are comfortable with them. Encourage the babysitter to get her fully engrossed in an activity before you go. When you leave, say a quick goodbye and head out the door. If your toddler gets upset, it will be easier to turn her focus back to the task at hand if she was already enjoying herself. Another great way to make leaving your toddler with a babysitter easier is to have them leave your home at the same time. Suggest that the babysitter take her out for a walk or to the park, but tell her you're leaving too so she doesn't get upset when she gets home to find you're not there.

Establish a consistent pattern in the way you say goodbye and the way you greet her when you return. This will make her confident that you will always come back when you go away. Even games like leaving the room and popping your head around the corner with a big smile can show your toddler that when you leave, you will soon be back again. A transitional object like a favourite toy or blanket, or a reminder of her parents, like a photo or a piece of your clothing, can be a source of comfort for her as you leave.

Sweet Sleep

At this point, you're probably convinced that the old cliché "sleep like a baby" is some kind of cruel joke, but don't worry—it gets easier from here. By 12 months, many toddlers are sleeping soundly through the night, although many still have a hard time sleeping for long periods. At this age, your toddler needs about 13 hours of sleep in a 24-hour period; usually 10 or 11 hours at night and a 2-hour nap during the day.

The importance of routine

One of the most important aspects of promoting good sleep habits is a bedtime schedule with a consistent routine. A routine signals when it's time to sleep, and helps your toddler wind down from his busy day. Many toddlers become quite attached to this bedtime routine—they gain a lot of comfort from knowing what's coming next—so try not to vary it too much, even if you're not at home. The routine can involve whatever you and your toddler enjoy, as long as it's quiet and relaxing.

Dr. Sacks Says

Even at this age, toddlers are very good at sensing your ambivalence. If you put him to bed, mean it.

Bath

Most bedtime routines include a soak in the tub. The combination of warm water, fun bath toys, and a snuggle in the towel as he's dried off is a soothing way to end the day both for parent and child. Also, his body temperature drops after he is out of the bath and in his pyjamas, which encourages sleep. If your toddler becomes agitated in the tub, though, save bath time for the morning and try other routines before bed.

Brushing teeth

From the time those first little teeth appear, and even before, brush or wipe your child's gums and teeth before bedtime. The sooner you start, the more comfortable he will become with the idea. Try to brush twice a day, or at least before bedtime. Use a pea-sized amount of a non-fluoridated toothpaste up until age two. Once children have closely spaced teeth, you should floss them daily.

Quiet games

A quiet game of peekaboo or This Little Piggy on your toddler's bedroom floor is a fun way to wind down together. Just make sure it doesn't make him overly excited—the idea is to calm him down and relax him.

Bedtime stories

A story is the staple of many bedtime routines. Snuggling in a chair or on the bed and reading is a great way to bond from the time your child is a few months old. Reading is important because it exposes him to new words and increases his language skills.

Sing songs

Don't worry if you don't think you can sing. Your toddler's favourite sound in the world is your voice, no matter how out of tune. Quiet singing is a wonderful way to calm him down, whether it's lullabies, folk songs, or just a favourite tune. Ending with the same one every night is a great way to signal to your toddler that it's time for sleep.

Transitional object

A transitional object is a favourite item that your toddler forms an attachment to and draws on for a source of comfort. Think of Linus's blue blanket, or your favourite stuffed animal when you were little. After your toddler turns one year of age, you can put a transitional object in the crib with him to get him to sleep.

Put your toddler down while he is awake

Almost all experts agree that you should put your toddler down to sleep when he is sleepy but still awake. This will encourage him to soothe himself to sleep. Then when he wakes up during the night, he'll be able to get back to sleep on his own. Don't lie down with him until he falls asleep. You could easily become his permanent transitional object, making bedtime a never-ending struggle for babysitters.

NO BOTTLE IN BED

Putting a child to bed with a bottle might seem like a soothing way for him to fall asleep, but there are three problems with this. First, it can cause massive tooth decay. When a child falls asleep with a bottle in his mouth, the sugars from the milk, juice, or other fluids pool in his mouth and cause rapid breakdown of the enamel. Second, it can cause ear infections if fluid flows through to his ear cavity. Even more dangerous, children can inhale fluid and choke if they fall asleep while sucking a bottle. This is a particular danger for babies because they aren't as good as adults at waking up if something interferes with their breathing.

Many toddlers use physical movement like rocking in their cribs or banging their heads as a way of getting themselves to sleep. While this can be a bit unsettling for parents, it's nothing to worry about as long as your toddler isn't hurting himself. These types of rhythmic movements are just a way to release pent-up energy at the end of the day before he drifts off to sleep.

MAKE A NOTE, MAKE AN APPOINTMENT, OR GO TO THE HOSPITAL?

If you have concerns about your toddler's soothing methods, **make a note** to mention it to his doctor at his next appointment.

Night waking

Some toddlers will still wake in the night between 12 and 24 months, even though they don't need to eat and should be able to soothe themselves back to sleep. In fact, most babies past the age of six months no longer need to eat at night. Try to separate sleep from eating so that if he does wake up at night he won't need your breast or a bottle to get back to sleep. Everyone—even adults—wakes up several times during the night, but adults learn to roll over and get back to sleep. The key is teaching your toddler how to settle himself back down using self-comforting techniques like cuddling a stuffed animal. One caveat: try not to let those soothing methods be external ones, like playing music. If he becomes dependent on them, he will need them in order to fall back asleep every time he wakes up—which means you'll have to wake up and turn on the music. Don't put him down later at night thinking he will be more tired and sleep more soundly; this can result in sleep deprivation, which will actually make him wake up more frequently at night, not less.

Napping

Sometime during their second year, most toddlers go from two naps to a single afternoon nap of about two hours. It takes some toddlers most of the year to adjust to the one-nap schedule, so let him set the schedule. He may have one nap when he is at daycare or with a caregiver, and two naps when he's home with his parents on the weekend. By the time they are three, many toddlers have given up their naps entirely, but some will still need a nap for months after that.

Try to put your toddler down to nap in the same place that he sleeps at night, and at the same time every day. Make sure his room is cool, quiet, and dark. Don't let him sleep past 4:00 in the afternoon, or he may have trouble getting to sleep at night. There should be at least three hours between when he gets up from his nap and when he goes to bed for the night.

If your toddler is not sleeping through the night but is taking three- or four-hour naps during the day, it may be time to try to adjust his internal clock a little bit. Wake him up from his long naps, keep him active during the day, and put him down for his nap earlier in the afternoon.

Bedsharing

The controversy over bedsharing, also referred to as co-sleeping or "the family bed," does not die down even when your child's a toddler. The experts' opinions vary widely. Some strongly advise against it, saying that your child will never learn to sleep independently and soothe himself to sleep if you are there with him. Others are major advocates of the family bed, saying that both parents and children sleep best when they are beside each other. If you decide to bedshare, make sure everyone involved is happy with the arrangement, and decide from the very beginning when it will stop. If you allow your toddler in your bed for too long, it may be more difficult for him to make the eventual transition to his own room. Don't forget that you need a proper, restful sleep and a bit of privacy too.

Discipline

The thought of disciplining a one-year-old seems a bit silly to some people, but parents discipline their toddlers all the time, sometimes without even realizing it. When a toddler grabs something that's unsafe, her mom gently takes it away; when she starts to whine and fuss, her mom picks her up and takes her to another room to play with something else. Distraction, redirection, and setting limits are all forms of discipline.

In fact, discipline is more about teaching than punishment. The goal of discipline should be to keep your toddler safe, limit aggression, and prevent destructive behaviour. It is about teaching her self-control and appropriate behaviour, helping her to understand her feelings and emotions, and providing guidance to gently direct her along her way. Toddlers don't misbehave intentionally, although they certainly come to understand when they're doing something you don't like. At this stage, she's experimenting, exploring, and testing her limits—and yours. She'll do things that are dangerous or disruptive, like throwing food on the floor, pulling the cat's tail, or turning on the TV to full blast. The most important thing is to keep calm during these episodes and not let her push your buttons.

Dr. Sacks Says

The best way to teach is to mentor, so set a good example.
Don't "whiiiiine" when you tell your child not to whine.

A safe home to explore

You can use several discipline strategies at this age. Childproofing, which you've already done, is one way to control her exploring. Because toddler hands are naturally curious, it is important to remove objects that are bound to cause problems. Providing her with things she can freely explore in a safe home environment eliminates everyone's frustration.

No matter how childproof your home is, there will always be things that your toddler shouldn't touch or play with, like lamps (and their cords), televisions, and ovens. Yet having to say "no" all the time can quash your toddler's sense of independence and self-confidence, not to mention drive you crazy. To avoid being a constant naysayer, find alternatives that you can say "yes" to. When your toddler reaches for the lamp cord, gently remove her and redirect her to something else that's safe for her to play with. It's all right to say "no" at the same time to start teaching her what it means, but focus more attention on the positive, which is the new plaything. If she returns to the lamp cord, gently but firmly redirect her again. She'll soon get the picture.

Remember, though, that the more child-friendly your home is, the less you'll be fighting with her to keep her away from special things and places. Make sure there are lots of toys and books within her reach, low cupboards she's allowed to open and empty, and spaces in which she can play freely. Your ultimate goal should be to allow your toddler to explore and to develop a healthy sense of independence in a safe environment without constantly engaging in a battle of wills.

Winning the war with words

Toddlers respond well to gentle but firm vocal disapproval. Get close and look her in the eye, speak sternly, and use brief, declarative words like "stop." So your child learns more than "no," try to think of other words you can use to direct her behaviour, like "hot," "gentle," and "danger." Vary the intensity of your voice according to the situation. She doesn't yet have the language skills to understand long explanations about why she can't or shouldn't do something, and her attention span is shorter than your lecture.

Don't overreact; toddlers thrive on attention, whether it's positive or negative, so yelling can just reinforce the behaviour by giving her the attention she wanted in the first place. Reinforce your words with your body language by pointing or shaking your finger and keeping your face very serious to let your toddler know you mean business. Above all, don't smile or laugh, no matter how funny the situation might actually be.

Dr. Sacks Says

Discipline should be balanced with fun. Don't neglect discipline, but don't forget to enjoy your toddler's explorations and her personality. Let her have her fun and you'll have fun too. And you may just delay the day when you realize you sound like your parents.

Positive reinforcement works wonders, so when your toddler is playing well with a friend or touching a sibling gently, encourage her with big smiles, a loving touch, and positive words. She understands more than you think, and she certainly knows from your reaction that what she is doing is good.

Sometimes toddlers need to be physically removed from a place or situation against their will. A change of scenery can do wonders to calm a cranky child. Try to gently take her by the hand or forearm and walk her to another place. If she refuses, don't force her by pulling her, just pick her up and carry her.

TO SPANK OR NOT TO SPANK

Should you spank your children? The short answer is no. The Canadian Paediatric Society strongly discourages the use of any type of physical punishment on children, including spanking. The goal of discipline should not be to punish children, but to change their behaviour, help them develop self-control, and foster their self-esteem so they can make good decisions. Discipline or guidance will be most effective if it's given with respect and love, and in ways that are consistent and reasonable.

Research has shown that spanking doesn't work, and it may even be harmful. It can harm your child emotionally, causing her to be fearful, anxious, and distrustful. If done in anger, it can escalate physically. Even parents who don't mean to can hurt a child by spanking if they hit harder than they realize. Spanking can also make aggressive behaviour worse because it teaches a child to lash out physically when she is angry. Some experts believe that children don't actually learn a lesson about bad behaviour and consequences, but see spanking as a debt to pay for what they've done, and believe the slate is wiped clean after the spanking is over. Other forms of discipline can be more constructive, leaving a child with a sense of guilt and helping her form a conscience.

The toddler years can be a bit baffling for parents, so keep your expectations realistic and understand normal toddler behaviour. Your toddler is growing and developing both physically and intellectually in huge leaps right now, and it's important that your little explorer have room and freedom to find out what she is capable of. It's your job to give her that freedom inside a safe, supportive, and loving environment. Your toddler is watching you and learning from you all the time. Do your best to remain loving and patient to provide a solid example for her.

Keeping Your Toddler Busy

During the first year of his life, your baby focused all of his attention on his parents and maybe a regular caregiver. You were his first playmates, and your reactions to him and his antics were crucial in his physical, social, and intellectual development. As he enters his second year of life, he will learn to interact with others, such as grandparents, aunts and uncles, other adults, and even other toddlers. For the next year or two, he'll build on the skills you have taught him and learn to talk, play games, socialize, and make friends.

Between 12 and 24 months of age, your toddler is increasingly interested in the world around him. Seeing how others react to him is endlessly fascinating now, and he will really start to enjoy being in the company of other children. At this stage, however, toddlers mostly engage in parallel play—playing with toys or books in the same room, but independently. Once he hits 18 months, he will probably start to notice his playmates and interact with them a little more (often in a way you won't be particularly proud of). Toward the end of his second year, he will start to engage in imaginative play, creating his own little worlds and scenarios—often things he sees his parents doing, like housework and working with tools—and acting them out. As he becomes more independent and begins to develop a sense of ownership, he can become fiercely protective of his toys, and can start to bite, hit, or engage in other types of aggressive behaviour. You need to deal with all these nasty little tendencies so they don't get out of hand, but at this point they are completely normal.

Even as he reaches the age of two and is starting to seek out certain friends and interact with them more, the art of socializing is still a learning process. He has a limited sense of empathy, so be patient—and empathetic—with him. Because he lives in the moment, the idea of sharing and taking turns is almost meaningless. Slow, gentle guidance on your part will get the message through soon enough. Also, be patient with your toddler's anxieties around other adults. Some toddlers are outgoing, eager to show toys and smile at your adult visitors, while others may cling to their parents or even run out of the room in tears when people come to visit. Let him take it slowly, offer calm reassurance, and allow him to come to visitors at his own pace.

Learning through play

In the second year of life, learning is doing. Your toddler is going through a period of huge growth, and since much of his learning is done through touching and exploring, in his mind, nothing is off limits in your home. If you continually interrupt his exploration and say "no," you may undermine his self-confidence and make him doubt his abilities. Right now, his actions are not entirely separate from his thoughts, so if forbidden objects are within range, there is bound to be confrontation. Try to offer safe alternatives for him to play with that are just as attractive as the forbidden ones. There's no need to fill your home with hundreds of toys. Remember that you live there too, and toddlers prefer the boxes toys come in anyways. If people want to buy toys for your toddler, suggest they buy books or make donations to a children's charity instead.

MYTH BUSTERS

Myth: "Educational" videos and TV shows are good for a toddler's development.

Fact: Everyday interaction with parents helps a toddler's brain develop. After all, Einstein did just fine without educational videos. A happy, well-attached child will learn to his maximum capacity.

—*Dr. Alyson Shaw, MD, FRCPC*

Some great playthings for this age include large plastic bottles with handles, old bracelets (as long as they can't be easily broken), and kitchen items, such as pots and pans, spoons, wooden utensils, rubber spatulas, pastry and vegetable brushes, plastic cookie cutters, and measuring cups and spoons. Shoeboxes or other large cardboard boxes are endlessly fascinating, as your toddler will like to empty things out of other things at this point, and will also love to drag things around behind him. Attach a string to a shoebox (be careful it's not too long), and he'll pull a stuffed animal around for hours.

By 18 months, your toddler will be fascinated with measuring and pouring, so sand and water play is great for this age. Funnels, plastic squeeze bottles, sieves and colanders, bulb basters, and eggbeaters are interesting alternatives to the standard shovels, cups, and pails. Your 18-month-old will also be matching and sorting, so shape-sorter toys—large plastic or wooden boxes with different-shaped holes and corresponding blocks—are wonderful now. With some guidance, he will soon be able to fit the square block into the square hole. Toddlers also enjoy simple arts and crafts, like drawing with large crayons on blank paper, playing with clay, and painting with large paintbrushes.

Your toddler is experimenting with cause-and-effect now. He likes to manipulate things that function, like zippers, snaps, hooks, and dials. Workbenches, blocks, toy telephones, musical instruments, and dolls with clothes that fasten with Velcro or snaps should stimulate his intellectual growth and fine motor skills. Simple puzzle boards with several pieces are also fun. Rolling maze toys and pound-a-ball toys, where your toddler drops a ball into the top of a maze and watches it pop out the bottom, are also great.

Keep on reading

After your baby's first birthday, his language skills will advance tremendously, and he will develop a sense of humour. Books become more important than they were during his first year of life, and he is no longer the passive baby who will sit quietly while you read to him. He wants to interact with books by turning the pages, examining the illustrations, and pointing out the objects he can identify. Some toddlers prefer books with photographs, while others like ones with built-in activities, like flap books or ones with images hidden behind sliding partitions. Make books part of your toddlers's daily routine by incorporating them into bedtime, mealtime, and any time.

Dr. Sacks Says

Decorate with precious books, not precious valuables. Put baskets of books in each room so that when your toddler wants to grab something, he'll grab a book, and when you need to clean up, you can just throw them back in the basket.

In the second half of this year, you can also begin to introduce concept books, which help toddlers understand numbers, letters, shapes, colours, textures, actions, size, direction, and parts of the body. Concept books make learning fun, and books with big, detailed illustrations captivate his interest. He will also enjoy books with singsong rhythms and playful rhymes, and he will enjoy hearing these rhymes while you are playing throughout the day as well. Introduce different types of books to your toddler every once in a while. Don't be discouraged by a one-year-old who wants to run around while listening to a story. Follow his lead if he only wants to listen to a few pages between laps.

By age two, most toddlers can follow a simple story in a picture book and are happy to flip through books on their own. The books he likes best now have images of children doing familiar things like sleeping, eating, and playing. They also have simple rhymes and predictable text, and they only have a few words on each page. He will also like books about saying hello and goodbye, and goodnight books for just before bedtime. Books for this age should be sturdy board books that are easy to handle and carry around.

Be a library regular and get to know your librarian. This is a great time to join a library storytime program. Storytime helps foster your child's love of books while getting him into a social setting. After storytime is over, let him help you choose some books to take home from the library. Encourage reading by responding when he wants to read. Don't force him to read in a logical, linear fashion. Let him control the book, and be comfortable with his attention span. Get him involved in the story by asking him to point out things. At 18 months, he may be able to tell you what something is when you point to it. By then, you can also help him compare stories to his own experiences.

Playing with others

Anything can happen when you put two or more toddlers together in the same room. From battles over a stuffed giraffe to idyllic moments of cooperative play, playtime can represent toddler togetherness at its best and its worst. Inviting a friend over is a great way to encourage your toddler's social and sharing skills. To make playtime a positive experience for everyone involved, schedule it for a time of the day when your toddler is normally in a good mood, such as the morning, right after a nap, or after he has been fed, so that he's more likely to have a positive attitude.

You'll increase the chance of success if you start with a snack—making sure everyone's well fed may help curb hunger-induced crankiness.

Dr. Sacks Says

Why are they called play dates? Remember when it was just called "playing"? Please don't rush your child—you don't want your two-year-old to start dating yet!

Keep playtime small and short. Invite one friend at a time, at least until your toddler becomes better accustomed to playing and sharing his toys with other toddlers. Plan for no more than an hour, and schedule visits only once or twice each week to give him something to look forward to. If he is forced to play with others too often, or if the visit stretches on for too long, it may seem more like work than play. Toddlers have short attention spans, so find fun activities and crafts that you can do together in a short period of time.

If you're having a friend over, put away your toddler's favourite toys to lessen the odds of a tug-of-war. Set out a few toys that he might not mind sharing with his playmate, or try having several copies of favourite toys so that they can easily mimic each other. If your toddler is still reluctant to share, reassure him that his friend won't be allowed to take any of the toys home with him. You or another adult should constantly supervise the toddlers so things run smoothly. It will also allow you to keep a dispute over a toy from escalating into a physical struggle.

Dealing with toddler aggression

It'll understandably come as a bit of a shock when your toddler hits or bites a friend—or even you—for the first time. Hitting and biting is very common toddler behaviour, especially between the ages of one and two, and it's a normal part of toddler development. Because one-year-olds lack the communication skills necessary to express themselves, have a fierce desire to be independent, and still operate on impulse reflexes, physical aggression is a normal way for toddlers to express themselves. That doesn't mean you should ignore it and just hope it will go away as he gets older. You need to let your toddler know that aggressive behaviour is unacceptable, and show him other ways to express his feelings. And you shouldn't ignore it, as there's a real chance that someone will get hurt.

Toddlers can lash out physically for any number of reasons, including fatigue, hunger, frustration, or even simple curiosity. Most of the time a toddler who hits his playmate is simply looking for a way to assert independence or get a reaction, rather than actually trying to hurt his friend. Since they don't have the verbal skills to communicate feelings and desires, frustration builds up and can culminate in a kick or a bite. In fact, since toddlers are also orally fixated at this stage, biting is an especially attractive way to communicate. Much of the time, toddlers tend toward aggressive behaviour when they are in a new situation or when they feel out of control, such as in daycare or a new playgroup. Adjusting to a major transition, like moving or the arrival of a new sibling, can also trigger aggression. Some toddlers are also just more physical and assertive than others. If your toddler is aggressive, you need to spend time working with him on this problem. Teach him other ways to express frustration or anger.

Be patient and consistent with your child when he's aggressive. Respond immediately; don't wait until the second or third time he hits another child. He needs to know right away that he has done something wrong. Then attend to the person who was hit or bitten first, and make sure your toddler can hear you when you apologize to the child. By focusing your attention on the other child first, your toddler receives the message that biting or hitting is not an effective way to get your attention.

Once you're sure the other child is okay, remove your toddler from the situation. Sit down with him and watch the other kids play, and explain that he can go back in when he feels ready to join the fun without hurting others. Toddlers don't possess the cognitive maturity to be able to imagine themselves in another child's place or to change their behaviour based on verbal reasoning, so don't lecture him. Calmly tell him in a firm voice that hurting others is not acceptable behaviour. Simply say, "You hurt Tom when you hit him. You must not hit people. You wouldn't like it if someone hit you." Once he has settled down, encourage him to say how he feels. Don't be too concerned about what happened. Instead, teach him to say simple things like "I'm mad" or "I'm tired" to get his point across. Then teach him to say sorry. It may start out as insincere, but he'll soon learn to apologize when he's hurt someone.

Throughout the whole episode, be sure to keep your cool. Your toddler is looking to you as a role model, and yelling at him or berating him will only reinforce the aggressive behaviour. Don't try to show him how it hurts when he bites or hits others by biting or hitting him back. Make your point verbally, not physically. Be consistent, and react the same way every time he acts aggressively. If he knows that when he hits, he has to stop playing, he will soon associate aggressive behaviour with an unwanted consequence: missing out on the action.

MAKE A NOTE, MAKE AN APPOINTMENT, OR GO TO THE HOSPITAL?

Physical aggression is a phase that generally starts to get better when your toddler's vocabulary has grown, but sometimes his aggression requires more intervention than a parent can provide. **Make an appointment** to see his doctor if

> ‣ he seems to behave aggressively more often than not;
> ‣ he seems to frighten or upset other children;
> ‣ your efforts to curb his behaviour have little effect;
> ‣ his daycare complains; or
> ‣ he frequently bites other children.

Child Care

Unless one parent will be staying home with your child, you'll have to find dependable child care. Do this early, months before you go back to work or (in some cities) even before your baby is born. Deciding on child care is probably one of the most difficult tasks of parenthood. Choose a solution that works for both you and your child; if your toddler is safe and happy but you have to rush there from work every night to avoid paying additional fees, you won't be happy for long.

Child care isn't just about babysitting. Your child will spend a lot of time in child care, so she should get as much support, stimulation, and nurturing as possible. Good caregivers understand how children develop, provide them with opportunities to learn, and know how to respond to a child's emotional needs. They are also willing to cooperate with you and address any concerns or goals you have for your child. The relationship between you and the caregiver is extremely important. If you don't trust or respect a caregiver after interviewing them, or you feel that they don't respect you or are not going to cooperate with your requests, it's not going to work.

A good childcare setting is clean and safe and has a small number of children per staff member. Staff members are qualified and have had security checks. The facility or house has areas for indoor and outdoor play, as well as a quiet space for naps, and is smoke-free outside as well as inside. The routine is flexible but regular, and it includes a variety of activities. Your child should have access to a variety of toys and equipment and be provided with nutritious foods. Most importantly, a good childcare setting allows you to visit unannounced for short periods of time.

Centre-based programs and home-based programs

Provinces and territories license childcare programs in Canada. Centre-based programs must be licensed and, depending on the province, must employ qualified staff. Home programs don't need to be licensed, although some may be licensed and supervised by provincial home childcare agencies. Unlicensed home programs are often just as good as licensed ones, but your child is not protected by provincial regulations, such as ones that require that fire safety and playground equipment standards be met.

Centre-based programs are often in convenient locations, you can easily check their reputations and references, and they are obligated to meet safety and qualification standards. Home-based programs provide more individualized attention and a less structured environment, and they might be next door or down the street. The best way to ensure your child will get quality care is to visit during operating hours and to talk to other parents.

Part-time care

One option you might consider is a combination of types of care. If you work part-time or have a flexible schedule, you can consider options like putting your child in a play group or nursery school for part of the day and caring for her yourself for the rest of the day, or sharing a nanny with another family. Or your child could have in-home care for part of the day and attend nursery school for the other part so that she gets both individual care and an opportunity to socialize. Keep in mind that if your child is being shuttled around constantly, you'll all be exhausted. Avoid more than a couple of arrangements, and try to avoid frequent changes to her schedule. Also, make sure that wherever she goes, she receives high-quality care. If she attends a great playgroup but goes home to a neglectful caregiver for the rest of the day, the benefits of the quality care could be lost. Pay attention to her comfort and happiness with each situation, and to how well she is learning and growing.

Choosing child care for your needs

To find the perfect child care for your family, think about your own needs and priorities first. The following are some questions you should consider, adapted with the permission of the Canadian Child Care Federation.

- How old is your child?
- Do you have more than one child requiring care?
- Are you eligible for a government subsidy?
- What fee can you afford?
- Do you prefer a centre-based setting or a home-based setting, and do you prefer licensed or unlicensed care?
- What hours of the day do you require care?
- Would it be more convenient near your home or your work?

Finding child care

Because provincial governments regulate and license centre-based and home-based facilities, check your provincial or territorial government's website for information about childcare centres. You can also check the Yellow Pages under Child Care or Day Care, your municipality's website, your local child or family services office, local not-for-profit agencies, and community information centres, and talk to friends in your area. For information on Canadian childcare options from the Canadian Child Care Federation, see "Child Care" in Resources.

Make a list of candidates and phone them or check out their websites to answer any easy questions you have. Ask about availability (or the length of their wait list), the cost, their hours, what they charge for late fees, how they deal with discipline, and their policies on sickness, vacation, and parent involvement. Then visit the candidates that fit your criteria. When you visit a location, look carefully to see if it's clean and safe. Watch and listen to the activity that's going on, and pay attention to how comfortable the children seem. Visits are important because they allow you to get a sense of the atmosphere. It's also important for your peace of mind to be able to visit the home or centre whenever you want once your child is attending. If they say they do not allow unannounced parent drop-ins (some claim it's disruptive for the children), knock them off your list.

A SAMPLE OF QUESTIONS TO ASK WHEN INTERVIEWING A CHILDCARE PROVIDER

- ‣ Is your facility or home child care licensed, or is your home child care supervised by an agency?
- ‣ Can I dropped by unannounced to see my child?
- ‣ What are your qualifications, or the qualifications of your staff? Does everyone have first-aid training, and have they had security checks?
- ‣ How many staff members does your facility have? If it's a home-based child care, will anyone else have access to the children?
- ‣ How much does it cost? Are there any additional charges?
- ‣ Will I be charged if I'm late picking up my child?
- ‣ Do you have a waiting list?
- ‣ What are your hours?
- ‣ What is your illness policy? What is your vacation policy?
- ‣ How many children do you care for? What are their ages?
- ‣ Do you have separate areas for indoor play, outdoor play, and naps?
- ‣ What kind of toys do you have?
- ‣ What kind of activities will my child take part in?

> ‣ How do you discipline children?
> ‣ What kind of snacks and meals do you serve? Do you prepare a weekly menu?
> ‣ Is the facility or your home smoke-free?

Before making a decision, check references for the daycare centre or caregiver. Talk to other parents who have used the care for a while rather than just reading a list of references handed to you. If you live in a small town, your childcare options may be limited, so keep an open mind and some flexibility for arrangements that might not be your first preference. When you have decided on a childcare provider, sign a contract with them to prevent future misunderstandings.

Your responsibility doesn't end once you've found good child care. Keep in touch with your caregiver so you can agree on goals and expectations for your child, and so you can listen to and express any concerns about your child or the arrangement. Talk to your child each day about her experience so you have a sense of how well it's going. It could take her weeks or even months to adjust to a new situation, so don't worry too much if it's not going well, but keep your parental instincts alert for signs of a bad fit.

Plan the gradual transition to daycare a few weeks prior to your return to work so your child is comfortable there before your first day. These trial runs will be a chance for you to prepare for your return to work too.

Dr. Sacks Says

In 35 years, I've yet to see a child fall in love with a caregiver in the same way she loves a caring parent.

Back to Work

Returning to work after parental leave can bring up a host of emotional issues for parents. You may feel sadness about leaving your toddler with someone else, anxious about her well-being…and guilty for actually wanting to be back in the world of grown-ups. It can also bring up other issues—mainly, how to juggle all the duties of parenthood with your work schedule. To help make the transition back to work easier, accept that you may be a bit emotional at first, and be realistic about what you can accomplish. Divide up the chores, keeping those you enjoy for yourself and looking for volunteers for (or, even more realistically, assigning) the rest. If they don't get done, focus on the long term. Remember that it's more important to spend time together than to live in a spotless home.

Choose a return day that's later in the week so your first week back to work is a short one. Talk to your manager about your job duties and schedule so you'll know what's expected of you upon your return. Know your company's sick day policy, and prepare a plan for when your child is ill. Ask about flexible hours or working from home on occasion. You might be surprised at your manager's flexibility if you offer suggestions for making a more flexible arrangement work.

Breastfeeding for the working mother

If you are going back to work and don't want to wean your child yet, it is possible to continue to breastfeed. Get a good electric pump, as they're more effective than hand pumps for expressing milk. Double breast pumps allow you to express your milk more quickly than single breast pumps. Let your manager know that you plan to continue to nurse and will have to pump while at work. You will only need two 15-minute pumping breaks during the course of an eight-hour workday, so you won't be taking time from your work schedule. Try to space the breaks evenly throughout the day if you can. If you can't space them out, try to at least keep up the frequency (twice during an eight-hour workday) to maintain your milk supply.

Ask your employer to recommend a private room with a lock where nursing mothers can express their milk. The bathroom isn't it; a good rule of thumb is not to pump breast milk in an area where you wouldn't eat your lunch. Also, find a place in your office where you can keep your supplies: your breast pump, breast pads, empty containers for expressed milk, and extra blouses in case you have milk leakage during the day. If you don't have an office, ask your employer if a locking cabinet or closet is available for you and any other nursing mothers to use. To store your breast milk at work, use an insulated bag with cold packs. Breast milk will stay fresh and safe for up to 10 hours at room temperature or eight days in the refrigerator. Take your milk home in the insulated bag.

When you get home from work, nurse your child immediately to help maintain your milk supply. It's also a great way to bond with your child after spending the day apart. Ask your caregiver not to feed your child right before you're due to pick her up. Of course, if your child is fussy or hungry at the end of the day, give the go-ahead to your caregiver for a feeding, but suggest that it be a smaller portion than usual.

If you can't express your milk at work, pump just before you go to work and after you return home. You could also pump one or two times a day on weekends to have a supply of extra breast milk for the week. Pumping any breast milk your child doesn't drink in a 24-hour period will help keep your milk supply going steady.

HEALTH

Common Problems

After his first birthday, your toddler may start going to daycare, attending classes, and socializing. This means he'll be exposed to a whole new world of fun and adventure…and a whole new world of germs. If he wasn't sick very often in his first year of life, which can happen with your first child, it's almost guaranteed that he will have many colds when he starts interacting with other children. Many children have between 8 and 10—yes, 10—colds a year, especially between the ages of one and two years. Colds and other upper respiratory infections are most common during the fall and winter, from October through March. Ear infections may also continue to be a problem for your toddler. If he was susceptible to them in his first year of life, he may continue to get them, particularly when he has a cold.

MYTH BUSTERS

Myth: If you don't dress warmly when you go outside in the winter, you'll catch a cold.

Fact: Colds and ear infections are not caused by going out in the cold without your hat and mitts, they're caused by germs spread by our fellow human beings.

—*Dr. Ken Schelberg, MD, FRCPC*

Now that your toddler is eating new and different foods and is out and about in new settings with other children, gastrointestinal infections are more likely, especially if he's in daycare. Gastroenteritis is quite common in babies and toddlers, and is usually spread from person to person. Symptoms are a sudden onset of diarrhea, vomiting, and abdominal cramping. It is caused by a virus that infects the bowel and results in inflammation, and does not respond to antibiotics. Gastroenteritis may last 7 to 10 days, and most of the time requires no medical intervention as long as the child is kept well hydrated. Oral rehydration solutions, taken in small amounts frequently, work very well. You may also continue breastfeeding while your child has gastroenteritis.

To prevent colds and gastrointestinal infections, make sure everyone in your home washes their hands. Many of these minor infections may cause fever, but if your toddler remains active and drinks enough fluids, there is probably little to worry about. For more information on hand-washing and fever, see Chapter Six.

Dr. Sacks Says

Over-the-counter medications for colds don't work at this age and can be dangerous. They are not recommended for children under six.Save your money for a book to read to your toddler.

MAKE A NOTE, MAKE AN APPOINTMENT, OR GO TO THE HOSPITAL?

Make a note to mention it to your toddler's doctor at his next scheduled visit if he has

- ▷ frequent colds with a lingering cough;
- ▷ frequent episodes of diarrhea;
- ▷ frequent skin infections; or
- ▷ frequent episodes of fever.

Make an appointment to see his doctor if

- ▷ your child becomes listless;
- ▷ he is losing weight;
- ▷ he has diarrhea (8 to 10 watery stools, or 2 to 3 very large stools per day) for more than a few days, even if he stays active;
- ▷ there is blood in his stool;

- he seems to have cramping with his bowel movements;
- he seems to have discomfort with urination, or has foul-smelling urine;
- he is vomiting frequently and seems unable to keep any fluids down;
- he develops severe abdominal pain;
- he has a fever for more than 48 hours without any other symptoms; or
- he has been diagnosed with more than 4 to 6 ear infections (keep a record of all doctors visits).

Take your toddler to the hospital immediately if he

- has vomited more than four times in 1 or 2 hours;
- appears to be dehydrated—he looks pale and thin, his eyes are sunken, his hands and feet are cold, he's drowsy, and he's not urinating;
- is wheezing or having trouble breathing;
- is eating poorly and has fewer wet diapers than normal;
- has bouts of prolonged crying, or says he's in pain; or
- has a purpuric rash—a cluster of red skin lesions about 2 millimetres (⅛ inch) in size that do not fade when pressure is applied to them. To test for purpuric rash, press a clear glass against the skin to see if the lesions fade.

Happy Feet

Orthopaedic problems

Once your toddler starts to walk, you may notice orthopaedic problems like bowlegs, flat feet, and in-toeing. In most cases, these conditions are nothing to worry about. Flat feet and in-toeing are commonly observed once toddlers start to walk, but are rarely significant. If you notice that your toddler's legs curve outward at the knees, he has bowlegs. Most cases of bowlegs are also of no concern, and many toddlers between the ages of one and two have legs that appear bowed. Most of the time their legs straighten out completely by age 10, but if the curvature is extreme or only one side is affected, bowlegs could be caused by a more serious problem and should be checked out by a doctor.

Baby's first shoes

Shoes are selected for protection, not correction. Physically normal children rarely need corrective shoes. The Canadian Paediatric Society no longer accepts the old belief that a baby must wear shoes soon after birth. In fact, there is some evidence that wearing shoes in early childhood might actually hurt the development of their feet. Walking barefoot develops good toe gripping and muscular strength, so keep your toddler out of shoes in warm, dry conditions.

Until toddlers have been walking for at least a few months, the only purpose of footwear is to protect their feet and to offer some grip on a smooth surface. Before your toddler starts walking, all he needs is soft-sole footwear for warmth. Never buy shoes unless he is there to try them on, and never buy used shoes that have lost their shape. Shoes must fit the foot properly at the heel and allow enough room for the toes, leaving about 1.25 centimetres (½ inch) between the longest toe and the tip of the shoe when measured standing up. This allows enough room for wiggling toes and for growth, although only so much growth. Your toddler's feet are growing quickly, and he'll need new shoes every three to six months.

NUTRITION

In her second year of life, your toddler's adventure with food continues. You'll both discover more foods that she loves and some that she doesn't. Her growth will slow down after her first birthday—she will only gain about three pounds this entire year, and only grow about three inches to her height—and her appetite slows down with it. Being mobile, she is more interested in doing and exploring than she is in eating. Some days she'll hardly eat anything, and others she'll eat as much as you do. Unlike adults, toddlers know how much food they need and will eat accordingly, so don't worry about this variance in appetite. Just offer her a variety of nutritious options, and she'll take care of what, when, and how much of it she eats.

Toddlers don't actually need very much food—about a quarter to a half of an adult's needs. It's better to offer small servings and let your toddler ask for more. Since her stomach is small and she's not able to eat much at one time, she needs two to three snacks during the day in addition to her meals. Feed her when she's hungry or thirsty—not as a reward or bribe, or for entertainment. Between 18 to 24 months, toddlers prefer to drink rather than eat, but be careful to limit her fluids or she won't get all the nutrients she needs. Beverages with caffeine or added sugar, like tea, coffee, pop, and energy drinks, are never appropriate for a toddler, and juice should only be given in small amounts.

At 12 months, your toddler will probably enjoy playing with a spoon, but may spend more time banging it around and making a mess than getting food into her mouth. Over the year, she'll get better at feeding herself, so encourage her to use a spoon or fork when appropriate. Sometime this year your toddler will also be ready to start drinking from a cup, but introduce it slowly. Baby cups with lids and spouts may limit spills while she becomes familiar with the sensation of holding and drinking from a cup. Start by giving her water in a cup, or try serving milk in a cup at one meal. If she shows no interest in it, dilute the milk you put in her bottle with water so that she will prefer it from a cup, and then gradually increase the amount of milk in the cup.

Tips for Feeding Your Toddler

If your toddler refuses a certain food, respect her wishes and remove it after a reasonable length of time. Don't get angry or try to force her to eat it; it only reinforces the behaviour. Instead, try the food again a day or two later, and be patient. It may take several tries for her to actually accept a new food. It's also a good idea to introduce a new food along with familiar foods when your toddler is hungry and in good spirits. Let her smell, touch, and examine the food, and encourage her to taste one bite, but don't pressure her if she's not interested. Food likes and dislikes change over time, so she may love it the next time you give it to her. Just as her food dislikes may seem random and strange, she may become suddenly hooked on a certain food. If she only wants to eat bananas, don't worry about it. It's normal, and it won't last long if you don't make an issue of it.

Eating with your toddler is important because she'll learn to eat by watching others, so have her sit with the rest of the family at mealtime and turn the television off. Seat her at a comfortable height relative to the table, and make sure her feet are supported. Serve food in bite-sized pieces or as finger food so that she can handle it. Go easy on seasonings and avoid adding salt. Most toddlers don't like their food to mix or touch, so keep foods separate from one another.

A caution about choking

Foods that are small, hard to chew, or round or oval in shape can choke a toddler by lodging in her throat and blocking her airway. Toddlers often swallow without chewing enough or at all, so cut things into very small pieces. Remove pits from fruit before giving it to your toddler. Some foods that are choking hazards include popcorn, nuts, peanut butter (if spread too thickly), whole grapes, raw carrots, hard candies, and hot dogs. Stay with your toddler while she eats; make sure she sits, and doesn't walk, run, lie down, or talk with food in her mouth. Learn what to do when she chokes—take a first-aid course.

What to Feed Your Toddler

By 12 months, your toddler has likely tried lots of fruits, vegetables, cereals, meats, and dairy products like cheese and yogurt. After her first birthday, she can also have whole cow's milk. If she drinks vitamin D–fortified whole milk, she no longer needs a vitamin D supplement. Your toddler can eat many of the same foods the rest of the family is eating as long as they are mashed or in bite-sized pieces. In addition to the foods she's already eating, other great food ideas for this age include the following:

- New fruits like melon, papaya, mango, and citrus fruits
- New vegetables like well-cooked broccoli and cauliflower, asparagus, and eggplant
- New dairy products like cottage cheese
- Vegetable juices
- Baked beans
- Grain products like barley, unsalted pretzels, rice cakes, and ready-to-eat cereals (not sweetened with sugar)
- Combination foods like macaroni and cheese, casseroles, and lasagna
- Dried fruit like prunes, dates, raisins, and apricots that have been soaked until they're soft

Your toddler can also have honey and egg whites now. Introduce new foods one at a time, with at least three days in between, to be sure she is not allergic to them. If you have a family history of allergies, you may want to wait until she is three years old before introducing peanuts, tree nuts (such as pecans or walnuts), or shellfish. Do not introduce her to junk foods—she'll catch on to what the colourful wrappers and intriguing advertisements represent soon enough. In the meantime, keep her in the dark for as long as you can.

Iron deficiency anemia

After 12 months of age, your toddler should not take more than 750 millilitres (3 cups or 24 ounces) of milk per day. In addition to filling up her stomach, suppressing her appetite, and replacing her consumption of iron-rich foods, too much milk can lead to iron deficiency anemia. Milk provides many important vitamins and minerals, but it is low in iron and it interferes with the body's absorption of iron from other foods. Typical signs of anemia are pale skin, fatigue, irritability, loss of appetite, and a swollen tongue, but some children with anemia exhibit no symptoms at all. If untreated, anemia can cause mental and physical problems.

MAKE A NOTE, MAKE AN APPOINTMENT, OR GO TO THE HOSPITAL?

Make an appointment to see your toddler's doctor if you suspect she has anemia. A simple blood test can tell whether she is anemic. If she is, the doctor will likely advise an increase in iron-rich foods like lean meats, poultry, fish, legumes, eggs, and iron-fortified grain products, and may also recommend an iron supplement.

Food Allergies

Certain foods seem to disagree with some children, so there's a chance your child could be allergic to or intolerant of a food. Food intolerances and food allergies are not the same thing; food intolerances are common, while actual food allergies are rare. With a food allergy, an immune system reaction is triggered when you eat a certain food or food additive. A food intolerance is different from an allergy in that it doesn't involve an immune reaction. Often the reason for the food intolerance is unknown. A child who has an intolerance may have bloating, loose stools, gas, or other symptoms after eating the food. In most cases, the solution is to just avoid the food.

Any food can trigger an allergic reaction, but common trigger foods are cow's milk, nuts, eggs, fish, and shellfish. Children with food allergies may develop wheezing, hives, vomiting, or diarrhea. In severe cases, an allergic reaction can be triggered by eating just a tiny amount or by just being in contact with the allergen, and can happen very suddenly. Reactions can be serious, and can even be life threatening. A severe reaction is called anaphylactic shock, or anaphylaxis.

The diagnosis of food allergies is difficult to make and requires a doctor. Often a child needs to eat a food more than once before a parent knows he is allergic. The first time your child is exposed to nuts, he will probably have no reaction, but if he develops an allergy to nuts, subsequent exposures could be serious and even fatal. The initial allergic reaction acts like a warning signal for later reactions.

Signs and symptoms of an allergic reaction

Respiratory problems	coughing	wheezing	shortness of breath	voice changes	choking
Skin symptoms	hives	swelling (of the face, lips, or tongue)	itching	eczema	
Nasal symptoms	sneezing	blocked nose	runny nose		
Eye problems	itchiness	redness	watery eyes	swelling	
Gastrointestinal problems	diarrhea	stomach cramps	vomiting	problems swallowing	
Cardiovascular problems	pallor	dizziness	loss of consciousness		

Source: Adapted from *Well Beings: A Guide to Health in Child Care*, 3rd Edition. Canadian Paediatric Society, 2008.

> ## MAKE A NOTE, MAKE AN APPOINTMENT, OR GO TO THE HOSPITAL?
>
> **Make an appointment** to see your toddler's doctor if you suspect he has a food allergy. The doctor may refer him to an allergist.

If your child has a food allergy, you must take every reasonable precaution against exposing him to the trigger food. You and anyone else caring for him must learn how to use his emergency medication. Keep a dose with your child and one on yourself at all times. Many children outgrow food allergies, especially if the allergies start before age three, but some allergies will not disappear. An allergist can let you know if and when your child can have the food again.

For a list of organizations that can give you more information on allergies, see "Allergies" in Resources.

The Weaning Process

Weaning is a natural stage in your child's development, but many mothers have mixed emotions about it. It's normal to feel excited at the new independence you can both enjoy, but you'll probably also feel some sadness as he moves to another stage in his life. There is no right or wrong age to wean, but the Canadian Paediatric Society recommends breastfeeding for at least the first year of your baby's life, and you can breastfeed even past the age of two.

When you and your child are ready to wean, the experience will be a more positive one if you keep a few things in mind. It's easiest for both of you if weaning is done gradually over several weeks, months, or even longer. A sudden, abrupt wean should only be considered in extreme circumstances. The transition to weaning may be easier if you first introduce your child to a cup instead of a bottle. Breastfed babies easily learn to drink from a cup as early as six months of age, so start by using a cup for his least favourite feeding of the day. Someone other than mom may need to offer this feeding for him to accept it. Watch the cues you give to your child: if you sit in the same chair you usually use when you're nursing, he'll likely want to breastfeed, and he probably won't be satisfied with just a cup or a cuddle.

When you're ready to wean even more, substitute the next least favourite feeding at the opposite time of the day. Continue this way, substituting one feeding at a time. The pace of weaning is up to you and your child, but the slower the better. Wait at least a few days in between each change. An abrupt wean can be uncomfortable for you and upsetting for your child, but sometimes you may have no choice. If you are very sick, if you and your child have to be separated for a long time, or if you have to take certain drugs, you may have to wean abruptly. If your breasts get uncomfortable, express your milk to avoid blocked ducts, mastitis, or a breast abscess. Children who are sick should not be abruptly weaned.

Don't bind your breasts or drink less fluids while you're weaning. If your breasts are uncomfortable, try expressing enough milk so that you are comfortable. Over-the-counter painkillers like acetaminophen or ibuprofen can also help, as can cold compresses or gel packs applied to your breasts. Check your breasts regularly to make sure you aren't developing a blocked duct, which will feel like a firm, tender area of the breast. If you do, see your doctor or lactation consultant. These problems are more likely to occur during an abrupt wean.

You may want to try a partial wean, where you substitute one or more feedings with a cup or bottle but continue to breastfeed for other feedings. This can work well if you are going back to work but still want to breastfeed. If you do this, check your child's weight gain regularly. Some mothers choose infant-led weaning, which means watching your child's cues and weaning at his pace. Mothers who practise infant-led weaning never refuse to breastfeed, and may continue to breastfeed for two to four years, but they also do not offer the breast when their child isn't interested. This type of weaning is practised by many non-western cultures.

Sometimes your child may go on a "nursing strike" and suddenly refuse to breastfeed. This doesn't mean he is ready to wean, though. It can be caused by many different factors, such as teething, an ear infection or other illness, the onset of your period, or a change in your diet, soap, or even deodorant. If this happens, be sure to pump your milk so you don't develop a blocked duct. Try making feeding time quiet, and spend more time cuddling your child. Don't starve him; instead, try offering your breast when he is sleepy. If you can't figure out the reason for the strike, see your child's doctor.

Substitute foods

Appropriate substitute foods for breast milk depend on how old your child is when you start to wean. If your baby is under 12 months, you should give him iron-fortified infant formula. Between 12 and 18 months, give him follow-up formula or whole cow's milk (3.25 per cent). Between 18 and 24 months, give him whole milk. Once he's older than two, he can drink 2 per cent milk instead of whole milk. If your child has a milk allergy, talk to his doctor about appropriate substitute foods. After 12 months of age, your child should not drink more than 750 millilitres (3 cups or 24 ounces) of milk per day, or he'll fill up and won't want to eat solid foods, and he may develop iron deficiency anemia.

Your weaning experience is ultimately up to you and your child, so try to follow his cues whenever possible. However, your doctor, lactation consultant, or breastfeeding clinic can give you guidance and answer any questions you have about weaning.

MAKE A NOTE, MAKE AN APPOINTMENT, OR GO TO THE HOSPITAL?

If the weaning process has you feeling blue, **make an appointment** to see your doctor. If your child doesn't seem to be taking in enough substitute foods, **make an appointment** to see his doctor.

Feeding the Vegetarian Child

When properly managed, vegetarian diets are safe for children and may reduce the risk of certain conditions such as obesity. Vegetarian diets have long cultural traditions, and adults who provide a vegetarian diet for their families are often very knowledgeable about nutrition and serve well-balanced meals. The three main types of vegetarians are vegans, who eat non-animal foods only; ovo vegetarians, who eat non-animal foods plus eggs; and lacto-ovo vegetarians, who eat non-animal foods plus eggs and dairy products.

A vegan diet may compromise the growth of infants and children. Babies of most species, including humans, are meant to have milk as their staple food for the first 6 to 12 months. They may not get enough energy, protein, iron, calcium, vitamin D, vitamin B12, and riboflavin from their food. Malnutrition can result if a child's parents are not familiar with children's minimal nutritional requirements, or if they don't put enough care into meal planning and preparation. The same problems can occur with a vegetarian mom: breastfeeding is the best source of nutrition for your baby, but lactating vegetarian women sometimes need counselling to learn how to meet their protein, calcium, iron, and vitamin B12 requirements when foods from animal sources have been eliminated.

If you're going to feed your child a vegetarian diet, educate yourself first. Children eating an ovo vegetarian or a lacto-ovo vegetarian diet will have less trouble meeting their nutrient needs than vegans. Vegetarian children should be fed the same variety of vegetables, fruits, and cereals as other children, but alternate foods should be added to replace meat, fish, poultry, and, if necessary, dairy products. They should receive plant proteins such as legumes, mild milk cheese, tofu, and meat-like products made from vegetable protein. After 9 months of age, infants on a lacto-ovo vegetarian diet can have egg yolks, and they can have whole eggs after 12 months. The texture of foods needs to be modified for toddlers, so cook foods well, purée them, or put them through a sieve, blender, or grinder. Since nuts are highly allergenic, it's best not to introduce them until your child turns three years old.

Vitamin Supplements

Vitamins are necessary for the normal functioning of the body, but children don't need to take vitamin supplements on a regular basis if they're eating a diet containing all four food groups. Breastfed children need a vitamin D supplement, but once a child is drinking whole milk, it's no longer necessary as vitamin D is added to all commercial liquid milks. It is more important for children to get their vitamins from eating a variety of good foods rather than taking extra vitamins "just to be sure." Vitamin popping encourages sloppy eating habits, and it may give children the idea that they have to take a pill every day just to stay well. It is also expensive, and, without careful management, taking too many vitamin supplements can actually cause disease.

Dr. Sacks Says

Unnecessary vitamins make for expensive pee.

INJURY PREVENTION

Childproofing for a New Walker

Now that your toddler is up on her feet, or pretty close to it, it's time once more to check that your home is childproof. Walking legs can take her all kinds of new places, and increasingly dexterous hands can do more and more things as the months go by. Toddlers have trouble remembering rules, so don't be surprised if you tell her not to do something and she does it again the next day (and the day after that, and the day after that...). Be gentle but firm, and try to provide as safe an environment as possible for her to play. Creating a safe environment for your toddler doesn't mean stopping her from playing, it means allowing her to play safely.

Dr. Sacks Says

If your toddler is properly immunized, the biggest threat to her life in her second year is injury. Be vigilant with your childproofing so she can have a safe place to explore and grow.

Some things that might pose a danger to your toddler you can't possibly remove from your home, like lamps and stoves. This means you may have to constantly guide her behaviour for a little while, gently steering her away from them. She will see you touching them, of course, so be a role model. If you show her how to touch and handle these things gently, she will start to understand the concept of "gentle."

While serious injuries are most likely to occur in the kitchen and bathroom, they can happen anywhere and at any time. Throughout your whole home, continue to be vigilant about sweeping the floors and getting down on your hands and knees to check for choking hazards. Learn the names of all your houseplants and get rid of any that are poisonous (for a list of poisonous plants, see page 423 in Chapter Seven. At stairway openings, install safety gates that are fixed securely to studs in the wall. To block access to rooms, such as the kitchen, use pressure gates. Ensure that your windows cannot open more than 10 centimetres (4 inches), as toddlers can be injured falling out of windows.

Consider creating a separate, safe play space for your toddler, such as a separate room or an enclosed space in a room. Keep older children's toys, which often have small parts, out of reach of your toddler. Drill breathing holes into any trunk or box you're using as a toy box, and install safety hinges on it. Out of doors, keep her away from the barbecue at all times. Even when it is not in use, it can stay hot for a long time, and curious hands can loosen fittings to a gas or propane tank.

In the bathroom, always empty bath water immediately after a bath so she won't drown if she accidentally falls in. When running bathtub water, be sure to turn off the hot water first so that if she accidentally turns on the water, she won't be burned by the water left in the faucet. Remove all poisons from any place your toddler can reach, and ask grandparents and other relatives you visit frequently to do the same.

Changing the car seat

Once children are over one year of age, or when they exceed their rear-facing seat's height and weight limits, they can start to use a forward-facing car seat. Don't be in a hurry to move to a forward-facing seat if your child still fits into her rear-facing seat after her first birthday, though. As long as she meets the seat's guidelines, the longer she's in a rear-facing seat, the safer she'll be.

Once again, make sure that your toddler meets the new seat's weight and height requirements, that the seat fits securely in your vehicle, and that you follow the manufacturer's instructions when you install it. To secure your toddler in a forward-facing child seat, adjust the harness straps to the slot positions that are at or slightly above her shoulders.

She should be in an upright position with her back flat against the back of the car seat. The chest clip should be positioned at her armpit level to hold the harness straps in place. Check that the harness straps are fastened tightly so that only one finger fits between the straps and your child's chest.

Your child will stay in this seat until she is ready to move to a booster seat, which is usually around the age of four.

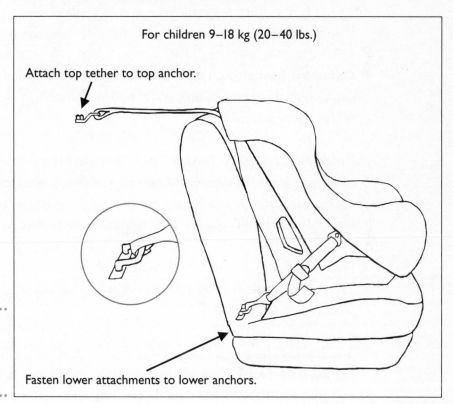

For children 9–18 kg (20–40 lbs.)

Attach top tether to top anchor.

Figure 3.1: Forward-facing car seat

Fasten lower attachments to lower anchors.

Source: *Well Beings: A Guide to Health in Child Care*, 3rd Edition. Canadian Paediatric Society, 2008.

The Babysitter Checklist

By now you're probably ready to leave your child with a babysitter for the evening—and you and your partner could probably use the time alone.

When you're looking for a babysitter, choose someone with whom you feel comfortable. Ask friends and family for the names of babysitters they've used, and if the sitter is a young teen, make sure she has taken a babysitting course or has experience taking care of young children. Prepare information so your babysitter knows your child's routine and what to do in the case of an emergency, and so that you can be confident that your child is safe, even in emergencies. The better informed your babysitter is, the more enjoyable your evening will be.

Below is essential information to leave for the babysitter.

- **Contact information.** Leave both of your cell phone numbers, work numbers (if applicable), and the name, number, and address of the place you'll be.

- **Emergency contact information.** In case the babysitter can't reach you, leave the names and numbers of close family members or friends, as well as emergency numbers like the police, the hospital, your child's doctor, and the poison control centre.

- **Food and drink.** Leave a list of your child's preferred foods and beverages, as well as foods that are off limits due to allergies or potential choking hazards.

- **Medical information.** If your child has an illness or medical condition, if she takes regular prescription medication, or if she has any other health problem, even diaper rash, let the babysitter know. Leave a signed and dated medical authorization note (see page 183) that gives the babysitter the power to make medical decisions for your child if you and your other contacts can't be reached.

- **A fire escape route.** In case your babysitter needs to evacuate the home for any reason, make sure she knows how to get out, as well as the locations of the fire extinguisher, the first-aid kit, and flashlights.

Sample information form for babysitters

INFORMATION FOR THE BABYSITTER	
Where we will be	
Name:	Location phone number: ( ) –
Address:	Our cell phone numbers:
	( ) –
City:	( ) –
Who to call if you can't reach us	
Name:	Name:
Relation:	Relation:
Phone number: ( ) –	Phone number: ( ) –
Emergency numbers	
Police: 911 or ( ) –	Ambulance: 911 or ( ) –
Fire Department: 911 or ( ) –	Poison control: ( ) –
Doctor's name:	Doctor's phone number: ( ) –
Address/fire number of this house	
Address:	
Closest intersection:	
City:	Phone number: ( ) –
Fire number:	
Location of emergency items	
Where the emergency escape plan is kept:	
Where the fire extinguisher is kept:	
Where flashlights are kept:	
Where the first-aid kit is kept:	
Our child's medical information	
Illnesses or conditions our child has	
Medication our child takes	
Where it is kept:	Where it is kept:
Medication name:	Medication name:
When to give it:	When to give it:
How much to give:	How much to give:

Where it is kept:	Where it is kept:
Medication name:	Medication name:
When to give it:	When to give it:
How much to give:	How much to give:
Where it is kept:	Where it is kept:
Medication name:	Medication name:
When to give it:	When to give it:
How much to give:	How much to give:

WHAT TO FEED OUR CHILD

Foods our child likes	Foods our child doesn't like

Foods our child shouldn't eat	Food allergies or intolerances our child has

Where our child's epinephrine device is kept [if applicable]:

SCHEDULE

When we will be home:

When our child should eat:

What our child is not allowed to do:

What to do if our child misbehaves:

Our child's bedtime routine:

Our child's bedtime:

Sample medical authorization note

Date: ....

If, at any time, due to such circumstances as an injury or sudden illness, medical treatment is necessary, I, ... [parent's name], give permission for .... [caregiver's name] to take whatever emergency measures he/she deems necessary for the protection of my child .... [child's name] while my child is in his/her care.

I understand that this may involve contacting a doctor, interpreting and carrying out the doctor's instructions, and transporting my child to a hospital or doctor's office, including the possible use of an ambulance.

If possible, the hospital will be ....[name of preferred hospital] or the doctor contacted will be .... [name and address of doctor].

I understand that this may be done prior to contacting me, and that any expense incurred for such treatment, including ambulance fees, is my responsibility.

Parent's signature: ....

Source: Adapted from *Well Beings: A Guide to Health in Child Care*, 3rd Edition. Canadian Paediatric Society, 2008.

The Wonder of Water

Water is an endless source of fun and fascination for toddlers, but it can also be very dangerous, whether it's in a pool, bathtub, bucket, or puddle. Toddlers not only drown when they become submerged in water that is too deep, but also when just their faces are covered in water and they can't get out. According to Safe Kids Canada, at least one child drowns every two weeks in Canada between June and August, and there is a near-drowning incident almost every day (see "Injury Prevention" in Resources for information on Safe Kids Canada). Toddlers are at risk of drowning because water is appealing to them but they don't understand the danger.

There are two key ways to prevent drowning. First, always supervise your toddler when she's around water. Whether she's at the beach, splashing in a kiddie pool, or having her evening bath, never take your eyes off of her, even for a minute. If the phone rings while she is in the tub and you absolutely must answer it, wrap her in a towel and take her with you. Or just let it ring—there are very few people who can't wait 10 minutes to talk to you.

Second, remove or protect your toddler from any standing water in or around your home. Don't leave water, cleaning solutions, or any other liquid in buckets anywhere she might have access to them. Put a lock on your toilet lids, and keep toilet lids down and the bathroom doors shut when they're not being used. Don't leave your child standing beside the bathtub while the water is running, and always drain the bath immediately after she gets out. Cover the bottom of the bathtub with a non-slip mat to provide some extra traction for her while she's in the tub.

Although infants naturally hold their breath under water, they may still swallow some, so don't let a baby younger than six months old go under the water. Empty wading pools after each use, and if you have an in-ground pool, follow legal guidelines regarding safety, and lock the gate after each use. Pools must be enclosed by a fence at least 1.2 metres (4 feet) high that has a childproof gate. Make sure there is appropriate and easily accessible rescue equipment by the pool. For extra protection, put kids in a lifejacket any time they're around a pool or at the beach, and take an infant/child CPR course so you're prepared in the event of an emergency.

Common Toddler Injuries

Falls

As your toddler learns how to walk and run, she will inevitably do her share of falling. At first, little things like uneven ground, attempting to stop quickly, or even turning a corner can cause her to land on her bottom or even fall and bump her head. This is all part of the learning process, and it should rarely elicit more than a momentary cry before she's up and off again. If you have a choice, use soft floor coverings in your home to cushion her fall.

If she takes a more serious tumble, like from a tabletop, down some stairs, or off a piece of climbing equipment, check her thoroughly for injuries. Falls of this nature can result in serious lacerations and bruises, broken bones, or even concussions, which obviously need to be tended to immediately. If she looks and acts okay, the fall likely didn't cause any serious damage. Even a large goose egg on the head is rarely an indication of anything serious, although it can look awful. Swelling protrudes outward when a child bumps her head because her skull is right under the skin, leaving only one way for the swelling to go. An ice pack or a bag of frozen peas wrapped in a towel and held over the area for 10 or 15 minutes will usually reduce the swelling. Pay close attention to her for the next 24 hours, though. It is fine to put her down to sleep after she's had a fall, but it's a good idea to wake her up twice a night for the following two nights just to make sure you're able to rouse her.

MAKE A NOTE, MAKE AN APPOINTMENT, OR GO TO THE HOSPITAL?

If your toddler is vomiting, groggy, confused, acting irritable, or exhibiting any other unusual behaviours after a fall, **take her to the hospital immediately.** If everything's fine, getting a clean bill of health will at least give you peace of mind.

To prevent the likelihood of serious falls, never leave your toddler unattended on any surface from which she can fall, such as a change table, a high chair without straps, or a crib with the sides down. Adjust the height of your crib mattress as she grows, and move her out of her crib before she is tall enough to hook her leg over the side. Do not leave anything in the crib that she could use for climbing out.

Pulled elbow

If your toddler is favouring one arm—holding it close to her body and not putting any weight on it—she may have a dislocated elbow joint, a common condition called pulled elbow. Often, pulled elbow occurs when a child is picked up by one arm, grabbed by the wrist, or swung around by the arms, causing the radius bone to pop out of the elbow joint. Your child may cry at the time this happens and hold her bent arm tightly by her side. She may soon stop appearing to be in pain, but will continue to protect the arm and refuse to use or move it.

MAKE A NOTE, MAKE AN APPOINTMENT, OR GO TO THE HOSPITAL?

If you suspect your child has a pulled elbow, **take her to the hospital.** A doctor will examine her and try to pop the elbow back in place. She will be fine immediately afterward and her arm will return to normal.

TRAVELLING WITH YOUR CHILD

Now that your child is over a year old, you may finally feel that the time is right to take a family vacation. Family vacations are the stuff memories are made of—both good memories and the "someday we'll look back and laugh" variety. Travelling with children can be a rewarding, eye-opening experience if you start with realistic expectations, prepare for any outcome, and follow some simple guidelines.

Pick a destination that's family-friendly. If you choose somewhere that is used to catering to families with young children, half the work will be done for you, and everyone will be more relaxed. Family resorts and campgrounds are your best bet. Family campgrounds usually have a shaded playground and a supervised beach, and most have a general store on-site in case you run out of sunscreen or diapers. Family resorts often let children stay for free in their parents' rooms, or at least eat for free.

Travel can be tough on your toddler's constitution, but making an attempt to keep to his regular schedule—even to a small degree—will help him adjust a lot easier. Try to keep mealtimes, naptime, and bedtime relatively consistent. You don't need to be stringent about it, but an attempt to keep his routine in place will keep him much happier. If your child is old enough to sleep in a bed, get him his own bed, if you can. You'll have a hard enough time getting him back into his sleep routine once you're back from vacation without having to break any new habits.

While trying to keep up your routine is important, it's also crucial to be flexible when travelling with a toddler. This is not a vacation for sightseeing, so keep your itinerary simple. Spend half the day on one outing or activity a day, and the rest of the day relaxing. If you factor in time to just hang out, it can make for serendipitous results. The best memory of your entire vacation might be the hour you spent splashing in the wading pool or playing hide-and-seek in the hotel room. Your toddler is at his best in the morning, so plan outings and sightseeing before lunch. Accept the fact that this is not going to be a vacation of intimate late suppers and lazy mornings in bed.

If you're planning a long trip, try taking a few short trips first to get your child used to long car rides and sleeping away from home. A day trip or an overnight visit can help you figure out what works and what doesn't when you're on the road: what to pack and what to leave behind, what toys your toddler likes, and how long he is happy in his car seat.

Getting There

If you're driving to your destination, factor in several stops during the day so your toddler can get out of the car, get some fresh air, stretch his arms and legs, and work out any pent-up energy. Provincial travel websites can help you locate parks and great picnic spots along your route. Try not to schedule too much driving in one day. Quit early so you can check in, relax, and have some family time before your toddler goes to bed. With a 12- to 24-month-old, plan to stop every couple of hours. Consider starting a long car journey early in the morning or at naptime, when your toddler may sleep for a few hours. Once you're at your destination, don't coop him up for too long either. Toddlers don't take well to being in confined spaces for too long, whether it's the car, the stroller, or anywhere else. Try to get outside as much as possible, and make sure there is some space for him to run around a bit wherever you go. Or set aside a good chunk every day for him to splash about in the pool or race around the local park. He'll be happier for it, and he'll probably sleep better, too.

If you aren't driving to your destination but will be once you get there, find out whether a safe car seat will be available. Those offered by rental car agencies or by family or friends may not meet current safety standards. Or if you're going to be taking a taxi, you will need to provide the car seat yourself. Often it's easiest to take your own when you travel.

Air travel

Air travel is not recommended for babies younger than seven days old because cabin pressure in an airplane changes often, and newborn babies' systems may have trouble adjusting. Airlines have different policies about age of air travel, so check before you make plans. Air travel will expose your toddler to hundreds of people in an enclosed space, so make sure all immunizations, including the flu vaccine, are current. Children travelling abroad should have documented proof of immunization and should have a list of medical conditions and contact numbers for health care.

Toddlers under two years old usually fly for free when they sit on a parent's lap. If you've ever experienced sudden turbulence, though, you know how hard it can be to hold on to your book, your MP3 player, and your beverage all at the same time. If you can afford it, the safest way for your toddler to fly is in his own car seat. An active toddler will also appreciate the comfort of his own space, and you'll have more room to store your travel gear. Check that your car seat has a national safety label that indicates it is certified for use on aircraft. Car seats must be placed in the window seat to allow for safe emergency clearance of the row. If your toddler is on your lap, a flight attendant should direct you on how to hold him securely during takeoff. You should not use a sling or front infant carrier to hold your child on an airplane. If possible, have children seated away from the aisle to avoid potential injury from service trolleys, passengers walking in aisles, and hot meals or liquids being passed over the aisle seat. Select your seats early, and try to get bulkhead seats, which have more legroom, or to be seated in a row with an empty seat if the flight isn't sold out.

Plugged ears and air sickness are no fun for adults, but they're even worse for children. Changes in cabin pressure can be especially painful for toddlers because they have small Eustachian tubes, the part of the ear that helps even out pressure. For babies and toddlers, breastfeeding, or sucking from a bottle or on a pacifier, may offer some relief. For toddlers, the swallowing action of eating healthy snacks such as crackers or sliced grapes may help. If your toddler is bothered by plugged ears, help him hold his nose and encourage him to exhale gently from his mouth. Placing hot washcloths in plastic cups and putting them over your child's ears may also help relieve the pressure. Children shouldn't fly within two weeks of having an ear infection, if possible. Some children are more sensitive to motion sickness than others, but they shouldn't be given anti-nausea medication when they're younger than two years of age. Try pain medication (acetaminophen or ibuprofen; **never** aspirin) instead.

Many airlines can accommodate specific dietary needs if you let them know in advance. If you are concerned that any of the airline food may not be safe for your child, bring your own food on board. If your child has a severe peanut allergy or any other serious health concerns, you should alert the airline and flight personnel in advance. Although many airlines no longer offer peanuts as snacks, some passengers may bring them on board. If you think your child is having an allergic reaction during the flight, alert the flight personnel and administer the emergency medication as your child's doctor has shown, and seek medical attention when you land. It is possible that an allergic reaction can occur for the first time during a flight. You may need a note from your child's doctor to carry epinephrine or other medications on board, so check with the airline in advance.

MAKE A NOTE, MAKE AN APPOINTMENT, OR GO TO THE HOSPITAL?

Make a note to ask your child's doctor the following questions at an appointment before your vacation.

- ▷ Is your child well enough to travel?
- ▷ Do you need a medical letter?
- ▷ Does your child need a prescription for any medication?
- ▷ Does your child need any immunizations before travelling?
- ▷ Is there anything you should do to prepare your child for flying?

Like adults, children can suffer from jet lag. To minimize his jet lag, make sure your child is as well rested as possible before you leave. Plan to arrive at your destination in the evening and assume your child's usual bedtime routine. Adjust immediately to the local time; if it's nighttime when you arrive, put your child down to sleep at the time you normally would. Just like you, it will take him a few days to adjust his body clock.

What to Pack

By now, you no doubt feel a bit like a packhorse anytime you go somewhere with your child, no matter if it's to the grandparents' home or to the beach. Going on a long vacation means increasing that load exponentially, but being organized can help. A couple of weeks before you go, start compiling a list of everything you're going to bring, and continue to add to it as you think of things. Save a master list of basics that you can use for future trips. Find out as much about the place you'll be staying at as you can before you go: Is your brand of formula available? Can you get diapers easily? Will a safe crib and high chair be available? If you're flying, you'll also have to carefully plan your carry-on luggage needs. Rules about carry-on luggage change frequently, so before any flight, and especially when you're travelling with children, contact your airline to find out what you are allowed to carry on board. Consider the list below.

- **Well-stocked carry-on luggage.** Pack a change of clothes for your child and an extra shirt for you in your carry-on bag or diaper bag. You never know what will happen en route or when you get there. Plan for lost luggage and travel delays by making sure you have enough supplies in your carry-on bag to get you through 24 hours without your suitcase.

- **Diapers and wipes.** Put several in your carry-on bag or diaper bag, and pack a good number in your suitcase as well. Find out where and when you can purchase more when you get to your destination.

- **Pain or fever medication.** Pack it in your carry-on or have it readily accessible in the car for on-board crying bouts.

- **Sample sizes of baby skin products.** Pack small containers of diaper cream, baby wash, shampoo, and any other products you normally use in zip-lock bags to protect against spills. Using the same brands you do at home can prevent skin rashes and irritation while you're away.

- **Plastic grocery and zip-lock bags.** Put several in your carry-on bag and in your luggage so you have a place to store soiled diapers and clothes.

- **Blankets.** Pack one or two in your carry-on bag to keep your child cozy on the air-conditioned plane, or to drape over the stroller for shade while you're on your trip.

- **Lots of clothes.** Count on one or two outfits per day. Find out if there is laundry available where you're going; if so, you might not need to bring as much. And to make those clothes go even further, pack dark clothes—they don't show dirt as much.

- **Bathing suits.** Even if you're not going somewhere warm, you never know when you might come upon an indoor pool along the way. Remember, hot tubs are not for children.

- **Sun hats and sunscreen.** If you're going somewhere sunny, your child will need them, and so will you.

- **Insect repellent.** Check with a travel medicine clinic or the Public Health Agency of Canada (see "Travel" in Resources) to find out if you should also pack mosquito netting.

- **Laundry soap and stain remover.** If laundry is available where you're going, take small containers of your child's usual brand of soap.

- **Night light.** If you use one at home, bring it; if not, buy one for the trip. It will make late-night diaper changes in a strange room a bit easier.

- **Portable playpen.** Check if the place you're staying can arrange to have a crib in your room, and ask if they use standard-sized fitted crib sheets. If not, bring your own sheets. If they can't provide a crib, a portable playpen is a good substitute.

- **Bibs and toddler utensils.** For use in restaurants that don't supply them.

- **Car seat.** If you're flying, you can check your car seat or use it on the plane if your child has his own seat. Ask the rental company if it will fit into your rental car before you go.

- **Lightweight stroller.** You can take your stroller right to the door of the airplane and leave it there to be checked. Strollers can be damaged in flight, so don't bring your expensive jogger. An inexpensive umbrella stroller is best.

- **Your child's favourite toy.** For the sake of everyone's sanity, this may be the most important thing on your packing list. Do not forget your child's teddy bear, blankie, or whatever his comfort object may be. It will help him feel more secure in a new place. Blankies notoriously get left behind on trips, so you might want to buy a couple of the exact same comfort object in case the original gets lost.

- **First-aid kit.** Always carry a first-aid kit with you when you travel, and make sure it's easily accessible. Pack fever and pain medication, antibiotic cream, gauze, bandages, a plastic bag or towel for sickness, any medication your child is taking (antibiotics, asthma puffers, etc.), a small ice pack, and hand sanitizer. If there's a chance your child might need epinephrine for allergy emergencies, pack more than one in your carry-on luggage. Bring a list of medications that anyone in your family is taking and the dosages.

- **Passports.** Even babies need passports to travel outside of Canada. Obtaining a birth certificate, which you need to get a passport, can take time. So can getting an open-eyed, non-smiling photo of your child. Start early and plan your trip accordingly.

- **A list of consulate numbers.** Canadian consulates abroad can provide numbers for local doctors (see "Travel" in Resources).

- **Familiar foods.** While you may be excited to sample the local cuisine, your child probably isn't. Plus, you don't want to discover he has an allergy to something when you're miles away from home, so introducing exotic foods isn't a great idea while you're away. Bring some of his favourite foods with you—fruit bars and cereal both pack well—and take them with you when you go out to restaurants or on day trips. If he's not happy with the local selection, he'll still have something familiar to eat.

Put together a big bag of toys, books, and games to amuse your child along the way. Start pulling things together several weeks before your trip. Include lots of things he's never seen before, and plan to bring much more than you need. When he starts to fuss or get bored, pull something new out of the bag. Also pack a bag full of lots of drinks (water and formula or breast milk) and nutritious snacks that travel well, like crackers, bananas, little bags of whole grain cereal, and canned fruit. Like adults, children can get very dehydrated when flying, and they get hungry before the airline provides food (*if* the airline provides food).

FLYING WITH FORMULA

As important as they are, airline security measures can seem a bit much at times. For a little while, it was a challenge to carry bottles of formula and milk in carry-on luggage. Fortunately, the United States Transportation Security Administration has since instituted a common-sense approach. As long as you tell the customs officer that you are carrying breast milk or formula, you should not have a problem carrying amounts greater than 90 millilitres (3 ounces), whether you are travelling with your child or not. Canada, on the other hand, will only allow you to carry these items if you are travelling with an infant under two years old, and only in "reasonable" amounts (see "Travel" in Resources). Airlines are usually accommodating, and many will refrigerate breast milk, formula, and certain medications during the flight if you ask.

Carry an oral rehydration solution in case your child gets diarrhea during the trip. If your child is breastfeeding and has diarrhea, continue to offer breast milk. Over-the-counter medications to stop diarrhea aren't recommended for children of any age. To stop harmful germs from spreading, wash your hands often and carry a hand sanitizer product when travelling. Keep children well away from stray or sick animals while on vacation, and seek medical advice without delay if any illness persists while you are away or after you have come home.

Immunization for Foreign Travel

If you're travelling to certain countries, you and your child may require special vaccinations or medications. Many of the diseases prevented by these vaccines are rare or nonexistent in Canada but are still common in other parts of the world. Common vaccinations are hepatitis A for developing countries, yellow fever for Africa and South America, Japanese encephalitis for Asia, and typhoid for Asia, Africa, the Caribbean, Central America, and South America. The vaccinations you require will vary according to the time of year, your destination, the ages of travellers, and the current situation at your destination, so ask your doctor or a travel medicine clinic what vaccinations you will need for your particular vacation. Because the vaccination schedule can take months, do this well in advance of your trip. Find out the schedules for adults and for children, as they can differ. A list of travel medicine clinics is available from the Public Health Agency of Canada (see "Travel" in Resources).

Childproofing While You're Away

Childproofing may be second nature to you now, but it won't be for some of the people you visit. Some hotels do provide childproofing equipment, so if you're staying in a hotel, ask before you leave. If not, or if you're staying in a home that doesn't have children, it's a good idea to bring some childproofing equipment with you, such as outlet and doorknob covers, a toilet lid latch, and table corner covers. All of these items are easily packable, but if you're really pressed for space, just throw a roll of masking or painter's tape in your bag. It can do a number of child-proofing jobs, from attaching electrical cords to the floor, to covering outlets, to securing drawers and cabinet doors so they can't be opened.

When you get there, inspect the room carefully and check that nothing has been left in drawers or cabinets that could be harmful to your child. Get down on all fours and look for any choking hazards that may have been missed by the cleaning staff, such as coins or buttons.

ooooo

By now your child will be such a forceful presence in your home that you won't be able to imagine what life was like without her. The years of walking and talking will be filled with challenges, but those challenges will be completely offset by your amazement at how quickly she learns and develops. Her smile is no longer just for you, and it's exciting to see her warm to new people and make new friends. Your attention still makes all the difference in her development. She may be becoming her own person, but she still needs all the cuddles her parents can give.

4

CHAPTER

Your Toddler in Transition: Ages Two and Three

Your child, who seemed only yesterday to be sleeping swaddled in your arms, is now on her way to becoming a preschooler. As her intellectual, physical, and emotional skills improve, there are days when she will no longer seem like a baby, but a little person with a fully formed personality. She has definite likes and dislikes—even if they change every day—and is able to express her opinions and wishes. Some days, her new-found independence may astonish you, while other days, when she clings to you as you try to leave the room, you'll be reminded that she still relies on her parents completely. The frustration and fear that comes with learning to master her environment can put the "terrible" in the terrible twos. Her remarkable successes, on the other hand, put the "terrific" in the terrific threes. Although she may test the limits of your patience while she is testing her own limits, you'll watch her blossom as she starts to discover the world on her own terms.

INCLUDED IN THIS CHAPTER

GROWTH AND DEVELOPMENT

Your toddler will spend her third and fourth years of life improving her coordination—and burning off that enormous reserve of energy—by taking part in all kinds of physical activity, so let her run, play, and explore. She'll get some of the exercise and experience she needs just going through her daily routine of going up and down the stairs, climbing on the furniture, racing around the backyard, and doing all the other things active toddlers like to do. And you'll probably get a complete workout just trying to keep up with her. It's just as important, however, to get outside, even in the winter, so she can run and explore in a park and climb and swing in a playground. Remember, she still needs constant supervision as she explores and experiments.

Your two-year-old will still have a very short attention span, but over the next couple of years her ability to concentrate for long periods will get better and better. At two she can memorize short rhymes and songs, do simple puzzles, and flip through a book by herself, and by her fourth birthday she may be able to have prolonged conversations with you and sit still while you read her a long story. You can help her increase her attention span by gradually reading longer and longer stories to her and engaging her in extended conversations.

She will also begin to understand that she can make things happen, that events occur in the world because of something she has done. In fact, she may think that everything that happens is because of something she's done. Even some two- and three-year-olds have trouble understanding that some sad or upsetting events, like illness and divorce, are not their fault. Learning about cause and effect and understanding when things are beyond her control are important steps in her emotional development, and they begin in these important years.

Mastering Motor Skills

Now that your child is comfortable walking and has started to run, the next two years will see her master these skills. The stiff-legged toddler walk will slowly be replaced by a more mature heel-to-toe walking motion, and by age three, she will be walking backwards and sideways, turning sharp corners, and easily going up and down stairs while holding the handrail. She is now standing more erect, losing her slightly curved spine and "toddler tummy." Her increased muscle control and stronger, leaner body mean she is becoming ever more agile. With new agility comes new skills, so now's the time to teach her about safety, such as wearing a helmet when she rides her tricycle, as she develops these skills.

Her fine motor skills are improving, too. By the end of her third year, she will be using a spoon and fork, building block towers, turning the pages of a book one by one, and holding a crayon or pencil properly and making vertical, horizontal, and circular strokes with it. She will become increasingly adept at turning handles, opening jars and boxes, and using scissors, so you must continue to be vigilant to prevent injuries. Interlocking blocks, toy workbenches, and things that can be taken apart and put back together will encourage this development. By her fourth birthday she will likely be able to put on her own socks and shoes (sometimes elegantly backwards), do up buttons (when she feels like it), and pour liquid from a pitcher with only minor spills.

Dr. Sacks Says

Compare your child to herself, not to the neighbour's kids.
Make sure she is progressing in the right direction.

Language Leaps

By the age of two, most children have a vocabulary of about 50 words, and that number will increase to about 300 by their third birthday. During that year, your child will begin to use pronouns (such as "I," "me," "you") and will start stringing together simple three- to five-word sentences ("I get down"). He will also start to answer simple "who" and "where" questions, and to use language to describe how he is feeling ("I hungry"). Many of the harsh or vulgar expressions adults use will mysteriously start to appear in your child's vocabulary, so better watch what you say! Children this age can understand about three times as many words as they can say—and they hear everything.

Around age three, he will know the names of most objects, and when he doesn't, he'll gladly ask. This is also when the infamous "whys" begin. He'll start to use "why" in a repetitive manner, and you may find it a bit of a challenge to pay attention and answer every question. He'll be able to answer simple questions, so ask him lots of questions too. If he tells you about a dragon he saw in a dream, for instance, ask him about it: What colour was the dragon? What did his body look like? Was he a nice dragon or a mean dragon? Not only will your questions encourage him to use and expand his vocabulary, they will spark his imagination and show him you're interested in hearing about his thoughts and feelings.

In the year between three and four, your child's vocabulary will increase exponentially. By four, he may know 1,500 words and be speaking in four- to six-word sentences. Most of what he says by this age should be understandable to strangers, although his enunciation may not be perfect and he may mispronounce certain words or consonants. He may also go through periods when he chatters non-stop—an annoying but crucial way for him to improve his ability to use and understand language.

Reading and talking to your child are the most important things you can do to encourage his language development. Reading helps him learn new words and associate those words with pictures, and talking helps him practise his language skills. Meals, bath time, and quiet time before bed are ideal times to ask him about his day and how he is feeling. Be sure to pause and wait patiently for an answer, as he may have to take some time to think about the question before he comes up with an answer.

Misspeaks

The language skills of two- and three-year-olds are developing every day, and in the process they commonly mispronounce words, use the incorrect word, or have difficulty with certain sounds. Most of the time it's nothing to worry about; it's just your child learning the intricacies of language and developing the oral control to be able to master it. Some hard consonant sounds like "g" and "k" are pronounced at the back of the throat, so children cannot see how to actually make the sound. As long as your child's speech is improving over time, it doesn't need to be perfect at this stage. You may find his mistakes cute, but make sure you respond to him with proper pronunciation rather than baby talk or mimicking. By the age of three, his speech should be clear enough that even strangers can understand most of it.

Up to the age of five, common misspeaks include dropping syllables in longer words ("amal" instead of "animal"), mispronouncing words ("bisketti" for "spaghetti"), and substituting an "f" sound for "th" ("frow" instead of "throw"). Incidentally, parents inadvertently teach their children the power of certain words by how they respond to misspeaks. We don't giggle when they say "goggie" instead of "doggie," so be careful not to giggle if he substitutes an "f" for the "tr" sound in "truck" (as hard as it may be).

MYTH BUSTERS

Myth: Talking to your toddler in more than one language may confuse or slow his language development.

Fact: Children exposed to two languages from birth do not get confused, and their language development is normal.

—*Dr. Shirley Blaichman, MD, FRCPC*

Pronouns like "I" and "you" may also be confusing to your child now because they are constantly changing, even in reference to the same person. Daddy might say "I want to do this," but another person talking to him says "You want to do this." Help your child to learn how to use pronouns correctly by not talking about yourself in the third person: say "I want you to do this" instead of "Mommy wants you to do this." A common problem for children exposed to two languages is that they may use the syntax of one language with the vocabulary of the other. With enough practice, however, they are able to sort the languages out on their own.

MAKE A NOTE, MAKE AN APPOINTMENT, OR GO TO THE HOSPITAL?

Make a note to mention to your child's doctor at his next appointment if he has trouble with vowels (says things like "hoo" instead of "how") or if he talks mostly in vowels and can't say consonants (says only "a" for "bat," for example). He may not be hearing all the sounds that make up words, so the doctor may recommend a hearing test. Also mention to your doctor if your child cannot make you understand what he is saying.

Lisping

If your child lisps at this age—pronounces the "s" sound like a "th," for example, the word "sister" becomes "thithter"—it's usually not cause for concern. Many children lisp, and most outgrow it completely by the age of seven. Pointing it out to your child and trying to get him to stop will only draw his attention to it and make him ashamed. However, there are certain things you can do to minimize the factors that might be contributing to his lisp, such as not allowing him to use a soother during the day. Since mouth breathing flattens the tongue and pushes it forward, make sure he can breathe through his nose; have him blow his nose if it is stuffed up.

Your child should be off bottles and sippy cups and onto regular drinking cups by now; if he isn't, making the transition will help him improve his oral motor strength. Teaching him to use a straw and having him do exercises like blowing bubbles or blowing into a party horn or a whistle will also strengthen his lips and cheek muscles and push the tongue back in behind the teeth.

Stuttering

As children's language abilities rapidly develop, it's normal for them to stumble over words from time to time. Children often repeat words or parts of words, or hesitate while speaking, when they are excited, tired, anxious, or not feeling well. Your toddler's thoughts and ideas may be outrunning his ability to express them; he may just have so much to say that his mouth can't work fast enough to keep up. These types of occasional missteps are very common and are different from true stuttering. In fact, about one in 20 preschoolers (and four times as many boys as girls) will suffer from true stuttering at some point—holding or repeating the first sound or syllable of a word, or opening their mouths with no sound coming out. Most children simply outgrow it by about age six without any intervention.

MAKE A NOTE, MAKE AN APPOINTMENT, OR GO TO THE HOSPITAL?

If your child's stuttering is accompanied by tension in his jaw or cheeks, if he grimaces or clenches his fists when he speaks, or if he is so self-conscious that he avoids talking to prevent the stuttering, **make a note** to mention it to his doctor at his next appointment. The doctor may refer your child to a speech therapist, although many experts suggest waiting until a child's language abilities are fairly well developed—at about age three or four—before seeking help for stuttering.

Stuttering can be extremely frustrating for a child who knows what he wants to say but just can't get the words out, and the more upset and anxious he becomes, the worse the stuttering may be. You can help him out by not making a big deal of the stuttering. Don't finish his sentences for him, try to rush him along, or tell him to relax or slow down. If you talk slowly and with a calm and pleasant expression on your face, he will pick up on that and relax too.

Regardless of whether your child engages in speech therapy, you can practise some therapeutic techniques at home with your child. Set aside some time each day for quiet, uninterrupted conversation. If he's having trouble with a sentence, repeat it in the correct tone and rhythm when he's done, but not in a way that suggests you are correcting him. Try singing or reciting simple songs, rhymes, and finger games with him. He may find the rhythm easier to handle than unstructured conversation.

MAKE A NOTE, MAKE AN APPOINTMENT, OR GO TO THE HOSPITAL?

Make a note to mention to your child's doctor at his next scheduled appointment if any of the below describes him.

Two years

▷ He has a vocabulary of fewer than approximately 50 words.

▷ He hasn't started speaking in two- or three-word sentences.

▷ He is not speaking or imitating others.

▷ He doesn't react when you call his name.

▷ He doesn't point to body parts or objects when asked.

▷ He doesn't respond when you point to things for him to look at.

▷ He doesn't seem to understand what you say to him.

Three years

▷ He can't say vowels (he says "dug" instead of "dog").

▷ His speech is very unclear, and strangers cannot understand him.

▷ He can't name most household objects.

▷ He constantly struggles to get words out.

▷ He gets frustrated while trying to speak and gives up.

▷ He doesn't seem interested in talking or communicating.

▷ He doesn't follow your instructions.

Make an appointment to see his doctor if your child's verbal skills are deteriorating or he is losing verbal skills he previously had.

In any of these cases, your child may have a speech, hearing, or development problem. If he has had frequent and recurring ear infections, it may have resulted in some hearing loss. His doctor may refer him to an audiologist or speech therapist for further evaluation. You'll need to address a speech or hearing problem as early as possible to prevent possible social, emotional, behavioural, or learning problems that can result from poor communication skills, so be completely frank when you talk to the doctor about your child's speech development.

Sleep Issues

A good night's sleep is essential for your toddler's health and for her ability to learn. By age two, most toddlers sleep for 10 to 13 hours in a 24-hour period and have only one nap a day, usually between one and three hours long in the early afternoon. Some give up napping entirely by age three, while others will continue to need a siesta until they are five. How much sleep your child needs during the day may depend on how long she sleeps at night. If she sleeps fewer than 13 hours a night, she will probably need to get some rest during the day.

Of course, she may not see it that way. Trying to get some toddlers to nap can be a Herculean task. If she doesn't want to nap, don't force it. As long as she's not irritable or falling asleep in her dinner, she probably doesn't need one. Instead, encourage her to rest her body with some quiet time in the afternoon. Turn off the television and dim the lights to help her relax. Try to get her to spend this time alone, but if that doesn't work, spend time together doing something relaxing like reading. Even if she doesn't sleep, it will still help her recharge her batteries.

The resistant sleeper

No matter how tired, your toddler may resist going to bed, crying when you leave the room or popping up like a jack-in-the-box time and time again after you tuck her in. She may insist she's not tired, try to make a game out of it (peeking down the stairs and saying "Hi Mommy," with a big smile on her face), or beg to join in with whatever the rest of the family is doing. And then there's the classic "I need to pee" ploy, which children learn so quickly—even if they're still in diapers!

Toddlers usually resist bedtime because of two conflicting factors: their new-found independence, and lingering separation anxiety. Your child wants to take control of her world, so she may say "no" to anything you tell her to do, and she's also afraid of being left alone. Children usually outgrow this phase on their own, but there are some things you can do to try to make bedtime easier. If your child feels that she has some control, she may be less likely to try to assert herself when it's time to turn out the light. Let her make simple choices, like which pyjamas to wear, what books to read, or which teddy bear she wants to sleep with. Don't ask her certain questions if you don't want to hear the answer, though. If you ask her if she's ready for bed, there's a pretty good chance the answer will be no. Instead, say something like, "It's bedtime now. Do you want to wear your red or blue pyjamas tonight?"

You can help her be ready for bed by making sure she's active during the day but quiet before bedtime. If she gets plenty of fresh air and exercise, she's more likely to be too tired to argue. Create a relaxing environment in the evening by eliminating TV after dinner and playing quietly instead. Try to keep your own stress out of the end of your child's day, and spend quality quiet time together. Play with puzzles, talk with her about her day, and listen to what she has to say. You'll be giving her the attention she needs, and helping her to relax and dispel any fears she has. To help ease her anxiety over being left alone, let her sleep with her favourite blanket or stuffed toy, and put a night light in her room if she wants one.

Dr. Sacks Says

A pleasant end to the day helps parents and children look forward to the next one.

Bedtime routines should be consistent and calming for both of you. Do your best to maintain the same routine every night. Start to help her wind down about half an hour before bedtime, at the same time every night. Give her a little bit of warning before each step of the routine ("Five more minutes and then we're going to get out of the bath"), don't let her delay too much, and don't grant her unusual requests, like a bout of jumping on the bed or a second glass of water. In fact, avoid giving her water just before bedtime so that she isn't woken up by a full bladder.

MAKE A NOTE, MAKE AN APPOINTMENT, OR GO TO THE HOSPITAL?

Make a note to mention to your child's doctor at your next scheduled appointment if she refuses to sleep in her own bed or wakes up frequently during the night.

From crib to bed

There's no right or wrong time to move your child from her crib to a bed, but most parents do it when their child is outgrowing the crib and is able to climb out of it on her own, or there is a new baby on the way who will need to use the crib in the coming months. If you are expecting another child, move your older child to her bed at least eight weeks before your due date so she doesn't feel resentment toward the baby who took her crib.

Some children take to their new bed right away, while others have a very difficult time adjusting to it. Children who are generally resistant to change or are very attached to their crib might find the move to a bed unsettling, especially if it also coincides with other major changes like starting toilet learning or daycare. Firstborns may have a little more trouble than subsequent children, who tend to want to be like their older siblings. To make the transition from crib to bed a little easier, put the bed in the same place the crib used to be, and give her sheets and blankets in her favourite colour or with her favourite animals or characters on them. For the first while, allow her to sleep with her crib blanket, and give her a stuffed toy or blanket to take to bed with her. Maintaining your regular bedtime routine will give your child a sense of security and consistency, despite the change in sleeping arrangements.

If your child is nervous about being up high in her new bed, it may be less intimidating for her to start with the mattress on the floor. When she is more comfortable, you can place the mattress on the bed frame. Close baby gates at the top of stairs, and lock all exterior windows and doors in case she gets up in the middle of the night and wanders around while everyone is sleeping. Do not use bunk beds for children this young; even if she sleeps on the bottom bunk, she'll be tempted to climb the ladder and try out the top bunk.

Knowing your child's temperament will help you plan for the change. Some children accept change easily, while others are slower to adapt. If after a few nights she is still very resistant to the new arrangement, there's nothing wrong with bringing back the crib for a while and trying again in a few weeks or months. Just be sure that she doesn't think that she did something wrong or that you're bringing back the crib as punishment. Stick as closely as you can to the routine—try to keep her in her own bed when she is ill or has a nightmare, rather than allowing her to sleep in your bed, even if she shares a room with others. If she needs to share your bed when you're travelling, return to her old routine as soon as you get home.

Sleep disturbances

Nightmares
Children of all ages can have nightmares, but they are particularly common in kids aged two to four. At this age, their imaginations are

blossoming, and normal childhood fears—like monsters, the dark, and abandonment—start to develop. They have not yet fully grasped the difference between fantasy and reality; if they see something scary on TV or hear a scary story, they may not understand that it isn't real.

Nightmares most often occur in the second half of the night, during REM sleep, when most dreaming occurs. Your child may remember the dream the next day and continue to be afraid for several nights to come. If she has a nightmare, hold her and comfort her until she calms down. Gently encourage her to talk about the nightmare if she can, as sometimes just talking about it can ease her fears. Reassure her, tuck her in with her favourite stuffed toy, and leave a light on and the door open if she wants. Try not to send conflicting messages, like saying there's no such thing as monsters and then checking under the bed, or telling her that her teddy bear will protect her.

There's no surefire way to prevent your child from having nightmares, but you can try to help ward them off. Limit television after dinner, and make sure the programs your child watches at any time of day do not contain violent or scary images. Even if a program doesn't seem scary to you, it might to her, so watch it with her and pay close attention, or screen shows carefully before she watches them. Often children don't seem scared while they're watching, but will have difficulty with the images later. Keep the bedtime routine calm and pleasant. Play quietly and read upbeat stories that don't contain any potentially frightening imagery. It might help to read stories that demystify monsters and similar make-believe creatures. A warm bath, lots of hugs, soothing music, and a quiet talk should ease her mind and body into sleep. Talk about some of the pleasant plans for the next day. Remind her that sleep helps her grow and keeps her healthy.

Children have nightmares more frequently when they are anxious or under stress. Things like toilet learning, changes in childcare arrangements, transitioning from a crib to a bed, a new baby in the home, or even sensing parents' stress can all be very upsetting to them. Whenever possible, make changes gradually. If your child starts having frequent nightmares, try to determine what might be causing them. Talk to your child about her fears and reassure her. If possible, you may even want to back off whatever it is that is causing her tension—maybe take some time off from the toilet learning process—until she is better able to deal with it. If she's spending time in two homes, try to keep the bedtime routine consistent in both homes. Children are pretty flexible, so the routines don't have to be exactly the same between homes, as long as they are consistent in each home.

MAKE A NOTE, MAKE AN APPOINTMENT, OR GO TO THE HOSPITAL?

Make a note to mention to your child's doctor at your next scheduled appointment if the nightmares persist, and if she becomes extremely fearful of going to bed or is anxious or agitated during the day. The nightmares could be a sign of a larger emotional issue, such as anxiety or experiences at daycare, that may need to be addressed.

Night terrors

Night terrors are different from nightmares, and are mercifully less common. During a night terror episode, your child may appear to be awake and extremely agitated, sitting bolt upright in bed, and crying, screaming, thrashing, or moaning. She may have her eyes open and even be talking, saying things like "no" or "stop it," but will not respond to you in any way. In fact, she may push you away and get even more upset when you try to soothe her.

Night terrors usually occur in the first third of your child's sleep cycle, within the first few hours after bedtime. Some researchers believe that night terrors occur when there's an unexplained glitch in the transition between sleep stages. Children having a night terror actually remain fast asleep throughout the episode, which can last anywhere from 2 to 40 minutes. After it's over, she'll fall easily back to sleep and will have no memory of the incident in the morning. In fact, that may be the easiest way to determine whether it was a nightmare or a night terror—if you are more upset about it the next day than your child is, chances are it was a night terror. As many as 15 per cent of children will have a night terror. Some will have just a single episode, while others will experience them on and off for several years.

If your child is having a night terror, do not try to wake her. Just stay with her to ensure she doesn't hurt herself, speak quietly and calmly to her, keep the lights dim, and wait for the storm to pass. Most children outgrow night terrors by age seven. There's not much that can be done to prevent them, since no one really knows what causes them in the first place. Some parents find that waking the child up 30 to 45 minutes before it usually occurs helps avoid an episode. One thing we do know about night terrors is that children who are overtired or who have erratic sleep schedules are more prone to them. Make sure your child is getting enough sleep (at least 10 to 12 hours a night) and has a consistent and calm bedtime routine.

MAKE A NOTE, MAKE AN APPOINTMENT, OR GO TO THE HOSPITAL?

Make a note to mention to your child's doctor at her next appointment if she is experiencing frequent night terrors. In certain cases, they may be caused by sleep apnea, a condition in which enlarged adenoids and tonsils block airway passages during sleep and cause your child to stop breathing for a few moments and continually awaken. This type of sleep apnea can be serious, but is easily corrected through minor surgery to remove the adenoids or tonsils or both.

Sleepwalking

As with night terrors, sleepwalking usually occurs within a few hours of your child falling asleep. She may appear to be awake—her eyes may be open and she may even talk to you—but she is actually fast asleep. She may wander aimlessly around your home, mumble incoherently or say things that don't make sense, and do repetitive things like turning light switches on and off or opening and closing doors.

No one knows what causes sleepwalking, although a great deal of research is currently being done in the field of sleep disturbances. Sleepwalking does appear to have some genetic component—kids whose parents were sleepwalkers are more likely to sleepwalk as well—and it is more common in boys than girls. Between 10 and 20 per cent of all children will sleepwalk at some point, some only a few times and some on a regular basis for a period of time. Most outgrow it by puberty. Triggers for sleepwalking may be a full bladder, sleep deprivation, stress, and anxiety, so restrict fluids before bedtime, make sure your child uses the bathroom right before going to bed, keep a consistent bedtime routine, and try to minimize things that will give her stress or make her anxious.

If your child is sleepwalking, your only concern is to keep her safe, so do everything you can to prevent her from hurting herself. Keep the floor of her room tidy so she doesn't trip on anything. Make sure safety gates are closed securely and all windows and exterior doors are locked. If her sleepwalking persists, consider moving her bedroom to the main floor of your home, if necessary, to eliminate the possibility of falling down stairs or out a window. Don't ever let a sleepwalker sleep in a top bunk. If you wake during the night to find her sleepwalking, don't try to wake her up as you could scare her. Just gently guide her back to bed. She will have no memory of the episode the next day, so don't mention it to her.

MAKE A NOTE, MAKE AN APPOINTMENT, OR GO TO THE HOSPITAL?

Make a note to mention to your child's doctor at her next appointment if she has frequent and persistent sleepwalking episodes.

Toilet Learning

Most children are ready to begin toilet learning between the ages of two and four years, but every child is different. Take your cues from your child, not from your neighbours' kids, through each step of the process. He is probably ready for toilet learning when he can stay dry in diapers for several hours in a row, follow one or two simple instructions, and walk to the potty, and when he wants to be independent but also wants to please you. He should also be able to let you know when he needs to use the potty, and should be steady and balanced when sitting on it.

Dr. Sacks Says

Look at your list of priorities for your child's most important milestones—toilet training by age three shouldn't be on it.

Toilet learning starts with a relaxed attitude. It usually takes between three and six months before your child is out of diapers for good, so don't expect it to happen overnight. Pressure and stress can cause much more harm than good, so make sure you have enough time and patience to give your child the attention he needs during each day of the process. Before you start, decide which words you are going to use to refer to body parts, fluids, and functions. Just be direct, and try to use polite names, not silly ones. Do not use negative words like "dirty" or "stinky," as you may make him feel self-conscious, which won't help the toilet learning process. If other people care for your child, talk to them about your plans for toilet learning. It helps the process if his learning experiences with his different caregivers are consistent.

Your child will be more secure and stable on a potty chair than on a regular toilet, as his feet need to be supported. (If you don't use a potty, you'll need a toilet seat adapter and a footstool.) Put the potty in a place that your child can get to easily. Start by letting him get used to the potty. Have him sit on it while he is fully dressed, then after you've taken off his wet diaper. You may even want to put the dirty diaper in the potty to show him what it's used for. When your child is ready, take him to the potty several times each day and encourage him to sit on it for a few minutes without wearing a diaper. Develop a routine by having your child sit on the potty at specific times during the day, such as after getting up in the morning, after meals or snacks, before naps, and before bedtime. Watch your child for signs that he is ready to move from one step to the next.

Encourage your child to tell you when he needs to use the potty. Tell him that regular bowel movements are normal and healthy, and that he should go when he's ready. Be sure to praise him each time, even if he tells you after the fact. Also watch for signs that he needs to go. Expect accidents, and do not punish your child when they happen. Be patient, and praise him often. When he has used the potty successfully for at least a week, suggest that he try cotton underpants or training pants, and make this a special moment.

Toilet learning may not work the first time, but that just means your child isn't quite ready yet. If your child refuses to use the potty, take a break for one to three months. Another issue that might come up is that your child may not want to pass a stool in the potty, especially if he doesn't have good support for his feet. In the meantime, let him have bowel movements in a diaper so he doesn't get constipated, which can make going to the bathroom painful and the toilet learning process take even longer.

Dr. Sacks Says

Along with toilet learning may come constipation. Pressured or premature toilet learning can result in severe constipation. Use patience and fibre.

MAKE A NOTE, MAKE AN APPOINTMENT, OR GO TO THE HOSPITAL?

Make a note to mention to your child's doctor at his next appointment if

- he refuses to use the potty after several tries at toilet learning;
- he is older than four and is still not toilet trained;
- he was toilet trained for several months, but is now having frequent accidents; or
- he is withholding stool, has pain on defecation or urination, or has blood in his stool.

Social and Emotional Development

Discipline issues

We've all seen the children who whine and beg for candy in the grocery line, throw their cutlery while sitting in a restaurant, and don't wait their turn at the playground. We've all vowed to ourselves that our children will never act that way, and then one day it happens—an unexpected meltdown while you're shopping, or rude behaviour at a birthday party. The truth is, all children will present discipline challenges at times, but they will be much easier to deal with if you feel well equipped to handle those challenges.

Disciplining a child is one of the most important jobs of a parent, and probably one of the most difficult, but healthy discipline is part of a comforting family environment. Effective and positive discipline teaches and guides children—it doesn't just force them to obey—and it provides a foundation for self-discipline throughout life. It provides structure and boundaries that will help your child feel safe and secure throughout her childhood and adolescence. Discipline should protect your child from danger, help her learn self-control, help her develop a sense of responsibility, and instil values.

Effective discipline is consistent and fair, it should relate to a specific incident, and it should happen immediately. If your child doesn't heed your first warning, you need to act. Inconsistent discipline, such as giving multiple warnings or sometimes giving in to tantrums, confuses children and makes it hard for them to follow the rules. It can also reward children for unwanted behaviour, making it more likely that they'll do it again. Talk to your child's grandparents and other caregivers about how you discipline her and encourage them to do the same when they're caring for her. Although it may be unrealistic to expect grandparents or separated parents to have the same rules (everyone has a different level of tolerance for bad behaviour), each home should have consistent discipline.

Fair discipline means that the consequences of your child's actions are proportionate to what she's done wrong, and that the same rules and disciplinary measures apply to each child in your household in equal measure. "It's not fair!" is a common grievance of young children, and while most of the time they're probably overreacting, they can quickly lose respect for your authority if they think they can't trust you to be fair. The best you can do is to dole out appropriate discipline when your child misbehaves, praise her when she has made an effort to be good, and try to keep any promises you've made to her. If you can't keep your promise, explain to her why plans had to be changed.

If discipline isn't consistent and fair, not only will your child have a hard time respecting your authority, but she may not respect the authority of other adults or the rights of other children. Harsh discipline, such as name-calling, shouting, and humiliation, also makes it difficult for a child to respect and trust a caregiver. Children should be able to maintain their own self-respect while being disciplined. You have a unique bond with your child, so if you teach her discipline with respect, it will have lasting positive effects on her relationships with authority figures and her peers.

Of course, it would be nice to be able to forego discipline entirely by preventing bad behaviour. That may be impossible, but you can do some things to keep it to a minimum. Look for opportunities to praise your child for good behaviour so that she knows she'll get attention when she does something positive, not just when she misbehaves. Give her lots of opportunities for fresh air and exercise so that she can run off some of her energy. Make sure she has a wide variety of toys that are appropriate for her age, but not too many. If her temperament demands it (and you'll know her well enough to be able to determine if it does), prepare her for situations by telling her what to expect. Try distraction or redirection tactics: instead of saying "no" to her all the time, give her something more interesting to do. For instance, if she is climbing a fence, say "Come play on the swings."

Children two years of age and younger have trouble remembering and understanding rules, so don't expect them to stay away from those tempting kitchen cupboards. Continue to childproof your home so that you're not constantly telling your child "get out of there" or "don't touch that." By age three, your child should be able to follow your rules. Prioritize the rules you make. Give top priority to safety, then to correcting behaviour that harms people and property, then to correcting annoying behaviour such as whining, interrupting, and throwing temper tantrums. Concentrate on just two or three rules at first, and ignore the little things. Before you raise your voice, ask yourself, "Is this important?" You should also ask yourself if her misbehaviour is deliberate, or if it's something she can't help. Become familiar with behaviour that is appropriate for your child's age. A toddler who accidentally spills a glass of milk is not misbehaving; she's still developing her motor skills. If your child is tired and cranky, she's more likely to act up, so be understanding and help her settle down.

Using time-outs

By two years of age, you can start to use time-outs to discipline your child. Children crave attention, whether it's positive or negative, so time-outs work by taking your child out of the limelight, away from the attention that is reinforcing her bad behaviour. When she is doing something that is unacceptable, sending her away from the trouble spot to sit quietly by herself can help stop the behaviour and change the situation. To use a time-out effectively, send your child to an isolated and uninteresting but safe area such as a chair, hallway, playpen, or quiet corner. Tell her what she's done wrong in a firm voice, using simple words such as "no hitting." If she doesn't go by herself immediately, lead her by the hand or carry her. The time-out should last for one minute per year of age, to a maximum of five minutes. Set a timer; don't let your child decide when it is over. Make sure she can't watch television or interact with other people—including you. Time-outs are not opportunities to lecture your child. When she is in time-out, she should be ignored.

Try to schedule the time-out strategically. Stay alert for situations that are about to get out of control, and impose the time-out as soon after the incident as possible, or tell her to go to her time-out spot even before she blows her top. It may make it easier for her to settle back down, and will teach her to pause before she loses control. Although you should be consistent with time-outs, be flexible too. You may find there's no way your two-year-old is going to sit still for two minutes. Instead of getting into a battle of wills, chasing her around and trying to force her to stay in her chair, it's okay to stand beside the chair while she's in it, or to limit the time-out to one minute instead of two. The point is to calm her down and divert her attention, not frustrate her to the point that she forgets why she's there. Once time is up, create a fresh start by offering a new activity. Don't discuss the behaviour or try to make her apologize; just reiterate the rule ("no hitting"). If she has hurt another person, simply ask her to apologize to them. If your child repeats the behaviour that led to the time-out in the first place, go through the whole process again.

Your child must understand that time-outs happen if she does something wrong. Explain them to her before you need to use them by telling her simply, "If you do something mommy and daddy don't want you to do, and if you don't stop when we ask you to, you'll have to go sit in your time-out chair all by yourself until you calm down." Demonstrating with a stuffed animal or doll might help her understand. When she is misbehaving, do not give endless warnings or empty threats before sending her for a time-out. Don't shout or show emotion, and make sure your voice and your face communicate the same message.

Give your child "time-ins" too. Reinforce good behaviour by giving her lots of hugs and praise when she does something you like, especially if it's the opposite of the bad behaviour that often gets her into time-outs. For example, if she gets frequent time-outs for hitting her sister, praise her for being a great big sister when you see them getting along. More time-ins may mean fewer time-outs.

Coping with tantrums

Being a two-year-old can be frustrating. Your child wants to be independent, yet her desires sometimes exceed her abilities. She understands almost everything you say to her, but she can't always come up with the language to express how she feels. Most tantrums are the result of a child's frustration at not being able to say or do what she wants. And unfortunately, they are a normal part of life for most toddlers. They are most common between the ages of one and three, and start to taper off in both frequency and intensity by age four.

When your child has a tantrum, remain calm and do not have one yourself. This loss of control is frightening to her, and she'll be even more frightened if you lose control too. Stay with her, as having you close by will be comforting to her. If you're in a public place, quickly and calmly take her to a quiet place until she settles down. You may need to hold her to keep her safe. Whatever you do to calm her down, do not give in to her demands. Tempting though it may be, it will only reinforce the idea that throwing a tantrum will get her what she wants.

While you can't prevent all temper tantrums, you can lessen their frequency. Make sure your child is well rested and has little stress. Kids who are overtired, don't have enough quiet time, or live in an overly stressful environment have more frequent tantrums. Most tantrums take a while to build up, so when you see your child becoming angry or frustrated, try to distract her with another activity or take her to another room. Pay attention to situations that may trigger tantrums in your child, and try to avoid them. If she loses it when she gets hungry, always have snacks on hand. If she gets upset when she has to leave the park, give her gentle warnings 10 minutes, 5 minutes, and 2 minutes before you start packing up.

Another way to cut down on tantrums is to pick your battles. You may find yourself saying "no" as a reflex, but if she wants to walk a different way home or wear the red socks instead of the white ones, why argue? Offer her choices when it seems reasonable. A sense of independence and control can calm your child and diffuse built-up frustration, although too many choices can add to her stress. Reminding her of all the grown-up things she does can also be effective for boosting her self-esteem and calming her down. Finally, avoid taking your child to those notorious trouble spots—like the supermarket—if you can, and make other arrangements for your child when you need to go to them.

MAKE A NOTE, MAKE AN APPOINTMENT, OR GO TO THE HOSPITAL?

Make an appointment to see your child's doctor if

▷ she is still having frequent tantrums after the age of four;

▷ her tantrums involve her causing harm to herself or others, or destroying property;

▷ the tantrums occur because your child doesn't understand what's expected of her or the consequences of not behaving;

▷ the tantrums are accompanied by headaches or stomach aches, nightmares, refusal to eat, clinging, or extreme anxiety or irritability; or

▷ you feel you are not able to cope with her tantrums.

The doctor can help you deal with the tantrums and make sure they are not due to a significant underlying physical or psychological issue.

Learning appropriate behaviour

It is always easier to teach a child proper behaviour early and gradually reinforce it over time, rather than to try to change it later on. If you giggle every time your one-year-old smears food into his hair but tell him to stop doing it when he turns two, he will be confused, so try to discourage inappropriate behaviour as early as possible.

The key to all good behaviour is modelling. The good news (and the bad news) is that your child will mimic your behaviour. Start small; as soon as your child is talking, encourage him to use "please" and "thank you" in daily conversation. He may not start to use it on his own for quite a while, but there's nothing wrong with the age-old question "What's the magic word?" Once he gets used to saying them at home, prompt him to say "please" and "thank you" to other family members and to strangers. The positive reaction he gets will be great reinforcement.

You can also encourage children of this age to extend polite greetings to friends and family members, saying "hello" when you arrive and "goodbye" when you leave. Depending on his mood and how well he knows the people, he may smile broadly and wave, turn away shyly and smile, or just burst into tears. Don't force him if he refuses; just gently encourage him again next time. Greetings are a great way to start to instil the idea of polite social interaction.

Like any behavioural issue, use positive reinforcement. Tell him how nice it was to hear him say please or to see him wait his turn for the slide. Instead of scolding him when he forgets his manners, praise him when he remembers. And be consistent—if he's always expected to say please before you give him something, make sure he does. If he thinks it only applies in certain situations, he may become confused. "Please" and "thank you" should be non-negotiable.

Childhood fears

It's normal for toddlers to have fears, although by age three, most children can separate from their parents with little or no crying. Instead, their fears are fuelled by their vivid imaginations, and they have a hard time distinguishing reality from fantasy. Children of this age are concrete thinkers, and they can become frightened by passing remarks or jokes from parents. With insight, understanding, patience, and unequivocal reassurance, adults can help children deal with their fears. However, it's always important to ask questions so you know the situation your child is afraid of is actually safe. His fears may not be unfounded if he's being bullied at daycare, for instance.

A toddler's active imagination will conjure up imaginary dangers out of shadows in a dark room or a mask covering a familiar face. Your child may be frightened by everyday situations, such as bedtime, bath time, or visits to the doctor. He may fear things that make a loud noise he cannot understand, like a vacuum cleaner or a flushing toilet. Some children may also become fearful when things aren't quite right—if the furniture has been moved, a cup or plate is cracked, or adults are angry or upset. To an adult, a child's fears may be rational (such as a fear of dogs) or irrational (such as being afraid of what's under the bed), but to a child they are very real.

To help your child deal with his fears, it's important that you take them seriously. Never make fun of him for being afraid. Identify his fears, and reassure him that there are no such things as monsters, but that you understand why he is scared. Be calm and empathetic with him, and help him feel physically secure by hugging him, holding his hand, and being close. You can also teach him to take long, deep breaths to reduce his anxiety. Offer small challenges to keep him learning to face his fears, but keep his temperament in mind so that you don't put him into a fearful situation before he's ready. If he's afraid of dogs, don't force him to pet one. Let him overcome his fear at his own pace. When he does, be sure to give him lots of praise.

You can help your child work through the fear by reading books, making up stories, or acting out situations that deal with his particular fear. Drawing a monster can help him express his fears and learn to differentiate them from reality. Playing with a toy fire engine can desensitize him and reduce his fear of the real one. Encourage him to share his fears with one of his stuffed toys. Limit your child's exposure to media that may create fears or make them even worse, such as television, movies, video games, the Internet, and even some books. Overprotection can also cause children to be unnecessarily fearful, so be careful not to reinforce the fear by being scared yourself. Most children's fears are temporary, so they will likely fade as he becomes more secure in himself and his environment.

MAKE A NOTE, MAKE AN APPOINTMENT, OR GO TO THE HOSPITAL?

Make an appointment to see your child's doctor if his fears are starting to interfere with his normal daily activities (for instance, if he won't step out the back door for fear of seeing a snake), if he seems unduly anxious, or if his fears seem to be intensifying over time.

Phobias

Toddlers' fears are usually manageable, and your child should outgrow them. However, if the fears persist and intensify, if your child cannot be consoled and reasoned with, and if the fears start to interfere with his schedule, they may need to be dealt with professionally. Your child may have developed a phobia, which is clinically defined as a noticeable and persistent fear brought on by the presence or anticipation of an object or situation.

One of the leading causes of phobias is a traumatic event. Often this event goes unnoticed to a parent. A toddler who gets some water up his nose while swimming for the first time might become extremely phobic of water. An important phobia that could affect his ability to thrive is the fear of eating solids, which is usually the result of a choking episode. Parents may encourage fears by mentioning a frightening event, like choking on a food, and passing that fear on to the child. Some research has shown that a propensity toward phobias may be inherited. If you or your partner have a family history of phobias, your child may be more likely to have one, so let your child's doctor know the emotional health history of your family.

Some early signs of phobia in your child may include specific, prolonged, and inconsolable fear. Your toddler may be afraid of a specific object, or may even be afraid of the possibility of seeing the object. If he is continually and consistently afraid of the same thing, this can indicate a phobia. Generally, a few minutes with mom or dad can help to calm a toddler's fears, but if your toddler has a phobia, you may not be able to console him. The treatment for phobias is usually behavioural therapy, in which the child is exposed to the feared object or situation gradually so that he learns to overcome his anxieties and manage his fears. The phobia generally disappears or decreases so that it no longer interferes with his daily activities.

MAKE A NOTE, MAKE AN APPOINTMENT, OR GO TO THE HOSPITAL?

Make an appointment to see your child's doctor if a phobia interferes with his normal functioning.

Dealing with aggressive or shy toddlers

Aggression

Upsetting as it may be for parents, aggression is a normal part of a toddler's development. Your child is learning myriad new skills—verbal, physical, and social—and it's only natural for her to become frustrated from time to time and take it out on those around her. She doesn't have the emotional maturity or self-control to know how to process or express her frustration or anger, so she'll often release it by grabbing a toy from a playmate or by hitting, kicking, or shoving. She may also lash out if she feels threatened or cornered by one of her peers. A new social situation, like daycare or preschool, can cause anxiety or stress, which can manifest itself in aggressive behaviour. Or the cause might just be something as simple as the fact that she's tired or hungry.

As their language skills get better, children tend to get less frustrated, and are able to express their frustration through words rather than actions. Until then, there are appropriate ways of dealing with aggression in your child. Responding aggressively is not one of them. Although you might be frustrated or angry yourself, yelling or responding physically to your child's aggressive behaviour will only reinforce the idea that that kind of behaviour is okay. Remain calm but firm, and try to keep your temper in check at all times. If you express your anger in quiet ways, your child will learn from your example. Respond the same way every time she acts aggressively and she'll soon discover the pattern: she hits; she gets a time-out. Use this strategy even if you're out in public—any parent will understand your situation, so don't be embarrassed.

Dr. Sacks Says

Trying to teach your child not to hit by hitting her will only confuse her.

If an argument between playmates is minor, let the children try to sort it out themselves. You don't always need to jump in right away. If it starts to get physical and they don't stop when they're told to, or if one child is getting out of control, step in and remove her from the situation, and put her into a time-out. Don't wait for it to happen a second or third time. She should understand instantly that her behaviour was unacceptable.

Whenever possible, tell your child what you expect of her rather than what she is doing wrong.

After the storm has passed, sit down next to your child and quietly discuss what happened. Avoid talking about the events, as each child involved will have a different version of the incident. Instead, encourage her to talk about her feelings. Explain to her that it's okay to be angry, but it's not okay to hit. Teach her to say "no" or turn away if another child is provoking her. If your child has broken something or hurt someone, have her clean up the mess or apologize to the other person. Let her know that this is what happens when people behave the way she has.

You can try to prevent aggressive behaviour by using positive reinforcement. If your child has sharing issues that often result in hitting or shoving, but you see her sharing crayons nicely with a playmate, comment on her good behaviour. She'll soon understand that she gets more attention by cooperating than by lashing out. Read stories that model good behaviour, and always supervise television viewing, as even innocent cartoons and children's programs can contain aggressive or violent scenarios. Limit television viewing to one or two hours a day, monitor what she's watching, and watch it with her whenever you can.

MAKE A NOTE, MAKE AN APPOINTMENT, OR GO TO THE HOSPITAL?

Almost all children act aggressively on occasion, but if your child seems unusually aggressive and is biting and hitting every time she plays, if her behaviour is interfering with school or other activities, if she causes physical harm to herself or others, or if you're afraid for the safety of those around her, **make an appointment** with her doctor. The doctor can discuss discipline strategies with you, and determine if the aggression may be caused by a deeper learning, behavioural, or emotional disorder.

Shyness

Most children experience bouts of shyness at one point or another. Your child may hide her face in your knees when someone comes up to say hello, or she may stand at the sidelines when approaching a group of kids already at play. However, some children are just naturally more fearful of new situations than others. Many experts now believe that a child's basic temperament is inborn; some are predisposed to approach new people and situations with confidence and joy, and others are genetically inclined to be nervous or wary.

Many toddlers will experience a shy stage that is brought on by normal fears of separation. If your two-year-old is suddenly clingy and tearful when placed in unfamiliar surroundings or with new people, it may simply be because she is afraid of being away from you. This shyness will pass as the separation anxiety does, generally before her fourth birthday. If your child has had this tendency from birth, however, she may have an introverted personality, and there's nothing wrong with that. Shy kids are just as happy and well adjusted as their more extroverted peers. She may just need a little encouragement from you to make her feel more secure.

MAKE A NOTE, MAKE AN APPOINTMENT, OR GO TO THE HOSPITAL?

Make a note to mention to your child's doctor at her next appointment if she does not become comfortable in a new situation even after an appropriate length of time. It may take her a couple of weeks to adjust to a new childcare situation, for instance, but it shouldn't take longer than a month or two.

Just because your child is introverted, however, doesn't mean you should label her as such. While her introverted tendencies may be largely genetic, how you respond to her shyness will also reinforce or diffuse those feelings to a certain degree. If you say "Oh, she's just shy" every time you walk into a new situation, she will start to think of herself that way. She may even perceive the label as negative, as though you're making excuses for her. Simply tell people that your child takes a while to warm up to new people and places, and try not to make a big deal of her behaviour. Never criticize her bashful behaviour—it's not something she can turn on and off at will, and negative comments may only cause her to withdraw even further.

It's important to know your child's temperament at this age so you know how much preparation she needs for certain situations. Let her socialize at her own pace, but keep trying new situations. Don't force her to interact with others or tell her not to be shy—let her feel out the situation in her own time, and stay close by to hold her hand or offer other support. Once she's engaged in an activity, back off slowly and let her carry on by herself. If that doesn't work, try getting engaged in playing with the other children yourself. That will often draw your child into the activity, and once she feels comfortable, you can withdraw from the group and let her continue on her own. Remember, most toddlers engage in parallel play—playing alongside their peers, rather than directly with them—so at this age, socialization is a relative concept. If she senses that you're okay with her behaviour, it will build her self-confidence and make her more comfortable the next time.

Don't avoid social situations just to keep your child happy. The more exposure she gets to new people and places, the more comfortable she will become. Start off with smaller gatherings or familiar social places, like the library, to boost her confidence. If you're going to a big party or gathering, try to get there a few minutes before everyone else to allow her time to get used to the surroundings. To diffuse a potentially awkward greeting, ask family members and friends not to push your child into interaction or pressure her. Encourage them to come down to her eye level when greeting her.

If your child is still exhibiting the same clinginess and fear of new situations when it's time to attend preschool, just keep quietly encouraging her. Introduce her to new friends one at a time, and expect it to take several meetings before she feels comfortable interacting with anyone new. Arrange short playtimes with children you think she may be comfortable with, and with just one child at a time. Exposing her to children of different ages may help as well. An older child may take the initiative to talk and play with her; a younger child may make her feel less intimidated and more confident.

Many shy children will outgrow this tendency as they develop social skills and move toward adulthood. If she feels comfortable and loved, she'll be confident in herself and her abilities.

MAKE A NOTE, MAKE AN APPOINTMENT, OR GO TO THE HOSPITAL?

If her shyness is preventing her from fostering any relationships outside the family, if it is chronic, or if it is getting worse, **make a note** to mention it to your child's doctor at her next appointment.

Gender identity: Who's a boy, who's a girl

Most children develop a clear sense of whether they are boys or girls at a young age. In fact, the idea of gender identity is established sometime between 18 and 30 months of age. Gender stereotyping also starts early in our culture. By age two, your child has already absorbed much of it. Even if parents and caregivers make a conscious effort to avoid gender stereotyping, children will still form their own gender identity. Conventional male and female role models abound, and friends and relatives may be innocently reinforcing them, buying dolls for your daughter and trains for your son.

Between ages two and three, children start to prefer to play with members of their own sex. They may start to strongly identify with the same-sex parent, as well as siblings, friends, and neighbours of the same gender. They might also begin to take their gender identification very seriously; girls may insist on wearing dresses and jewellery, and boys may act aggressively and carry around sports equipment. Often they will sense approval from others when they act in this manner, and disapproval if they start to stray from it. By the age of four, children of both sexes are aware that specific gender differences exist and that the ways boys and girls dress, play, and behave are quite distinct. By the time they reach kindergarten, their gender identities are well established.

There's nothing wrong with reinforcing these characteristics in your child, as long as it is not to the exclusion of opposite characteristics. Girls should be encouraged to be nurturing and empathetic, as long as they are also encouraged to play sports and act assertively when necessary. Boys should be encouraged to be adventurous and self-assured, but they should also be encouraged to express their feelings and emotions. Don't tell them what is acceptable for one gender or the other, and don't ever give your child the impression, even jokingly, that it is better to be one sex or the other, or that one sex has different talents or abilities than the other. Even subtle hints of these ideas can make an impression on a toddler.

Make sure your child has the chance to play with a variety of toys, and be cautious of gender stereotyping in television shows and books. If your child likes to do things that are typical of the opposite gender, it is not necessarily an indication of a gender identity problem or future sexual preference. Two- and three-year-olds love imaginary play, and if you've been open and supportive of experimentation with all kinds of toys, your child won't know the difference.

Playtime: Reading, Imaginary Play, and Other Creative Pursuits

The joy of reading

Reading with your child is one of the most important things you can do. When he's nestled close to you, listening to your voice and watching as the story unfolds through pictures, your child's brain is stimulated every time you read to him. At this age, your child is learning about how books work. He'll learn that they are read from front to back, one page at a time, and that they have a storyline with pictures and words. By describing the pictures, talking about the characters in the book, and labelling objects, you are promoting language development. Your child may start to incorporate reading and themes from his favourite books into his imaginary play, perhaps by reading stories to his teddy bear as he tucks it in for a nap.

Dr. Sacks Says

Read, read, read. Computer learning is nowhere near as important to your child's total development.

Toddlers love books about animals, the alphabet, and children their age. Rhyming books and flap books are also popular with this age group. They love repetition, which helps them relate the words they are hearing to the pictures they see. They're also fickle; suddenly, after insisting on the same book for weeks, your child may suddenly reject it and move on to another favourite. Older toddlers will be able to sit and listen to longer stories.

You can start to expose your child to different kinds of books, such as fairy tales and poetry. Librarians and teachers are good sources of advice for books that are appropriate for your child's age and reading level, and bookstore staff members are often quite helpful. Visiting your local library is an inexpensive way to introduce him to different books, so make a library visit part of your weekly routine. Preview new books before you read them to him. The more familiar you are with the text and storyline, the better you'll be able to anticipate your child's reactions to it, and to answer questions he may have. Read books that you enjoy too—if you're not enjoying a particular book, your toddler will soon pick up on it. Why not dig out some of the classics you loved as a child, such as Dr. Seuss, Curious George, Maurice Sendak, and others that have stood the test of time? They may become some of his favourites too.

Books aren't just for bedtime, so build reading into your day. Find some quiet time together after breakfast, while riding the bus, or while dinner is in the oven. Incorporating reading into your day firmly establishes reading as a part of your toddler's life. Try to eliminate distractions when you read (although that might not be so easy on the bus). Turn off the television and music while you're reading together, and find a place that's comfortable for both of you and has good lighting so he can see the pictures clearly. Make the story dramatic by reading slowly and using different voices and faces while you're telling the story to fully engage your child. Make sounds where appropriate, use accents for different characters—even sing. Your child will love it, and may even join in.

Take cues from your child. It's okay if he wants to skip pages, stop the story for a while and talk about the pictures, or make up his own story as he goes along. Encourage him to turn the pages or stop to draw a picture of something he sees that catches his interest. The most important thing is that you both have fun.

Point out words and letters in everyday life, such as on street signs and food packages. Through exposure to printed material, your child will become familiar with letters and signs. Alphabet books are also a great way to familiarize him with letters and the sounds they make. Talking about letters' shapes and sounds will teach your child about how these letters and their sounds go together. It's also important to be a good reading role model. When children see their parents and family members reading books, newspapers, and magazines, they learn that reading is important and valuable.

Toys

These years are ones of great learning for your child, and much of that learning takes place through play and exploration. Two-year-olds mostly engage in parallel play—playing alongside peers, rather than with them—but by age three, children start to interact and play together. They have seemingly limitless reserves of energy, and their developmental and intellectual skills are constantly expanding, so toys should challenge their developing minds and help them expend their energy. Their toys should provide a variety of experiences and challenges, they should be lightweight and easy to carry, and they should be safe. They still like bright colours, but toys that are realistic and that have working parts, like toy kitchens and lawn mowers, are increasingly interesting to them.

Children can learn an enormous amount from the everyday things around them, so don't overwhelm them with a lot of expensive, complicated toys. As always, your child can dream up hundreds of uses for the infinitely versatile cardboard box, and you'll find lots of things in your kitchen that are good for stacking and nesting, making noise, and playing with water. Limit the number of toys he has to a small variety of versatile, flexible toys. This may seem impossible when it's time for his birthday party, but birthdays are actually a great opportunity to teach your child the importance of giving to others. In the invitations, encourage gift givers to give your child two small, identical gifts so that he can give one to a toy bank, or ask for a book and a donation in your child's name to a children's charity. Every time your child makes a donation, mark the occasion in some way, such as with a sticker on a calendar. Instead of accumulating more toys, you can assemble many of them from objects around your home. Small plastic containers and wooden spoons can keep busy fingers and active minds occupied for a long time.

Children really enjoy active play toys at this age, such as ride-on toys, push and pull toys, and outdoor equipment. Your child should play outdoors whenever possible, but many of these types of toys can be used indoors as well. Realistic ride-ons like tractors or motorcycles, and ones with storage trays or bins, are great. When he is able to pedal, somewhere between two and three years of age, tricycles are appropriate. Push and pull toys include wagons, baby strollers, and pull toys with strings, as well as adult-style toys like shopping carts and lawn mowers. Appropriate outdoor equipment at the park and in your backyard includes tunnels, climbing structures and slides, and swings with restraining straps.

Opportunities to dig and pour with different types of textures are essential to children's development, and sand and water–play toys are ideal for that. Sterilized potting soil, clean play sand, or other shredded non-toxic materials can be used for this type of play. Clean water in water tables or dishpans is also appropriate for play as long as adults are directly supervising. Measuring cups, spoons, shovels, buckets, floating toys, and small cars and trucks are essential accessories in this play area.

Your child's hand-eye coordination and dexterity are improving all the time. Good toys to enhance his fine motor skills include nesting toys and cups, pounding or hammering toys, lacing cards, beading toys (check that the beads are big enough so your child won't choke on them), and blocks. Many of these toys can be assembled from household items or homemade. Block play also enhances social/emotional and language development. Try all different kinds of blocks: large cardboard blocks, soft blocks, and lightweight wooden blocks. In addition to stacking and sorting, your child may enjoy filling dump trucks and wagons with blocks and dumping them out. Construction toys like large snap-together block sets are great for hand-eye coordination skills, and they encourage your child to build higher and more complex structures than regular stacking blocks will allow.

By age two, your child will probably be able to solve pegboard puzzles with four to six pieces; by three he may be able to do jigsaw-type puzzles of 6 to 12 pieces. Look for puzzles with large pieces and a simple, easily recognizable picture. Intellectually challenging toys such as matching games, dominoes (especially giant dominoes), simple board games based on chance like Candyland or Snakes and Ladders, and games that sort letters, sounds, numbers, or concepts are also important for developing minds.

Art supplies allow your child to express creativity, enhance language development, explore various sensory and textural experiences, and begin developing fine motor skills. Set up an area in your home where he can make a mess while exploring with materials like paints and crayons. Keep everything contained in one place, and store it away from curious hands. Some good art supply choices are listed below.

- large crayons
- non-toxic paints (finger and tempera) and short-handled brushes with blunt ends
- modelling clay
- sturdy markers
- blunt-end scissors
- chalkboard and large chalk
- coloured construction paper
- non-toxic glue

Children this age love to make noise, so musical instruments like horns and whistles are great toys. Rhythm and percussive instruments, like bells, rattles, cymbals, drums, triangles, rhythm sticks, sand blocks, xylophones, and tambourines, are also a huge hit with kids. Not so much with parents, though—you may want to have pain relief medication on hand before striking up the band, since you'll have to listen to this symphony too.

Safe toys

Because toddlers are still exploring and examining their world through their senses, they are very likely to put toys and materials in their mouths. Materials that should not be used for play due to potential hazards include Styrofoam peanuts, small pebbles, dried beans, cornmeal, flour, and balloons. Young children are very attracted to balloons, but when balloons pop they become choking and suffocation hazards.

Check and maintain your child's toys regularly so you can avoid any toy-related injuries. Toys should be sturdy, not likely to break into small pieces, and strong enough for your child to stand on or in. They should be large enough so that they are not choking hazards and can't be pushed into your child's nostrils or ears, and they should be free of small parts. Dolls and stuffed animals should not have buttons, bows, eyes, noses, or other small parts that could be pulled loose by children, and they should be hypoallergenic and washable. Toys should have no sharp points or edges, detachable parts, or parts that can pinch or entrap fingers, toes, or hair. Children should not play with electronic toys unless supervised by an adult.

You may not read instructions on your own toys, but it's important to read the instructions on your child's new toys before you give them to him to check that they're assembled properly. Read the labels to check the recommended age level, to check for any warnings provided by the manufacturer, and to ensure they are made from non-toxic materials. Home lead testing kits do not reliably test for the presence of lead in toys, but new government regulations should increase the safety of the components of many toys. You can check Health Canada's website for a list of recalled toys (see "Product Safety" in Resources).

Imaginary play

Play is still your toddler's work—in addition to being fun and a physical release, the playing your child does at this age allows her to process the world around her and the emotions she's feeling. It helps her learn how to solve problems, to express herself physically and verbally, and to build all types of skills.

One of the ways your toddler does this is through imaginary play. At around age two, she will start to be able to create her own worlds, characters, and stories. She will take delight in realistic toys, like child-sized household objects (toy kitchens, vacuum cleaners, or dish sets), and will enjoy acting out scenarios from everyday family life, like making you a "meal" with toy food or putting her "baby" to sleep in her little crib. Even regular objects can be incorporated into her imaginary world—a cardboard box on a string becomes her pet dog, for example.

As she becomes more familiar with the world around her, she will also start to role-play, pretending to be a baker one day, a superhero the next, and mommy the day after that. This may all look like innocuous child's play to you, but in fact, it's her way of sorting through the complex rules and relationships she's beginning to understand. The sense of control she feels creating her own new world helps her to interpret all this new information, and even to work through something she may be struggling with, like the arrival of a new sibling. She may not be able to express herself through words, but she can do it through play.

It's important to encourage imaginary play. Let your child take the lead and create her own worlds and scenarios, as long as her play is safe. Her toys should help her extend her imaginary scenarios into real activities. If she invites you into this world, play along with her, but let her make all the decisions about the characters and scenarios. You may be in charge in the real world, but this is her world. Giving her this control and nurturing her imagination will build her self-esteem.

Remember, the cardboard box you and your toddler have decorated together is more precious than any manufactured toy. However, some good toys to encourage imaginary play are listed here.

- **Dolls.** All kinds, including realistic ones with hair and moving eyes, and doll accessories, like blankets, bottles, cribs and strollers, and simple removable garments (hook and loop, large snap fasteners).

- **Stuffed toys.** Plush ones, as well as soft, pliable animals. Parent and baby combinations are great. Toddlers prefer realistic animals and replicas of familiar characters.

- **Puppets.** Small hand puppets that are lightweight and sized to fit a child's hand (hand-and-arm puppets are too large). Puppets doubling as stuffed toys or that represent familiar characters are also good.

- **Role-play materials.** Dress-up clothes and costumes, child-sized equipment (stoves, ironing boards, refrigerators) and toys that can be pushed (vacuum, lawn mower, shopping cart). Put a full-length mirror at her level so she can see herself in dress-up clothes. Avoid toys inspired by war or violence.

- **Play scenes.** Familiar, realistic-looking scenes (playhouses, farms, garages, airports) that have multiple pieces but are not highly detailed. Toddlers prefer moving parts and parts that make noise. The interior of these scenes should be easily accessible.

Dr. Sacks Says

The toys your child will like best are not the most expensive ones, but the ones that you play with him.

Television: How much is acceptable?

Parents hear a lot about the negative effects of television, but if it's used correctly and sparingly, and with your active involvement, television can actually have a positive influence on your child's social, emotional, and mental development. The key is to be involved in her television viewing habits and to limit the amount she watches. Decide what your family's television rules are well before your child is ready for school. Once she starts attending school, she'll be influenced by the television habits of other children, but she'll be less likely to want to do what they're doing if you've already instilled a strong set of rules. Explain the rules of television watching in your home to caregivers such as nannies, babysitters, and grandparents. The Canadian Paediatric Society recommends that television viewing be limited to less than one or two hours a day. (For up-to-date information on television viewing from the Canadian Paediatric Society, see the Caring for Kids website: www.caringforkids.cps.ca.)

Let your child ask to watch television instead of automatically turning it on so you avoid sending the message that there are times when she "should" be watching TV. Choose a program, and when it is over, turn off the television. Break up your child's viewing into 10- or 15-minute increments. If you have a VCR or digital-recording device, record specific programs so they are available when your child wants to watch something. Only let your child watch programs you are familiar with. Calm, quiet programs are best; avoid lots of fast, random activity or scary images. Pay extra attention to ensure that your child does not watch programs that show violence, sex, and offensive language.

As frequently as possible, try to watch television with your child—do not use the television as a babysitter. Talk about what she learned from the show, such as the importance of sharing, giving, and loving, or the importance of learning the alphabet or numbers. Shows that encourage your child to say words, sing, and dance are ideal. Help her to continue learning from the program with follow-up activities that relate to what she saw.

Be careful with the example that you set as a parent, as children learn many of their values and ideas from their parents. Put the television in a place that's physically inconvenient—tuck it away in a den on the second floor instead of front and centre in your family room—and close the cabinet doors when you're not watching. Keep it turned off during mealtimes, and do not allow your child to have a television in her bedroom.

HEALTH

Now that your child is out in the world more often—at daycare or nursery school, classes or other group activities, birthday parties and all other kinds of gatherings—he will be exposed to an ever-increasing number of bugs. Don't be surprised if he seems to go from one cold to the next, especially if he is in daycare. More information on colds is provided on page 344 in Chapter Six. Most common toddler health issues require nothing more than basic care and remedies—and a lot of TLC from mom and dad.

Fever Phobia

Somewhere along the way we were taught to panic whenever a child has a fever. Fever in itself isn't dangerous; it just tells you that the immune system is reacting to an infection and fighting it. At this age, fever alone is not a reason to see a doctor, especially if your child is acting well and eating normally, and in any case it is often difficult for doctors to diagnose the cause of a fever in the first few hours. There's usually no cause for concern when your child has a fever—and certainly no cause to go to the emergency room. Fevers are very common in young children, and they usually go away after 48 hours. The most important factor in assessing whether your child needs to see a doctor is his level of activity.

Febrile seizures happen to many children of this age, and they can be terrifying for parents, but they will not harm your child. Since they are caused by a rapid elevation in temperature, they happen very quickly and are often the first sign of fever, so taking your child to the emergency room will not prevent a febrile seizure. For information on febrile seizures, see page 333 in Chapter Six.

MYTH BUSTERS

Myth: A high fever can cause brain damage.

Fact: High fever that comes on quickly may cause a seizure, but short (less than five minutes) febrile seizures do not cause brain damage.

—Dr. Diane Sacks, MD, FRCPC, FAAP

You can treat your child at home by keeping him comfortable and giving him plenty of fluids. Remove extra clothing or blankets to help lower his body temperature, but don't take off too much clothing because shivering could cause his temperature to rise again. You don't always need to give medication to reduce your child's temperature, but acetaminophen or ibuprofen used according to package directions (unless your doctor says otherwise) can help. **Do not give ibuprofen to a baby under six months of age without first talking to your doctor, and do not give aspirin (acetylsalicylic acid or ASA) to a child or teenager with a fever.** If the fever is due to chickenpox, influenza, or certain other viral infections, aspirin can increase the risk of Reye's syndrome, a very serious condition that can damage the liver and brain. For more information on fevers, see page 329 in Chapter Six.

MAKE A NOTE, MAKE AN APPOINTMENT, OR GO TO THE HOSPITAL?

If your child's fever lasts for more than 48 hours, or is accompanied by listlessness, vomiting, or pain, **make an appointment** to see his doctor.

Taking your child's temperature

Except in rare cases (very young infants, or children with certain conditions, such as sickle-cell anemia), an elevated temperature gives little information on how serious an illness is. Your child's level of activity and alertness are the most revealing indications of his health. Treatment decisions are rarely made on temperature alone, so it's useful information to give your doctor to think about, but that's about it.

Now that your child is over the age of two, you can use a digital ear thermometer to take his temperature. Non-mercury rectal thermometers are still the most accurate, but are probably less acceptable to your child now that he can voice his opinion on the matter. Let's face it: it's probably not a lot of fun for you either. For children between the ages of two and five, the most comfortable method of taking their temperature is by the ear. As digital ear thermometers improve, they become more accurate and reliable. Axillary (armpit) digital temperature-taking is less accurate, but it's okay if you just want to screen your child to make sure his temperature is in the ballpark, and there are specific thermometers for this purpose. Fever strips are not recommended because they do not give accurate readings. Whatever you do, do not use a mercury thermometer. If it breaks, you and your child might be exposed to this toxic substance.

Once you've taken his temperature, check the following chart to see whether your child has a fever. The normal temperature range varies, depending on what method you use. (If the manufacturer has listed normal ranges, refer to them rather than the chart.)

Normal temperature ranges

Measurement method	Normal temperature range
Rectum	36.6°C to 38.0°C (97.9°F to 100.4°F)
Mouth	35.5°C to 37.5°C (95.9°F to 99.5°F)
Armpit	34.7°C to 37.3°C (94.5°F to 99.1°F)
Ear	35.8°C to 38.0°C (96.4°F to 100.4°F)

Using Over-the-Counter Medications

Over-the-counter (OTC) medications are sold in pharmacies and other stores without a doctor's prescription. There are dozens of OTC medications on the market for common cold symptoms, such as a runny nose, congestion, sore throat, headache, or cough, but with the exception of pain and fever drugs, there is no proof that they work. There is also a risk of giving your child too much medication, such as acetaminophen on top of a cough syrup that already contains acetaminophen. The best treatment for a cold is still plenty of rest and liquids. Doctors do not recommend OTC cough and cold medications because they do not think they work, and they can actually be harmful. Do not give OTC cold medications to children under six years of age without first talking to your doctor. For current information from the Canadian Paediatric Society on OTC medications, see the Caring for Kids website (www. caringforkids.cps.ca).

Cough syrups

Coughing is stressful when it keeps children awake at night, but it can also be helpful. It can be a sign that the body is getting rid of mucus that irritates the airway. Syrups that stop this normal response can be harmful to children. Most studies of the effectiveness of these cough syrups have been done on adults, and the few that have been done on children show no benefits.

Decongestants and antihistamines

Decongestants and antihistamines are no longer recommended for young children.

Dr. Sacks Says ....

To no one's surprise, the best treatment for a cold is lots of TLC and not-too-salty chicken soup. Just ask grandma.

....

Saline nasal drops

Saline nasal drops can help your child breathe better when she has a stuffed-up nose. They contain a weak salt-water solution that will soften the mucus in her nose.

Pain and fever relievers

OTC pain relievers, such as acetaminophen and ibuprofen, can be given to a child to reduce fever, but should not be given for pain relief unless the situation is discussed with your child's doctor, except in the case of teething and ear infections. (For more on ear infections, see page 349 in Chapter Six.) Follow the manufacturer's directions regarding the proper dosage and frequency for your child's age.

Antibiotics and Antibiotic Resistance

Antibiotics are drugs that doctors use primarily to kill bacterial infections. There are many different kinds of antibiotics used to kill different bacteria, but in recent years the antibiotic resistance of bacteria that cause infections in children has become a major problem. Some medicines that used to kill certain germs don't work anymore, so many infections can no longer be treated with traditional antibiotics, and new (and often more expensive) drugs must be used.

There are many reasons why bacteria develop a resistance to antibiotics, including inappropriate use of medicines. Antibiotics may kill some bacteria, but not all, and when antibiotics are used for the wrong reason or for an incorrect length of time, more bacteria resistant to that antibiotic may be produced.

MYTH BUSTERS

Myth: Antibiotics are necessary for treating fever.

Fact: Fever often helps our bodies fight infection, so treating a fever could delay this process. To lower a high fever, use acetaminophen or ibuprofen. Only use ibuprofen on children older than six months.

—*Dr. Leona Fishman-Shapiro, MD, FRCPC*

You can try to avoid antibiotic resistance by trying to ensure your child only receives antibiotics when they are clearly for the treatment of a bacterial infection. Ask the doctor what the infection is that the antibiotic is for. Children with colds should not be treated with antibiotics. You should also try to have your child examined by her own doctor every time so the record of all her antibiotic use is in one place. Going to different walk-in clinics is not a good idea if you can avoid it.

Dr. Sacks Says

An unnecessary antibiotic used improperly is a dangerous thing.

If your child is prescribed antibiotics, be sure that they are administered properly at the prescribed dose and taken for the prescribed duration. Never give your child antibiotics prescribed for someone else, and never use antibiotics left over from an unfinished prescription.

MAKE A NOTE, MAKE AN APPOINTMENT, OR GO TO THE HOSPITAL?

If your child is taking antibiotics and she has a bad reaction, **make an appointment** with her doctor. The doctor can determine whether it's an allergic reaction or simply a side effect of the medication.

Common Respiratory Problems

Croup

Croup is a viral infection of the throat and vocal cords, or larynx. When children younger than five years of age have the infection, it is called croup; in those older than five, it is called laryngitis. Croup often begins like a cold, but then fever, cough, and difficulty breathing develop. The infection causes the lining of the throat and larynx to become red and swollen, and the child develops a hoarse voice and a cough that sounds like a bark. The air passage below the vocal cords may narrow, making it difficult for him to move air in and out, so breathing may become very rapid and noisy.

In most cases, croup sounds worse than it actually is. However, your child may become very tired because of the extra work it takes to breathe. In severe cases, his breathing can be obstructed. Some children become so sick that they have to be treated in hospital. Antibiotics are not effective because the infection is caused by a virus.

Mild croup is treated with cool air, hydration, and humidification. Moderate to severe croup may be treated by medication to decrease the inflammation. If your child's doctor prescribes medication, follow the directions. For cases of very mild croup, your child may continue attending a childcare facility or school if he feels well enough to take part in activities.

MAKE A NOTE, MAKE AN APPOINTMENT, OR GO TO THE HOSPITAL?

If your child has difficulty breathing that is not relieved with cool air or humidification in a few minutes, or if any of the signs listed below appear along with a croupy cough, **take him to the hospital immediately.**

▷ Fever higher than 39°C (102°F)
▷ Rapid or difficult breathing
▷ Severe sore throat
▷ New or increased amounts of drooling
▷ Refusal to swallow
▷ Discomfort when lying down

Asthma

Asthma is a chronic lung disorder in which the lining of the bronchial tubes becomes inflamed and swollen, affecting a person's ability to breathe. During an asthma attack, the muscles surrounding the bronchial tubes tighten, and the inflamed tubes produce an increased amount of mucus, causing the person to wheeze, cough, and breathe rapidly. A number of things can bring on an asthma attack, including upper respiratory infections, air pollutants or allergens, certain medications, cold air, cigarette smoke, and even physical exertion.

BRONCHIOLITIS

Bronchiolitis is a viral disease that causes the lining of small airways to swell, making it difficult for your child to breathe. The signs include coughing, wheezing, bluish skin, rapid and laboured breathing, and sometimes fever. It is usually not treated with antibiotics. Bronchiolitis is not the same as bronchitis, an inflammation and infection of the main airways. Bronchiolitis is more severe, and usually affects children under the age of two. Recurrent bronchiolitis could be an indication that your child may develop asthma.

If your child wheezes regularly or has a persistent cough that is worse at night, and he has allergies or eczema, or if either of his parents have allergies or eczema, he may be prone to developing asthma. There is no cure for asthma, although many children do outgrow its symptoms over time. For more information on asthma, see "Asthma" in Resources.

MAKE A NOTE, MAKE AN APPOINTMENT, OR GO TO THE HOSPITAL?

If you suspect your child may have asthma, **make an appointment** to see his doctor. If left untreated for a long period of time, asthma can cause permanent lung injury. It can be difficult to diagnose, so the doctor will give your child a thorough examination and take a family health history to determine if he has asthma. Additional breathing tests may be needed.

The goals of treatment are to lessen the frequency and severity of attacks, to eliminate symptoms wherever possible so that the child may participate fully in all his activities, and to have an action plan if an attack occurs. The plan should be followed accurately. The doctor will probably prescribe medication. Long-term inhaled steroids have been found to be quite effective in preventing recurrence of attacks, and do not significantly impair growth.

Precautions you can take to minimize the severity of your child's symptoms include making sure he gets a flu shot every year and avoiding exposure to airway irritants such as fireplaces, perfumes, and cigarette smoke. If you smoke, try to quit for your child's sake as well as your own; if you can't, don't smoke around your child. Don't let anyone else smoke when they're in a car with your child, and make sure his childcare situation is smoke-free. Limit his exposure to dust mites by removing carpeting, curtains, and anything containing feathers from his room, getting rid of stuffed animals, washing bedding once a week in hot water, using hypoallergenic pillows and bed coverings, and using a plastic mattress cover. In severe cases, preventing colds by changing his daycare situation to a smaller one may be necessary. Because asthma is chronic, parents and caregivers need to be aware of the treatment plan and stick to it.

MAKE A NOTE, MAKE AN APPOINTMENT, OR GO TO THE HOSPITAL?

Make an appointment to see your child's doctor if he starts to wheeze mildly, he's frequently using his inhaler, and your asthma action plan is not working.

Take him to the hospital immediately if he is wheezing heavily or having trouble breathing.

Dental Care

Good nutrition, appropriate cleaning, and properly timed dental visits are the key factors in ensuring a child's dental health. It's crucial for your toddler to begin to understand and practise the best ways to keep teeth strong, so talk to him about the importance of caring for his teeth. By the age of two, your child should be encouraged to try brushing his teeth by himself, with an adult completing the job, making sure that all tooth surfaces have been cleaned. You should also be flossing his teeth. Ask your child's dentist for help with flossing techniques, especially how to reach the back teeth. By age three, children usually have all 20 of their primary teeth, and proper dental care should be in full swing.

Teach a child "2 for 2," which stands for brushing twice a day for two minutes each time. Two minutes may seem like a long time, so playing music for two minutes may help him keep brushing. Begin by using a tiny, pea-sized smear of fluoride toothpaste, and teach your child to spit it out rather than swallow. Rinse the toothbrush well with water after each use and let it air dry, making sure it doesn't touch other toothbrushes. Don't share toothbrushes, and replace them every few months, when the bristles become flattened with use, or after a serious cold or sore throat.

Your toddler's eating habits can also promote healthy teeth. Between meals, quench his thirst with water. Encourage healthy snacking on fresh vegetables, fresh fruit, and cheese and crackers. Limit candy, dried fruit, and sugared drinks, and when he does eat something sugary or sticky, clean his teeth.

Children should visit the dentist every six months from one year of age onward. When you talk to your child about visiting the dentist, always keep the conversation positive. Role-play the visit with your child, or encourage him to role-play with a friend. Answer his questions in a very general way, and leave most of the explaining up to the dental professionals, who have special ways to describe procedures to children. For up-to-date information on dental care, see "Dental Health" in Resources.

Winning the brushing battle

You can lead a child to the sink, but you can't make him brush. Getting a toddler to brush his teeth can be a trial, and trying to force a toothbrush into his mouth will only upset and frustrate both of you. Make tooth-brushing more appealing by giving him a toothbrush in his favourite colour or with his favourite character on it, and toothpaste in a flavour he likes, or by allowing him to choose his own toothbrush and toothpaste. You can also try an electric toothbrush designed for children. The noise and action may hold his attention and keep him brushing longer, and may even calm him. Toddlers love to imitate, so show him how much you enjoy brushing your teeth. Look into the mirror together or directly at each other, and show him how you brush your teeth. You can even let him brush your teeth while you brush his at the same time.

NUTRITION

These years are a time of great change for your child. Her body is growing, she's mastering new skills, and her attitudes are forming. Her sense of independence means she's letting you know what she likes and doesn't like in no uncertain terms. All of these factors influence the way she eats.

Toddlers explore the world through all five senses, and the world of food is no exception. Squishing a banana before eating it is just too tempting for a two-year-old to pass up. Toddlers also need to control their world, so she may love bananas one day and refuse them the next, or eat nothing but bananas for several days. She may not be able to control when she goes to bed, but she can decide whether to eat, so her desire for independence is often expressed at the dinner table. As baffling or frustrating as these whims may be, they are all part of your child's normal development. Cajoling, bribing, or threatening won't work, and will make mealtimes an unpleasant struggle for everyone. While your child is young, she needs to develop good eating habits that will last throughout her life. Mealtime is the ideal opportunity to set an example by creating a positive atmosphere in which healthy food attitudes can be developed, and by eating healthy foods yourself.

Toddlers are fickle eaters. Their eating habits may seem bizarre, but the behaviours noted below are perfectly normal.

- Examining the chicken sandwich before she eats it
- Accepting toast only if it is cut in triangles
- Trying only a bite of squash today; maybe she'll try some more tomorrow
- Drinking milk only if she can pour it into her own glass
- Loving carrots on Tuesday, but refusing them on Wednesday
- Insisting that the apple be cut in slices
- Wanting a peanut butter sandwich for lunch every day of the week
- Gobbling up the cookies she helped make when they are fresh from the oven
- Drinking soup from a cup like mom

At first, she'll prefer simple foods she can recognize, but with time she'll become curious about new foods and ways of eating them. (For a list of cookbooks that include recipes for children this age, see "Nutrition" in Resources.) As long as her requests are reasonable, go with the flow.

Two- and three-year-olds like structure, so try to give her three meals and two snacks a day, as recommended by Canada's Food Guide, served at around the same time. By two, she should be able to use a spoon with some level of proficiency and drink from a cup with the occasional spill; by three, she should have mastered a fork and will spill her food and drink only rarely. If she's hungry, she will sit quietly at the table during mealtimes, but as soon as she's full, her attention will turn elsewhere. Keep your expectations relatively low. The "one more bite" battle is one you won't win if your toddler's already decided she's full. And she's unlikely to sit happily at the family dinner table for 45 minutes or leave behind a pristine high chair. As long as everyone's had enough to eat, the meal has been a success.

Making the Most of Mealtime

Mealtimes are a great opportunity to model good behaviour. Start by making sure everyone washes their hands before coming to the table. Use meals to teach the importance of saying "please" and "thank you" when your child would like something to be passed or when she would like more food. Make mealtimes short, and allow your child to leave the table before the family is done if she has eaten enough and she asks to be excused.

Dr. Sacks Says

*Family mealtimes are **not** optional. If one parent has to work late, at least gather everyone together for dessert.*

Ignore your child's awkwardness or messiness during the meal; it's just part of the learning process. Cleanup may be easier if you put some newspapers or a plastic mat under her chair. Have her eat a variety of finger foods and spoon foods at each meal so she can get enough to eat while she learns to use utensils. Don't allow her to bang or throw her utensils (or her food!), but let her practise her skills on her own—avoid watching expectantly and talking to her about what she is doing. If she drops food on the floor, don't get angry, but don't reward her behaviour by picking it up. Once she has learned the skill of dumping and spilling, it becomes a game. Often, it's a sign that she is full, so after a bit of time, just take the food away.

Encourage a child who eats very quickly to slow down by talking between spoonfuls. It also helps if adults eat slowly, use a calm voice, create a relaxed setting, put small amounts of food on the table, or use gentle reminders to chew food. You can also be a good role model for your child by keeping your culinary dislikes to yourself. Children learn by imitation and can pick up subtle messages about food. If dad says he doesn't like broccoli, your child may refuse to even try it. Sometimes you can get her to eat vegetables she doesn't like by calling them something more descriptive and fun. If she is interested in colours, have her try the "green balls" (peas) and "orange circles" (carrots) from a bowl of mixed vegetables. If she is interested in numbers, count the number of peas or carrots in a spoonful before giving it to her. Avoid substituting solid food with liquid calories, such as juice or milk.

Mealtime should be a happy time; it's not the time for lectures or stressful conversations. Include your child in the discussion, and praise her good behaviour at the table. Try not to get too hung up on formality. Just keep the mood light and your expectations realistic. The most important thing is to make mealtime an enjoyable family experience, and one that will encourage your child to behave respectfully.

What to Feed Your Child

Your child can now eat almost everything the rest of the family eats. You can continue feeding him baby cereal as long as he will continue to eat it, but offer him a variety of foods as well. At this age, it helps to think of a balanced diet as something your child eats over the course of an average week, not necessarily daily. He might eat a lot of meat one day, but then none for the rest of the week. This is fine, but gradually steer him toward a daily balanced diet. Make sure he gets enough calcium and fibre, and avoid adding salt to his food.

Offer your child a variety of foods from each of the four food groups set out by Canada's Food Guide—grains, meats, fruits and vegetables, and dairy products. The amount of food a child needs varies with age, body size and type, activity level, and appetite. For children two to three years old, the Guide recommends three servings of grain products, one serving of meat and alternatives, four servings of fruits and vegetables, and two servings of dairy products and alternatives.

Here are some examples of servings.

Grain products
- 1 slice of bread
- ½ cup cooked rice or pasta

Meats and alternatives
- ½ cup cooked fish, poultry, or lean meat
- 2 eggs

Fruits and vegetables
- ½ cup fresh, frozen, or canned fruits or vegetables

Dairy products
- 1 cup milk or fortified soy beverage
- ¾ cup yogurt

For more examples of servings from Canada's Food Guide, see "Nutrition" in Resources.

Preschoolers should drink 500 millilitres (2 cups or 16 ounces) of milk each day, as this is their main source of vitamin D and calcium. After the age of two, they no longer need homogenized milk, and can consume whatever type of milk the rest of the family is drinking. Foods that aren't in the four categories, such as butter, salad dressing, and jam, are fine in moderation.

Sample one-day menu for a child 3 years of age

	Recommended daily Food Guide servings			
	Vegetables and fruit	**Grain products**	**Milk and alternatives**	**Meat and alternatives**
Child 2 to 3 years of age	4	3	2	1

	Number of Food Guide servings				
Foods	**Vegetables and fruit**	**Grain products**	**Milk and alternatives**	**Meat and alternatives**	**Added oils and fats**
Breakfast					
½ bowl of whole grain cereal (15 g / ½ oz.)		½			
125 mL (½ cup) of 2% milk			½		
Snacks					
60 mL (¼ cup) carrot sticks and broccoli florets with salad dressing	½				√
water					
Lunch					
½ salmon sandwich on whole wheat bread (made with 30 g [1 oz.] of canned salmon and mayonnaise)		1		½	√
60 mL (¼ cup) red pepper strips and cucumber slices	½				
125 mL (½ cup) milk			½		
1 peach	1				
Snack					
½ bowl of oat rings cereal (15 g / ½ oz.)		½			

(continued)

(continued)

Foods	Number of Food Guide servings				
	Vegetables and fruit	Grain products	Milk and alternatives	Meat and alternatives	Added oils and fats
125 mL (½ cup) milk			½		
Dinner					
125 mL (½ cup) spaghetti with tomato and meat sauce (about 40 g [1½ oz.] of meat)	½	1		½	√
125 mL (½ cup) milk			½		
125 mL (½ cup) applesauce	1				
Snack					
½ banana	½				
Total Food Guide servings for the day	4	3	2	1	

Source: *Eating Well with Canada's Food Guide: A Resource for Educators and Communicators*, Health Canada. Reproduced with the permission of the Minister of Public Works and Government Services Canada, 2008.

What you shouldn't feed your child

Although your child's skills at the dinner table are improving, you should still be on the lookout for foods that are choking hazards, such as hot dogs (unless cut lengthwise and diced), whole grapes, popcorn, hard foods like candy, nuts, or raw vegetables, and sticky foods like peanut butter, unless it is spread very thinly on bread. Avoid giving your child processed foods or fast foods, as they tend to be full of unhealthy fat and salt and low in nutrients. Offer healthy snacks of fresh or canned fruit or small amounts of wholesome cereals, rather than packaged snack foods or drinks. Never give your child pop, and limit juice to ½ cup (4 ounces) a day. When he's thirsty, encourage him to drink water.

Introducing new foods

When you want your child to try a new food, be patient and encouraging. Introduce only one food at a time, and serve just a small amount with a familiar food that he likes. He may be more likely to try it when he's hungry, when he has a friend over for dinner, or when he sees that you are enjoying it. Don't coax him to eat it; if he rejects it, just accept the refusal calmly and try again in a few days. As new foods and new taste experiences become more familiar, he'll become more adventurous. Encourage him to ask questions about the food and help you prepare it. The more children know about a food, like where it grows and how to prepare it, the more they will enjoy eating it.

Is your child getting enough—or too much—to eat?

Adequate growth is a sign of appropriate nutrition. Your child's doctor will monitor his growth at his regular appointments and will alert you if there are any problems. However, children know how much food they need, and they will eat what their body needs if they're not pressured. Respect your child's ability to determine how much he should eat; don't force him to "clean his plate." His appetite can fluctuate from day to day, or even from meal to meal. Because he has a small stomach, he needs to eat small amounts frequently throughout the day, so give him small servings and allow him seconds if he asks. Set regular, frequent meal and snack times that work for the whole family. An ideal schedule is three meals and two snacks at approximately the same time each day.

Set aside enough time to prepare healthy meals and to eat them slowly in a quiet, comfortable setting. Not only does eating in front of the television take away from the experience of spending mealtime together as a family, but it can interfere with the signs of hunger and fullness. Children need to learn to listen to their bodies and know when they are full. Consider letting him dish up his own food, with your help. If he can't finish it all, don't make a big deal about it, especially if he's at least tried a bit of everything. It's not a good idea to use dessert as a bribe, but there's nothing wrong with a consistent rule that allows dessert if he's eaten a proper meal.

MYTH BUSTERS

Myth: It is normal for children to lose weight when they go through a growth spurt.

Fact: Rapid weight loss is often attributable to something more serious, and needs to be assessed.

—*Dr. Leona Fishman-Shapiro, MD, FRCPC*

INJURY PREVENTION

Childproofing for the Preschool Years

As your child becomes more and more coordinated and agile, your childproofing methods need to change accordingly. As she becomes increasingly comfortable with the stairs, for example, you may no longer need to be as vigilant about using your safety gate. However, she may also figure out how to get into things she wouldn't even attempt to investigate a few months ago. As always, the idea is to try to stay one step ahead of your child's abilities. It never hurts to regularly get down on your knees and wander through your home at your toddler's eye level. What's accessible to those little hands? What looks too tempting to pass by? You might be surprised by the things you see.

Toddlers still put things in their mouths, so constantly check the floor for small toys and other potential choking hazards. If you have older children, make sure their toys are inaccessible to younger ones. Unplug small appliances when they're not in use, and keep the cords out of reach. If your child is particularly dexterous and determined, she may be able to pull off the little plastic electrical outlet covers, exposing a threat from the outlet as well as the choking hazard of the cover itself, so invest in new outlet covers. There are now outlet covers available that have a sliding latch over the outlet.

Make sure televisions are pushed back from the edge of furniture and heavier items are placed in bottom drawers and shelves, making the furniture bottom-heavy. Bolt or tether large furniture and appliances to the wall, and keep all drawers closed when you're not using them—they make perfect steps for an eager climber.

Always lock windows and doors. Industrious toddlers may figure out how to open the window, especially after watching you do it. If you are replacing your windows, invest in some that are double hung; they can be opened from the top, so there's much less risk of your toddler climbing out. Windows opened from the bottom shouldn't open more than 10 centimetres (4 inches). You can buy special stoppers that prevent windows from opening any more than that. Make sure closets can be opened from the inside so that your toddler can't get locked in, and use wooden or plastic hangers instead of the wire ones, as children can be severely injured by wire hangers. Be vigilant about keeping poisons, cleaning products, and medicines in locked or inaccessible cupboards. Don't rely on "childproof" packaging—some toddlers can figure it out.

Be careful around water. You and your child may feel increasingly confident around water, but that confidence is unfounded. The Canadian Paediatric Society has found that swimming programs for children under four years of age are not an effective drowning prevention strategy. Children younger than four do not have the developmental ability to master water survival skills and swim independently. Don't ever leave your child unattended in the tub or wading pool, even for a moment— even if your toddler seems very coordinated. Always keep the bathroom door closed when it's not in use, and never leave any source of water where your child can get to it. A toddler can lose her balance and fall headfirst into a toilet or bucket and get stuck. Drain all wading pools immediately after use, and lock hot-tub covers at all times. Your toddler may be surprisingly strong, and if she gets the lid off even slightly, she may be able to get in, but not out.

MAKE A NOTE, MAKE AN APPOINTMENT, OR GO TO THE HOSPITAL?

Take your child to the hospital immediately if she has had any loss of consciousness or significant change in consciousness, whether from a fall, poison, a seizure, or anything else, or if she starts to vomit profusely after a fall.

Staying safe outside the home

If your child is spending much of her time outside the home, child-proofing your own home won't be enough. It's imperative you check that other places your child goes regularly are also adequately child-proofed. Most accredited daycare centres are up to code in terms of childproofing, but if you are sharing a nanny or putting your child in an unlicensed daycare, whether in a home or a small facility, take the time to visit before your child starts, talk to them about childproofing, and tour the premises.

A stickier situation may be ensuring grandma and grandpa's home is also safe for your child. Your parents and in-laws may not share your diligence when it comes to childproofing—"I raised several children of my own in this house and everyone survived" is a common defence. However, as a parent you have to feel comfortable that the same safety standards you're applying at home will apply at grandma and grandpa's. Take a walk through your parents' homes with them and gently explain the things that might be dangerous to their beloved grandchild, then go purchase the things you need and install them yourself. Install outlet covers, cabinet and drawer locks, and childproof doorknob covers so your child can't slip out if grandma is distracted. Put anything breakable or hazardous to little hands out of reach, such as figurines, candy dishes, picture frames, letter openers, and fireplace tools, and move all medicines and household cleaning products to inaccessible cupboards. Survey the backyard if your child is going to be spending any time out there.

If your child is going to be staying overnight at her grandparents' home, leave them a list of crucial phone numbers, including your cell phones, the phone number of where you're going, your child's doctor's phone number, and other emergency numbers, like poison control. Write a note empowering the grandparents to make medical decisions for your child, and sign and date it. Supply any medications or first-aid products that might be necessary, like pain reliever, bandages, sunscreen, and insect repellent. Make sure your parents know how to administer your child's medication (and remind them to keep all medication out of sight and out of reach). Give them a list of foods your child is allergic to and foods that are possible choking hazards, such as hot dogs, grapes, and raw carrots and celery. Write them down along with the list of phone numbers. If your child is going to be riding in their car, make sure there is a car seat in place and that it's properly installed. Show your parents how to put your child in safely.

Set up your child's bed before you leave. If she will be sleeping in a crib or portable playpen, bring the appropriate bedding and put it on. If she will be sleeping in a bed with a bed rail, check that the rail is in place and that the grandparents know how to move it up and down. Bunk bed safety rails are often dangerous; instead, put the mattress on the floor so no rails are needed.

Updating the First-Aid Kit

As your child gets older, it's important to update your first-aid kits, including the ones you may have at her grandparents' homes or your vacation home. Once your child is aged two and older, she may be able to take a number of over-the-counter medications that you should include in the kit, such as pain and fever medication (acetaminophen or ibuprofen), calamine lotion, and antibiotic cream for burns, cuts, and scrapes. Make sure that medications, including emergency medicine like epinephrine devices (if needed), have not expired, and that everyone still knows how to use them.

The Great Outdoors

Summer and childhood go hand in hand. Your memories of your own childhood are probably filled with endless days spent playing in the sun and splashing in the water. The hot summer sun can be very dangerous for children, however, and they're more likely than adults to lose body fluids and become dehydrated. Along with the fresh air, exercise, and opportunities to learn and explore that outdoor play provides, there are hazards from insects, water, falls, and the things you leave lying around outside. Just as you childproof your home, it's a good idea to look around your yard to check that it's safe too. Make sure barbecue supplies, like lighter fluid and matches, and lawn and garden supplies, like garden tools and chemicals, are inaccessible. For information on water safety, see page 317 in Chapter Five.

Sun exposure

Your child's skin can be burned by sunlight, but it can also be burned when he touches hot surfaces such as pavement, metal slides, or car doors. Bad sunburns and too much time spent in the sun without skin protection have been linked to a high risk of skin cancer later in life. As much as possible, keep your child in the shade or indoors during the hottest time of the day, between 10 am and 2 pm. Make sure that outdoor play areas have an area in the shade. Avoid long periods of exposure to the sun at the beginning of the summer, and get him used to being in the sun by gradually increasing the amount of time he spends outdoors over a period of several days. Dress your child in a sun hat, sunglasses, and a loose cotton T-shirt, and apply a sunscreen. Sun protective clothing provides even more defence, blocking out the UV rays that sneak through normal fabrics.

Sunscreen

Children over six months of age can and should wear sunscreen whenever they're out in the sun. Apply a sunscreen with an SPF (sun protection factor) of at least 30 on all skin that will be exposed to the sun. After your child has played in water, reapply his sunscreen, even if it is water-proof. Sunscreen can deteriorate over time, so check the expiration date. If the lotion has changed colour or consistency, throw it away. To be safe, buy new sunscreen at the beginning of every summer.

Sunglasses

Research now shows that sun exposure, even in the youngest children, can lead to eye damage over time, so infants and toddlers should wear eye protection when they're in the sun. Maximum UV blocking sunglasses are available for children of only a few months old, and many have bands on them to keep the glasses from falling off little heads. Just as you teach your child that he must always wear his seat belt in the car, teach him that if he is outside in the sunshine, he must always wear sunscreen, a hat, and sunglasses.

Heatstroke

Young children's bodies do not dissipate heat well, so on a humid day, they may not sweat enough to cool their body down, and heatstroke or heat exhaustion can occur. A child who has heatstroke may be weak and dizzy and have a headache. He may also have a high fever, and may be confused or lose consciousness. To prevent heatstroke on sunny days, especially humid ones, try not to spend too much time outside during midday, have your child play in the shade as much as possible, and encourage him to drink lots of water to replace the body fluids he loses in the heat.

Insect repellent

At best, insect bites are annoying; at worst, they can be dangerous. Mosquitoes and biting insects can carry disease, although cases are relatively rare in Canada. However, bites can cause allergic reactions or become infected. You can help your child avoid insect bites by dressing him in long pants and long-sleeved shirts outdoors, avoiding places where insects breed and live, like standing water, and staying inside during dawn and dusk, when mosquitoes are most active. You can also use insect repellent.

The active ingredient in most insect repellents is a chemical called DEET, although not all products have the same concentration or amount of DEET. Insect repellents that are used on children should have a small concentration of DEET, which is usually expressed as a percentage. Children between the ages of 2 and 12 should use repellent with no more than 10 per cent DEET. Products containing citronella and lavender oil are not considered safe for use.

Like any chemical, make sure you are using insect repellents safely, and read the entire label before applying. Always apply insect repellent on your child, rather than having him do it himself. Apply the product lightly, and do not apply it on irritated or sunburned skin. If you're putting sunscreen and insect repellent on your child, apply the sunscreen first. Put insect repellent on exposed skin and on top of clothing, but not under clothes. Be careful not to get it in your child's eyes; if you do, rinse them with water right away. So that he's less likely to get it in his mouth, don't apply it to his face and hands. If you are using a spray, be careful not to breathe it, and spray it in a well-ventilated place (not in a tent), well away from food. It's best not to use the product for too long, so don't apply it more than three times in one day, and when he doesn't need it anymore, wash it off your child's skin with soap and water.

MAKE A NOTE, MAKE AN APPOINTMENT, OR GO TO THE HOSPITAL?

If you think your child is having a reaction to an insect repellent, whether it's a local reaction like hives or a general reaction like facial swelling or breathing issues, wash his skin and **take him to the hospital right away.** Take the container with you so the doctor knows what you used.

Playground safety

According to Safe Kids Canada, falls from playground equipment are the cause of about 70 per cent of playground injuries, and nearly 10 per cent of those are head injuries. For kids under five, head injuries account for one in every seven hospital admissions due to falls from playground equipment. Children under five should play on equipment no taller than five feet, as the likelihood of severe injuries from playground falls doubles when children fall from heights greater than 1.5 metres (5 feet).

Choose playgrounds that fit your toddler. Children under five should only play in playgrounds designed for preschool children. Look for adequate surfacing, which is deep, loose fill. Good surface materials include sand, pea gravel (smooth, round, pea-sized stones), wood chips, and synthetic surfaces. Grass, dirt, asphalt, and concrete are not acceptable surfaces for underneath and around equipment. Notify your local playground operator if you have concerns about the safety of your local playground. Playground safety checklists have been developed for parents to evaluate basic playground hazards and are available at your local or provincial injury prevention centre or Safe Kids Canada (see "Injury Prevention" in Resources). Always supervise your toddler at the playground, and stay right beside the equipment he is climbing on, keeping an eye on him at all times.

ooooo

It may sound obvious, but by his fourth birthday, you should know your child. During these two years, you will get further insight into his personality, his temperament, and his likes and dislikes. You'll know how easily he smiles, how well he gets along with new people, what his favourite colour is (this week, at least), and whether he prefers running around outside all day or sitting quietly with a book. You'll need this information to make the transition to his school years easier for both of you, so spend lots of time really getting to know the complex person your child is becoming. Play together, hug him often, and encourage his sense of humour. The ability to laugh at situations and at his own antics is a tool he'll need later in life.

Of course, the appreciation should be mutual. He may not have a clear understanding of your personality, but your child should be well aware that you are confident in who he is and what he is capable of achieving. The school years will find him constantly compared to kids of varying abilities, so start him off on the right foot by letting him know that he has unique strengths that will carry him far.

5

Off to School:
Ages Four and Five

It's official: your little one is no longer a baby. As each week passes, she will want to take on responsibility, and will want to prove to you that she can do things herself. And, for the most part, she can, whether it's brushing her teeth and dressing herself, or playing a board game, or maybe even taking her first stab at reading and writing. This stage also presents its challenges. Four-year-olds can be bossy and belligerent, with a keen interest in "fairness" and an ever-growing (and more colourful) vocabulary. Although they can be aggressive with their peers, and are still learning about appropriate behaviour, they want to have friends, and they increasingly enjoy being with other children. By the time she turns five, your talkative, inquisitive, and energetic child will have mellowed a bit. She may seem grown up at times, but remember, she's still a child who needs your praise, guidance, and affection as much as she ever has.

INCLUDED IN THIS CHAPTER

GROWTH AND DEVELOPMENT

After the huge gains in the first two to four years of her life, your child's growth and weight gain will slow down now. Her intellect, on the other hand, continues to grow in leaps and bounds. School-age children love to explore, both physically and intellectually. She is increasingly interested in the function of everyday things, like money and machines. Museums, art galleries, parks, and libraries are great places to allow her imagination and curiosity to flourish—and, as a bonus, they're fun for you, too. Encourage her love of learning by giving her opportunities to find out more about the things she's interested in.

She will also start to understand how time works. By age four, she is aware that the day consists of morning, afternoon, and night, and that the year has different seasons. By age five, she may start to grasp the concept of time—that the day is made up of hours, and hours are made up of minutes—and that there are seven days in a week.

Motor Skills

Children of all ages have very individual patterns of development, and this pertains to their gross and fine motor skill development as much as it does to growth and language. The rate at which children reach motor skill milestones and how well they achieve them will vary, so don't worry about comparing your child with the neighbours' kids. Over time, however, he should gain skills and improve them—not lose them.

Gross motor skill development

Your school-ager has nearly the coordination and muscle control of an adult—or, depending on the adult, maybe even better. He is able to walk, jump, run, and hop with confidence, and he can skip, throw a ball, and swing without your help. His muscular strength is continuously improving, and he may love to test it by standing on one foot or trying to pull himself up a rope ladder at the playground. His hand-eye coordination is also improving, which means he may be able to catch a bounced ball and steer his bicycle by himself.

Encourage him to use these new skills and challenge himself through his daily play and physical activity. Simple outdoor activities, like playing in the playground, riding his bike, or building a snowperson, improve his gross motor skills and keep him fit and healthy. Toys that can help him improve his gross motor skills include balls, skipping ropes, pedal toys and scooters, crawling tunnels, and climbing equipment at the playground. Start to introduce your child to simple sports like swimming, dance, soccer, and skating. (See the Caring for Kids website at www.caringforkids.cps.ca for up-to-date information from the Canadian Paediatric Society on when to start sports.) Before you fill his schedule up with lessons, though, try teaching him yourself. Being your child's teacher as he learns these skills will be a rewarding experience for both of you.

Fine motor skill development

By the age of five, your child's fine motor skills are also almost fully developed. He can probably brush his teeth and hair, dress himself, and maybe even tie his own shoelaces. He has increased hand and finger control, so he'll soon be cutting on a line with blunt-edged scissors and using a fork and spoon with proficiency. As hand coordination increases, so does his interest in simple construction sets and more difficult puzzles.

His fine motor skills can be enhanced by doing arts and crafts, such as drawing, colouring, painting, and moulding. He may be able to take on more difficult creative projects, like simple sewing projects and cutting and pasting. Other toys that will improve his hand-eye coordination are sandboxes, water tables, building blocks, construction sets, and simple sporting equipment like baseball gloves and balls.

> ## MAKE A NOTE, MAKE AN APPOINTMENT, OR GO TO THE HOSPITAL?
>
> **Make a note** to mention it at your child's next scheduled appointment if you or a caregiver, such as one of his grandparents, are concerned about his development.
>
> **Make an appointment** to see his doctor if his gross or fine motor skills seem to be regressing.

Language Development

Your child's language skills are now exploding. Your four-year-old will have a vocabulary of about 1,500 words, and she should be talking in complete sentences. By age five, she should be able to tell you about actual events and describe people, things, and situations in detail. She is also able to explain things to you, and talk in past, present, and future tenses. She's expressing ideas now, not just labels, and can listen and react in a conversation. She's still not entirely certain about the difference between fantasy and reality, and will weave colourful tales limited only be her active imagination. Her increasing attention span means she is now able to listen attentively to longer stories.

Along with this increased vocabulary will undoubtedly come some words you wish she wouldn't say. Kids are bound to pick up a couple of curse words, whether from friends, media, or, most likely, their parents (oops!), and the reaction they get when they use them makes them all the more intriguing. To curb your child's use of bad words, be extra careful what you say around her, and when she does use them, don't overreact. If she doesn't get a reaction when she says them, the words will lose their appeal.

By five years of age, she will also start to ask you the meaning of words she doesn't know. Be patient with all her questions, including the ubiquitous "why?". It may be tempting to say "just because" or "I don't know," but attempting to answer your child's questions draws her into conversation and validates her thoughts and feelings. It's also a great opportunity to teach her how to solve problems by showing her how to look things up in the library and on the Internet. For more on problem solving, see page 446 in Chapter Eight.

You can encourage your child's language development by spending a lot of time talking with her. Help her learn to use words to express her feelings, not just describe events. Ask open-ended questions like "How did that make you feel?" and listen to her answer. Try to get her to expand her list of feelings from happy, sad, and angry, to other more complex feelings like surprised and confused. Reading with her will boost her vocabulary and grammar skills too, and it helps her to link meanings to pictures. The more she hears you speak using correct grammar and pronunciation, the better her language skills will be. She'll still make mistakes, so gently correct her speech so she'll see this as an important way to learn—it will prepare her for taking correction in school.

Does my child need speech therapy?

While your kindergartner may still mispronounce words, strangers should be able to understand most of her speech by the time she's five years old. Stuttering is a normal part of language development, but persistent stuttering past the age of four or five must be addressed. If you are concerned about your child's communication abilities, discuss it with her doctor. The doctor will likely rule out a hearing problem first by sending your child to an audiologist. The doctor or the audiologist may also refer you to a speech-language pathologist. (See "Special Needs" in Resources for information on audiologists and speech-language pathologists.) Speech therapy helps children who have articulation problems, so your child may need speech therapy if she is not always intelligible, or if she has errors in two or more speech sounds that are obvious enough to call attention to her speech.

In addition to articulation problems, however, speech therapy also helps correct language problems, such as mixing genders (your child says "she hit me" when talking about her brother), confusing pronouns (she says "her go outside"), forgetting words, and difficulty learning new words. Other common language problems include difficulty using descriptive words (she cannot describe what someone looks like) or difficulty retelling a story or explaining a situation (if you ask "What happened at school today?" she stares blankly at you and says nothing, despite prompting). She may also need speech therapy if she doesn't understand or answer questions like "What do you do when you're thirsty?" by age three or four, or if she makes so many grammatical errors by age five that it is difficult for an adult to understand what she's saying.

MAKE A NOTE, MAKE AN APPOINTMENT, OR GO TO THE HOSPITAL?

Make a note to mention it to your child's doctor at her next appointment if

- she continues to talk in "baby talk." This usually happens because someone told her it was cute. The doctor can suggest ways to gently encourage her to use her regular voice.
- she uses words hurtfully. If she hurls insults when she's angry, she needs to be shown how words can be positive, and encouraged to talk about her feelings in a calm way.
- strangers cannot understand her when she speaks. Her diction doesn't need to be perfect at this age, but what she says should be intelligible to others most of the time.
- she is not speaking in phrases or short sentences, doesn't initiate conversation, or still points to things instead of speaking.

Make an appointment to see the doctor if

▷ your child loses words or regresses verbally;

▷ her speech is slurred;

▷ she is teased because of her speech;

▷ she stutters whenever she speaks; or

▷ you sense that something is just not right with the way she communicates.

Understanding Your Child's Sexual Curiosity

You've probably noticed that your child is an extremely curious little being, and it's only a matter of time before he starts to become curious about his body. A normal part of any child's development is discovering that touching his or her genitals feels good. Baby boys often pull and tear at their penises, which can be pretty disquieting for a parent. And your child may ask some alarming questions once he starts interacting with other boys and girls or wondering about his own provenance. As completely normal as all of this is, you're probably not going to feel comfortable dealing with it. Time to get over your squeamishness.

While you don't want to overreact or cause him to feel shame, let your child know what is appropriate touching and what is not. Tell him that touching himself is something that should only be done in private, and that no other person—except his parents or, if one of his parents is present, a doctor—is allowed to touch his "private parts." This is a good opportunity to teach him some lessons about preventing abuse: never do anything to yourself that hurts your body, never do anything to anyone else that hurts their body, and don't allow anyone else to hurt your body. This message is easy to understand, and it gives a child a strong foundation to learn to respect other peoples' bodies as well as his own.

Dr. Sacks Says

When you teach your child about his body parts, make sure it's all positive. Think of the message you send when you pull or slap his hand away from his favourite toy.

Your preschooler or kindergartner may start to ask questions about sexuality, like why his sister looks different or where babies come from. Answer him in simple, straightforward terms, and try not to seem embarrassed; you want to encourage him to ask questions, not avoid the topic altogether. Use a comfortable vocabulary when discussing sexual body parts. If you start out using cutesy labels for them, it will be difficult to have a serious and intelligent conversation about sexuality when he's a bit older. If you're more confident using books to teach, there are terrific books for children this age, and you will be able to find one that you're comfortable sharing with him. See "Sexuality" in Resources for a list of books for children on sexuality.

MAKE A NOTE, MAKE AN APPOINTMENT, OR GO TO THE HOSPITAL?

Make an appointment to see your child's doctor if his sexual curiosity

▷ becomes compulsive, or more frequent or intense;
▷ involves language or behaviour that is explicit or adult in nature; or
▷ continues in inappropriate places or times.

He may simply have a health problem that is causing him some discomfort, but it could also be a sign of an emotional problem, or even an indicator of possible sexual abuse.

Sexual abuse

No doubt you wonder if your child is safe while he is at daycare or school or with a babysitter, and in the vast majority of cases, children are safe with their caregivers. However, sexual abuse of children is not uncommon, unfortunately, and is far more likely to come from someone a child knows, like a caregiver or relative, rather than a stranger. Special needs children are particularly vulnerable. Becoming overprotective or making your child fearful won't help, but you can protect him by recognizing potentially dangerous situations and removing him from them, and by teaching him to protect himself. It's also important that you learn to identify the signs of sexual abuse.

Sexual abuse is any sexual activity that a child cannot understand or consent to, including voyeurism, exhibitionism, exposure to pornography, touching, and oral, anal, or genital intercourse. Be aware of any changes in your child's behaviour, his personality, or his body. Some signs that may indicate abuse include the following:

- bleeding or bruising in or around the genital area
- unusually fearful behaviour or withdrawal
- attempts to run away
- sexual knowledge, curiosity, or behaviour beyond his age (explicit language or behaviour; obsessive curiosity about sexual matters)

These signs could have causes other than abuse, but sexual abuse should be considered when you are investigating them. If you think that your child might be a victim of sexual abuse, the first thing you should do is talk to your child's doctor or ask for help from your local Children's Aid Society. They are very knowledgeable, and they will provide you with good advice. Also, some paediatric hospitals have abuse teams, which often work with community services such as the Children's Aid Society, that can direct you to the best place to get help.

Children are naturally sexually inquisitive, so exploration and masturbation are almost universal, and are rarely signs of abuse. However, abnormal sexual behaviour of a more explicit or adult nature, accompanied by other signs of abuse, indicate that a child may have been exposed to sexual acts. Many parents who witness signs of abuse of any kind, not just sexual, are often reluctant to investigate them because they can't bring themselves to believe it could happen to their child. This is a grave mistake; the longer the abuse continues, the greater the emotional and physical impact on your child.

MAKE A NOTE, MAKE AN APPOINTMENT, OR GO TO THE HOSPITAL?

If you think your child has been abused, **make an appointment** with his doctor as soon as possible.

You can help protect your child from abuse by making sure he is in a safe childcare situation. Never enrol him in a daycare that does not allow unannounced parental visits, and do make a point of dropping in from time to time. If something doesn't feel right about a childcare situation, pay attention to your instincts, and if your child says anything unusual or worrying about what happens at daycare or school, don't ignore him.

It's also important to teach your child basic safety rules. Remind him that his body belongs to him, and it is never okay for someone to touch him if he doesn't want them to, even if the person doing it says it's okay. He should be taught to say "no" if someone asks him to do something he's not comfortable with. When out in public or in unfamiliar places, he should keep close to his parent or caregiver, and should always be around other children when playing or walking to school. You need to nurture his increasing independence, but you also need to make sure he is never alone, and is supervised at all times. It's also critical to let him know that if someone touches him, or tries to, he needs to tell you about it. Make very clear that he will never get in trouble if he tells you something that makes him uncomfortable. The point is not to make him afraid, but to make him feel empowered, and to let him know that he can always count on you to support him and keep him safe.

Thumb-Sucking

Sucking is a normal reflex for babies, and many children turn to their thumbs or fingers when they are tired, sick, scared, or anxious, and as a way to help them fall asleep at night. Most children who suck their thumbs or fingers start as infants, or even in the womb. About half of them stop by about seven months of age, and many more stop over the following couple of years.

In almost all cases, there's no cause for concern until your child's permanent teeth start to come in, after about the age of five. Aversive treatments, like putting a bitter substance on her thumb or using a thumb guard (a plastic cylinder that goes over the thumb), can cause anxiety, so try gentle reminders or rewards before other methods of treatment. For instance, you can put a gold star on a calendar for every day that she doesn't suck her thumb, then reward her with a gift after she gets five gold stars in a row. Children usually stop this habit when they are ready—often when they start to spend more time with their peers, who may tease them or pressure them to stop.

MAKE A NOTE, MAKE AN APPOINTMENT, OR GO TO THE HOSPITAL?

If your child is still sucking her thumb at age five, **make a note** to mention it to her doctor and her dentist at her next appointments.

Toilet Learning Revisited

By now, your child is probably almost toilet trained, having occasional daytime accidents and wearing training pants at night, if not fully toilet trained. Continue to encourage her, and don't make a big deal when she has an accident, as accidents are very common at this age. Once your child is out of training pants, bedwetting may be a problem, but it is normal and your child should outgrow it by age six or so. (For information on bedwetting from the Canadian Paediatric Society, see the Caring for Kids website: www.caringforkids.cps.ca.) Never make her clean up as punishment for an accident. It's important to talk about cleaning up with her, but be matter-of-fact when you do so. Talking about it in a negative way or making her clean up as punishment will only lead to bigger problems, like withholding. In time, the accidents will become rarer until they disappear altogether.

If the process seems stalled, however, your child may have a toilet-learning problem. The most common cause of delayed toilet learning is resistance. Resistant children are those who are older than three years of age and know how to use the potty or toilet but choose to wet or soil themselves. This resistance can be due to a power struggle between a child and her parents against what she feels are excessive reminders to go to the potty, but it can also be caused by painful stooling. Your doctor can rule out any physical concerns and advise you on the best way to treat resistant behaviour. A step back from toilet learning is often in order.

Another common problem is daytime incontinence. If your child was previously dry during the day but starts to have frequent accidents, she may have a urinary tract infection, urethritis, or another medical condition that is causing incontinence. Withholding of bowel movements, also common, happens if a child feels shame or fear about having an accident; has passed a hard, painful stool; or is afraid to go on the potty or toilet away from home. This can cause constipation, and, in severe cases, impaction, which requires a bowel cleanout. Liquid around the impacted stool can leak out onto the child's underpants, and parents may mistake it for diarrhea. Stool withholding can cause poor appetite, and can begin a very vicious cycle of events. It's important to handle these challenges properly, before they make the problem worse. After the acute constipation is resolved, you'll need to change your child's diet and include more foods with fibre.

MAKE A NOTE, MAKE AN APPOINTMENT, OR GO TO THE HOSPITAL?

If your child complains of pain during urination, urinates while laughing or while running to the toilet, has constantly damp underwear, or is withholding bowel movements, **make an appointment** to see her doctor. In case your child isn't able to urinate at the doctor's office, bring a urine sample in a sterilized jar. Try to make it as fresh as possible by getting it shortly before the appointment or keeping it in the fridge until you leave your home. The doctor will have to take another sample if the result is positive, but a negative result will not require another sample.

At School and At Play

As your child grows out of his toddler years, he becomes increasingly social, preferring to play with other children rather than on his own. His language skills, emotions, and intellectual capacity will thrive when he plays with his peers. Giving your child opportunities to explore the limits of his imagination is the key to making the most of this highly dramatic and creative age.

Children need time for free, open-ended play. There will be plenty of time for hockey, swimming, piano, and ballet lessons as your child grows, but right now he needs some free time. Try not to enrol him in so many activities, groups, and teams that he doesn't have time to play on his own terms. It's okay to schedule playtime with other children, but keep it short, and preferably with one friend.

Dr. Sacks Says

Start a new trend: only two formalized activities a week. Save the rest of your child's spare time for family playtime that includes physical activity.

This is a good age to introduce simple board games, which encourage social skills, like taking turns, as well as language skills. Because the concept of fair play is important to them now, school-age children like structured games with defined rules, and they may become upset if someone is not playing by the rules. Participating in games is still more important than winning or even keeping score at this age, however. When playing games with your child, do not place too much emphasis on winning, and avoid violent or gender-based games.

Social development

By now your child should enjoy spending time with other children his age. Thanks to his increasing confidence and his improved language and social skills, your school-age child will like the company of other children and will seek out friends. Four- and five-year-olds can be aggressive and are still learning about taking turns and sharing, but they do want to have friends, and they enjoy being with other kids their own age. Observe your child when he is around children his own age, and ask his teacher if he is interacting with his classmates during playtime, not standing on the sidelines refusing to join.

MAKE A NOTE, MAKE AN APPOINTMENT, OR GO TO THE HOSPITAL?

Make a note to mention it to your child's doctor at his next appointment if you have any concerns regarding his socialization skills. If he doesn't interact with others, if he relates to them more as objects than people, if he is unwilling to make eye contact, or if he can't seem to be in a group without being aggressive or exceedingly anxious, you should discuss his behaviour with his doctor.

Bullying

Now that your child is starting school, there's a chance he'll encounter a bully. A bully is someone who uses aggression—physical, verbal, and psychological—repeatedly in order to hurt another person. Bullies have little regard for other children's feelings; they want attention and power, and they have no problem abusing other children to get it. Bullying is a serious problem that can have lasting consequences for a victim, so never discount it as "just kids being kids."

You can help protect your child by teaching him how to deal with bullies and by listening to him. Always be aware of where your child is, what he is doing, and who he is with. When you ask him about his day at school, listen carefully to what he says, and take his concerns seriously. If your child is suddenly afraid to go to school or refuses to go, if he starts asking for money for "things," or if he starts losing possessions daily, he may be being bullied. He can reduce his risk of becoming a victim of bullying by playing with friends rather than alone, keeping in sight of adults, and staying calm and confident when he's confronted by a bully. Teach him to "walk and squawk": to simply ignore a bully, walk away, and tell an adult. This may require some practice at home, so try role-playing situations with him. Reassure your child that it is not his fault he is being bullied, and that he has your support and the support of his teachers.

You should also be aware of how to tell if your child is a bully. If he often intimidates his siblings or friends and shows no remorse for hurting them, if he regularly disobeys his parents and teachers, and if he becomes angry or frustrated very easily, it's important that you observe his behaviour around others. You can help prevent him from becoming a bully by spending time with him every day, teaching him non-violent ways to handle frustration, anger, and conflict, and teaching him to respect others and see things from their perspective. Bullies often pick up their tendencies from their parents, so make sure your own behaviour is appropriate, and that your child only sees and hears you showing respect for other people.

Encourage your child's school and your community to take an active stand against bullying. His school should be paying more than lip service to a no-bullying policy. Your child should know who to tell if he is being bullied, and the school should talk to the bully and to his parents. For more information on bullying, see "Bullying" in Resources.

Let's pretend

Children love to pretend, creating their own make-believe worlds and scenarios. In fact, many conversations between school-age friends start with "Let's pretend…." Fantasy play is a normal, healthy part of a child's development, and it helps her prepare for growing up. Kids enjoy imitating adults and older siblings, so toys like medical kits, tea party sets, dollhouses, play kitchens, and cash registers are popular. Everyday household objects can also be used to create new worlds. A sheet draped over the kitchen chairs becomes a tent or a cave, and a large cardboard box becomes a playhouse.

To encourage pretend play, don't interfere too much or ask too many questions; it interrupts the fantasy. Make sure your child has some toys that don't excessively direct her play, but instead allow her to construct her own scenarios, like building blocks and dress-up clothes.

The imaginary friend

Your child's imagination is in full bloom right now, so don't be surprised if she introduces you to her pretend pal or pet. This is completely normal and is not a sign that she's lonely, shy, unhappy, or has any other emotional problem. Quite the opposite, in fact. Children who have imaginary friends are just looking for a creative outlet to express their ideas, feelings, and concerns, and they are just as happy and independent as kids who don't have an imaginary sidekick.

Show interest in your child's "friend," but don't overindulge the pretence (the imaginary pal shouldn't have her own seat in the restaurant, for instance). Join in the imaginary play if she invites you to, but let her control the scenario, and be careful not to ask too many questions or get too involved.

MAKE A NOTE, MAKE AN APPOINTMENT, OR GO TO THE HOSPITAL?

If the imaginary friend persists beyond the age of five or occupies too much of your child's time, **make a note** to mention it to her doctor at the next appointment. Her reliance on an imaginary friend past that age may be indicative of emotional problems.

Cognitive development

Many school-age toys and games are designed to stimulate your child's intellectual development. Common toys like puzzles and flash cards are good for developing spatial awareness and size, colour, and shape concepts, as are activities involving sorting objects according to their characteristics. Simple board games, like Candyland or Snakes and Ladders, and card games, like Concentration and Go Fish, are great for practising pre-math abilities. Find games that your whole family enjoys, as interacting with other people is a very important play lesson.

Perhaps no childhood toy encourages intellectual development more than a good book. Some four- and five-year-olds may want to start learning how to read on their own, but most won't show serious interest until a year or two later. If your child is interested in learning to read, you should encourage her. Point out similarities in groups of words with common prefixes (like wallet, walnut, and walrus) and ask her to tell you what they all have in common. Introduce the idea of creating her own words by asking her to draw a picture and then tell you something about it. Write what she has told you on the picture and ask her to try "reading" her story to you. If she's not interested in reading yet, don't push her into learning before she's ready. Let her set her own pace, and continue to read to her. The goal is to make books fun, no matter who is reading them.

To help your child develop a lifelong interest in reading, show her that reading is an important part of everyday life by being a good role model. If she sees her parents regularly reading books, newspapers, and magazines, she'll understand that reading is valuable. Show her that words are everywhere by reading to her from road signs, cookbooks, and flyers. Put labels on items in your home, such as toys, furniture, and food, and read the words with her and discuss what they mean.

Visit the library often, and create one at home. Great children's books can often be found cheaply at yard sales. If there are more books than toys in your home, a child is more likely to pick up a book when there's nothing to do. Four- and five-year-olds will sit and listen to increasingly longer stories, so expose her to books that might take more than one sitting to finish, such as short-chapter books, and to different kinds of books, such as fairy tales and poetry.

Behaviour and Discipline

Your child may no longer be having temper tantrums, but he has discovered defiance. Four- and five-year-olds will often assert their independence by talking back to you, wilfully disobeying the rules and ignoring your requests. As frustrating as this is, it's normal—and, in some ways, even healthy—behaviour. He is establishing himself as a distinct entity apart from his parents, and testing his limits is one way to do that. By reinforcing those limits through routines and rules, you help him feel secure and comfortable (despite all the evidence he'll provide to the contrary). Make sure he knows that you understand why he's upset, but that there are times when rules determine what is done. It might seem impossibly far away, but teaching him this lesson now will help set the stage for how you approach his next rebellious phase when he's a teenager.

Set rules and routines to help alleviate the anxiety that leads to defiant behaviour. Be clear and specific about the rules, and only set enough rules to help the day go smoothly, such as "no television after dinner" and "all toys must be picked up before bed." Too many rules, or rules that are inconsistently enforced, will only confuse him and make it more likely that he'll disobey. Maintain a steady but flexible routine from morning to night so that he knows what to expect and can take comfort in knowing what happens next.

Different homes may have different rules, as spouses who are separated and grandparents may have slightly different approaches to discipline and behaviour problems. The rules don't need to be the same in each home, but the rules in each home should be applied consistently. Conversations between your child's caregivers about discipline should never happen in front of him, and caregivers should never undermine each other's authority when your child is around.

Keep your expectations in tune with your child's age and maturity level—be realistic about what he is capable of so you can avoid situations that are bound to lead to defiance. Keep in mind that he's just a kid, so don't expect him to sit quietly through an hour-long church service, clean up the basement all by himself, or eagerly come to dinner when he's in the middle of his favourite game. Pick your battles, and don't bother pressing an issue if it's really not a big deal. Does it really matter if he wants to wear a green shirt with yellow pants? Giving him choices every once in a while won't hurt, and will help him feel he has some control, although offering choices too frequently may only overwhelm and frustrate him. Only offer him a couple of choices, and make sure both choices are acceptable to you.

When your child disobeys you, and he will, calmly remind him of the rule he's broken. If you overreact to bad behaviour, you may only reinforce it with negative attention. Be authoritative, but speak to him respectfully, and stay in control, even if you feel that he's pushing your buttons. Remember that you're his role model, so if you yell at him or belittle him with your words or gestures, he'll think that's acceptable behaviour. Similarly, never use physical punishment, or he'll think it's okay to hit others. Besides, you want him to behave because he knows it's the right thing to do, not because he's afraid of what will happen if he doesn't.

If he still won't obey, talk with him to try to find out why he's being disobedient. He may not want to go to bed because he just doesn't want to miss out on the action, but it may be because he's been having nightmares and is afraid to go to sleep. Or he may make a fuss when it's time to go to school because he is being bullied or abused. Talking about his concerns and knowing that you understand him may take away his need to disobey you. Sometimes he may act defiantly only because he doesn't know how to do what you've asked of him, so show him how to do things, and even do them with him at first, until he gets the hang of it. If he's defying you because you broke a promise, own up to it. You don't have to be perfect for your child; he's going to learn that adults aren't perfect soon enough. Children remember everything you say in their heroic quest for fairness, so if you are in the wrong, apologize and admit you made a mistake.

Dealing with bad behaviour is only part of the equation. Positive reinforcement works wonders—your child learns how rewarding good behaviour can be when he receives acknowledgement for behaving. He should hear "yes" more than "no." Instead of always saying no to him, offer alternatives, or talk to him about right and wrong. Try to "catch" him being good, and praise his behaviour ("It's great that you picked up your toys!") rather than him ("You're a good boy."). The goal of discipline is to teach your child how to change his own behaviour and to make him want to behave.

MAKE A NOTE, MAKE AN APPOINTMENT, OR GO TO THE HOSPITAL?

By age four or five, your child should be able to settle into a new routine within a few weeks. **Make an appointment** to see his doctor if, after a few weeks of going to school, he refuses to go without causing a big scene or showing signs of severe distress in the morning.

Sibling Issues

There's no relationship quite like that of siblings. They can be the best of friends, laughing and playing together, or the most bitter enemies, bickering and fighting with frightening intensity. And they can go from those extremes several times in the course of a day. Almost all families with more than one child will have to deal with sibling rivalry from time to time. In general, the younger a child is when her sibling is born, the more likely she is to be jealous. Toddlers and preschoolers are still highly dependent on their parents and crave their attention and approval, so when they have to share that attention with a newborn sibling, they can experience intense jealousy. While a certain amount of conflict is unavoidable, you can teach your children how to treat each other respectfully and resolve their own disputes.

One way to try to avoid potential conflicts is to set property boundaries. Separate the older child's possessions by assigning her a shelf that her younger sibling can't reach. If your children are close in age, give them their own shelves or boxes, and explain that they must ask the other's permission before taking a toy that is in the other one's special place, or before going into the other child's bedroom.

Treating each other respectfully includes not tattling. If one child tells you that her brother is throwing toys on the floor, let her know that her job is not to get her brother into trouble, it's to try to stay out of trouble herself. Make sure that she understands that there is an exception: if someone is in danger of getting hurt, or is hurting someone else, she must tell you right away.

Try to avoid getting involved in your children's quarrels. Left alone, they will probably come to a solution, or one will just tire of arguing and simply walk away. If things start to get violent, though, step in, but avoid taking sides. If both children are able to talk, ask each of them to describe how they feel, rather than what happened—they'll both have different stories anyhow. Empathize with their feelings, and encourage them to come up with a solution that benefits both of them. If emotions are running too high, or if you hear attacks on self-esteem (such as "you're ugly" or "you're dumb"), separate them for a cooling-off period and address the situation later.

Dr. Sacks Says

When your child is upset, it does a lot more good to talk about her feelings rather than the details of what upset her.

Children are sensitive of their status in relation to siblings, and any hint of favouritism will undermine their self-esteem and make them more likely to lash out. They're sure to accuse you of preferential treatment at times, no matter how hard you try to be fair, so it's pointless to worry about it too much. However, you can be careful to avoid it as much as possible. Although you can't help but compare your children at times, try not to do it out loud. Saying things like "Your sister is much taller than you were at her age" will only foster resentment. Try to praise both of them at the same time ("My girls are so pretty!"), or if you're praising one child's attributes, say something positive about the other too.

Spend time with each child alone. Kids love one-on-one attention, so if your child is having a difficult time dealing with her younger sibling, a trip to the park with just her can ease the tension at home. Encourage her to talk about her feelings toward her sibling, listen attentively, and tell her that her feelings are normal and that most brothers and sisters don't get along some of the time. Let her know that she can talk to you anytime, not just when you're alone with her.

Acknowledge your children's individuality by nurturing their unique qualities. If one loves to move, provide her with more opportunities for physical activity; if the other is passionate about drawing, encourage his inner artist. Never suggest that one child's talents or interests are more important or desirable than the other's. When the special talents of each child are recognized, it sets them apart from each other and builds their self-esteem.

See "Adoption" in Resources for books that provide advice on helping your child understand the arrival of an adopted sibling, and visit the Caring for Kids website (www.caringforkids.cps.ca) for information from the Canadian Paediatric Society on adoption.

HEALTH

As he gets ready to start kindergarten, a world of new experiences awaits your child—new friends, new routines, and a whole host of potential health issues. You may need to deal with everything from gastroenteritis, to lice, to the cuts and bruises that inevitably come with his increasing independence and agility (or lack thereof), not to mention the old standbys, like ear infections, diarrhea, and colds, which are constant throughout early childhood (see Chapter Six for more on these). Respiratory illnesses continue as well, but over-the-counter drugs are still of little help and are not recommended for children this age. Your approach to your child's illnesses should be based on his level of activity, his ability to drink, and the duration of fever (not just the fact that he has a fever). A child who has a low-grade fever (under 38.3°C/100.9°F) for a short period of time and is active and drinking will do best if his own immune system is allowed to do its job. It's hard for doctors to make an accurate diagnosis early in a child's illness anyway, and, in fact, you may be exposing your child to other infectious illnesses in the doctor's office.

MAKE A NOTE, MAKE AN APPOINTMENT, OR GO TO THE HOSPITAL?

Take your child to the hospital immediately if he is listless, refuses to drink (he may be dehydrated), or has a high fever that is unresponsive to ibuprofen or acetaminophen.

A healthy, varied diet, lots of exercise, good hand-washing technique, continued proper dental care (brushing twice daily for two minutes at a time, daily flossing, and semi-annual dental checkups), and a good sleep routine can go a long way to keeping your child healthy, but it won't make him invincible. Daycare and school will expose him to a whole host of communicable illnesses. Armed with a little knowledge and immunizations against serious viruses like chickenpox, measles, and meningitis, you can keep most of your school-age child's health problems minor and short-lived.

Common Conditions for School-Age Children

School brings a flurry of illnesses and injuries with increased interaction with other children, and a few illnesses more frequently than others. Lice, ringworm, impetigo, and pinworm are common conditions that your child can easily pick up from her playmates. They are a nuisance, but are rarely serious, and can usually be treated at home.

Head lice

Head lice are tiny insects that live on the scalp and lay eggs, called nits. They are very common in young children, and they spread easily among children who are together in one place, such as daycare centres and schools. They spread through direct head-to-head contact, or indirectly on items such as hats, combs, hairbrushes, and headphones. They don't fly or hop, but they can crawl very quickly. Although lice often make the scalp itchy, you can have them without having any symptoms. They can live up to three days off the scalp, but they need a warm environment to develop, so they aren't likely to hatch at room temperature, and they can't live on cats or dogs.

To diagnose a case of head lice, you need to find live lice. On average, children with head lice will have no more than 10 to 20. They move fast, and are only about the size of a sesame seed, so they can be hard to find. Finding nits (which are bigger and easier to see) on the hair close to the scalp suggests a possible case of head lice, but a child can have a few nits without actually having a case of head lice.

MYTH BUSTERS

Myth: Head lice is a sign of poor hygiene.

Fact: False. A clean head is not necessarily a lice-free head.

—*Dr. Alyson Shaw, MD, FRCPC*

If you think your child may have head lice, or if another child in his class or daycare has lice, check his hair for nits immediately, then again after one week and after two weeks. Good lighting is important when you're checking for nits. Part the hair in small sections, going from one side of the head to the other, and look close to the scalp, behind the ears, at the back of the neck, and at the top of the head. Only treat your child if you find live lice in his hair. If he does have a case of head lice, check everyone else in your home too.

Most of the treatments for head lice contain an insecticide that kills the lice, though in many cases the lice are becoming resistant to the treatment, which means they don't always work. In Canada, three insecticides are approved for use in treating head lice: pyrethrin (found in R+C shampoo/conditioner), permethrin (Nix or Kwellada-P), and lindane (Hexit or PMS-Lindane shampoo). Pyrethrin and permethrin are safe for humans, but lindane can be toxic and should not be used on infants or young children under two years of age. A non-insecticide product called isopropyl myristate/cyclomethicone (found in Resultz, for example), which kills lice by dehydrating them, is also available. It should be used only on children aged four and older.

You don't need a prescription for these products, but don't use them unless you find live lice. Follow the package directions carefully, and don't leave the shampoo or rinse in longer than directed. Rinse hair well after the treatment. It's best to do the treatment and rinsing over a sink, not in the bath or shower, so that other parts of the body don't come in contact with the product. Be sure to repeat the treatment in 7 to 10 days. Sometimes the treatments will make the scalp itchy, so if your child is scratching after treatment, it doesn't necessarily mean the lice are back.

There are also many treatments you may hear about that don't work. Trying to smother the lice with mayonnaise, petroleum jelly, olive oil or margarine may make it hard for them to breathe, but it probably won't kill them. There is very little evidence that combing wet hair with a fine-tooth comb works, and no evidence that tea tree oil or aromatherapy oils kill them. Gasoline and kerosene are just plain dangerous, so never use them to try to kill lice.

Since head lice don't live long off the scalp, and since the eggs aren't likely to hatch at room temperature, you don't need to clean your child's belongings too much. If you want to get rid of lice or nits from specific items, like hats or pillowcases, either wash them in hot water (66°C/151°F) and dry them in a hot dryer for 15 minutes, or store them in an airtight plastic bag for two weeks.

Children with head lice can attend school or daycare as usual, but they should avoid close contact with other children until the lice are gone. Let your school or daycare centre know if your child has head lice so that they can let other families know to check their children. "No-nit" policies, which keep children with head lice away from school, aren't effective because lice are common among young children, and because children may have them for several weeks with no symptoms. Rest assured that head lice do not spread disease, and having head lice does not mean your child isn't clean, so they are just a minor inconvenience rather than a threat to your child's health.

Ringworm (Tinea)

Ringworm—which has nothing at all to do with worms—is a skin infection caused by a fungus. The infection causes an itchy, flaky rash that may have a ring-shape with a raised edge. If the scalp is infected, there is often an area of baldness. Fungal infections of the feet, which are usually very itchy and cause cracking between the toes, are most often a form of eczema, and can be treated with moisturizers and mild steroids. If a foot infection persists, however, it could be ringworm.

Ringworm spreads from person to person by touch. When someone with ringworm touches or scratches the rash, the fungus sticks to their fingers or gets under their fingernails. Ringworm of the scalp can also spread through shared combs, hairbrushes, and hats. The infection can be cured with medication, either orally or by using ointments or creams that are spread on the affected area.

If your child has come into contact with another child who has ringworm, check for the telltale circular rash on his head or skin. If he has ringworm, have him wash his hands thoroughly after touching the infected skin. If he has ringworm on his scalp, make sure no one else uses his comb, hairbrush, face cloths, and towels. He should stay home from daycare or school until after treatment has started.

MAKE A NOTE, MAKE AN APPOINTMENT, OR GO TO THE HOSPITAL?

Make an appointment to see your child's doctor if your child has a persistent rash, or a rash that seems to be spreading.

Impetigo

Impetigo is a highly contagious bacterial infection that is very common among children. It occurs when one of two bacteria, streptococcus or staphylococcus, enters the skin through a cut or scrape, causing blisters that scab over with a yellowish-brown crust. The blisters can appear as red clusters filled with fluid, or larger ulcer-like sores. The sores commonly occur around the mouth and nose, but can also appear on the arms, legs, or elsewhere on the body. If your child has a scratch that is orange-red in colour with discharge, it may be impetigo.

The bacteria are most often spread by touch. Your child may pick up the bacteria by touching an infected child or something that child has touched, such as a toy or a piece of clothing. The bacteria enter her system through a cut, cold sore, insect bite, or other small lesion in the skin. Impetigo looks awful and is very itchy, but, with rare exception, it isn't serious. However, the infection can spread if it isn't treated. Your child's doctor will prescribe antibiotics; in some cases these are topical creams, and in others they will need to be taken orally. If they are oral antibiotics, your child must take the full course to ensure the infection doesn't return. In the meantime, wash the infected skin with soap and warm water, and thoroughly dry the area, using a clean towel each time. Don't forget to wash your hands after cleaning your child's wound. Keep your child's fingernails trimmed, and discourage her from scratching, as this may spread the infection. Your child will be contagious until 24 hours after starting treatment, so keep her home from school and away from other children during that time.

MAKE A NOTE, MAKE AN APPOINTMENT, OR GO TO THE HOSPITAL?

Make an appointment to see your child's doctor if you suspect that she has impetigo. Once treatment has begun, you should also make an appointment if she gets a fever; if the infected area enlarges rapidly or becomes inflamed, red, and tender; or if the infection doesn't seem to be improving after 72 hours.

Pinworms

Pinworms are whitish-grey, threadlike worms that cause itching and irritation around the anus, and in girls they can irritate the vulva and the vagina, often causing a lot of pain during the night. Your child becomes infected by getting pinworm eggs on her hands, either from scratching her anus or from an object touched by another infected child, and then putting her hands in her mouth. The eggs travel to the large intestine and hatch, and then the female pinworms travel out of your child's anus to lay their eggs. You can sometimes see the worms around a child's anus or in her stool. As alarming as pinworms can be, they are essentially harmless, and they are not a result of poor hygiene. Almost 10 per cent of children become infected with them. They are extremely contagious, though, and do require treatment.

If you suspect your child has pinworms but you haven't seen any, your doctor can provide you with a test kit. You press a small, sticky paddle gently on your child's anus and have the paddle tested for pinworm eggs. If the diagnosis is positive, your doctor will prescribe an oral medication to kill the worms, and may advise other family members to take the medication as well, since they may also be infected. There's a chance the test will be negative but your child will have pinworms, so if the symptoms persist, tell her doctor. Wash all her pyjamas, underwear, and bedding in hot water to destroy the worms and eggs, and to reduce the risk of re-infection.

To prevent pinworms, encourage your child to wash her hands after using the bathroom, before eating, and after touching family pets, which can carry the eggs in their fur. Vacuum and mop regularly to destroy eggs that may be on the floor. Check that your child's daycare centre washes toys frequently, especially if a number of children share them. Keep your child's nails trimmed and clean, and discourage nail-biting and thumb-sucking.

NUTRITION

Now that your child is school-age, he's practically eating like an adult. There may still be the occasional spill down the front of his shirt or argument over the necessity of eating peas, but at least he'll be close to mastering the fork, spoon, and cup (when he feels like using them), and is even learning to use a knife.

Your child should also be observing basic table manners now, like not talking with his mouth full, asking to have things passed instead of reaching across the table, and asking to be excused when he's finished eating. However, this increased maturity doesn't necessarily mean he'll run to the table when called, neatly eat everything he's served, and put his plate in the dishwasher when he's done. Try not to make an issue of little transgressions; all that matters is that mealtimes are pleasant.

He may also be a very picky eater, and have specific preferences when it comes to what he'll eat and how it has to be served, or have periods when he eats only a few foods and refuses to try anything new for a time. Monitor your child's nutrition to ensure he gets enough, but allow for his individual needs and preferences, and don't force him to clean his plate. The "one more bite" battle is one you can't win if your child has decided he's full. The eating habits your child learns now will last a lifetime, and healthy eating habits include eating as much as he feels he needs, not necessarily as much as he's given (of course, you'll be mentoring this behaviour by practising good eating habits yourself, won't you?). His refusal to eat now will seem idyllic in retrospect when he's 15 and vacuuming out your fridge daily.

The Basics: Your Child's Nutritional Needs

Your school-age child's nutritional needs won't change much from when he was a preschooler; only the quantities have changed. He should be eating a balanced diet that consists of foods from all four food groups, and he should have three meals and two snacks every day, at scheduled times. You may not always be able to get him to eat the recommended amount from each food group every day, but if you give him a good variety, he'll probably get what he needs over the course of a week or two. Meals should include at least three food groups, while snacks should include at least two. (For help with planning meals from the Dietitians of Canada, see "Nutrition" in Resources.) Snacks are important for keeping your child's energy up throughout the day, but they should never have more calories than meals, and they should always be nutritious.

According to Canada's Food Guide, children aged four to eight should eat the following number of servings per day:

- **Five servings of fruits and vegetables.** Choose at least one dark green and one orange vegetable or fruit each day.
- **Four servings of grain products.** At least half of those choices should be whole grain.
- **Two servings of milk and milk alternatives.** Dairy products fortified with vitamin D are essential. Milk and some yogurts have vitamin D added to them, but cheeses do not.
- **One serving of meat and meat alternatives.** Choose a variety of lean meats, poultry, and fish, as well as peas, beans, tofu, and eggs.

Use fats and sweets sparingly. Your child's diet should now be like yours when it comes to fat—no more than 35 per cent of his daily intake of calories should come from fat. Limit things like butter, mayonnaise, and salad dressing, and have sweets only occasionally, and after he's eaten other, more nutritious foods.

The best foods to give your child (and yourself, while you're at it) are whole, fresh, and unprocessed—whole grains; fresh produce, dairy, and meats; and home-cooked meals. When you're in the supermarket, show your child how you read ingredients in order to select foods. Keep processed foods to a minimum, but don't refer to them as "bad" foods. No need to make them any more intriguing than they already are! Instead, talk about "everyday" foods and "sometimes" foods. Foods that are high in sugar, salt, or fat, highly processed foods that include dozens of unpronounceable ingredients and that will last on the shelf or in the freezer indefinitely, and fast foods—which epitomize all of the above—can be occasional additions to a meal, not everyday fare.

By the age of five, your child should be getting between 1,200 and 2,000 calories a day, which seems like a huge range, but it will depend on his size and how active he is, and it can vary widely from day to day. Serving sizes for this age group can be very small—as little as ¼ cup of juice or ¼ of a bagel, for example—or nearly adult-size, although portion sizes generally increase with age. You can control *what* your child eats, but you should let him control *how much* he eats. The amount he eats is influenced by the amount he grows, not vice versa. If he's going through a growth spurt, he will be hungrier and will choose to eat more. Despite what your grandmother told you, he won't grow to be big and strong if you force him to eat more. He probably will grow—just not in the right direction.

Don't worry if your child doesn't seem to be eating enough. If he is on track in terms of weight and size, he's probably getting what he needs. Above all, don't convey your fears about food and eating to your child. If you're constantly hovering and cajoling at mealtime, he's likely to dig in his heels even more. Children are influenced by talk about dieting at a younger age than you might think, so be careful that you're not sending the message that dieting is a normal and necessary aspect of eating. If your child learns proper eating habits young, he may never have to worry about dieting.

MAKE A NOTE, MAKE AN APPOINTMENT, OR GO TO THE HOSPITAL?

If you feel that your child really isn't eating enough, or is eating too much, **make a note** to mention it to his doctor at the next appointment.

Limiting sugar and fat

Honey, molasses, syrups, raw sugar, and refined brown and white sugars all have similar caloric content and promote tooth decay, which is the main danger of eating too much sugar. Artificial sweeteners are not good alternatives for children, so don't use them as a way to avoid sugar. Instead, limit candy and junk food, and also limit fast foods, which can contain sugars in unlikely places. If your child wants something sweet, teach her to opt for fruit (but not fruit juice) by keeping it on hand instead of junk food and by making that choice yourself.

Some fat is necessary in a child's diet, but it should come from foods with healthy, unsaturated fats, like those in fish and in vegetable oils such as canola and olive oil. Minimize saturated fats and avoid trans fats, which are produced when foods are processed and have been shown to be harmful to heart health. Read the labels of processed foods carefully to check for these fats. Serve high-fat salad dressing, mayonnaise, butter, and soft margarine in small amounts. Limit fried foods and processed meats, such as wieners and luncheon meats, which are also high in nitrates.

Getting enough fibre

Dietary fibre—the part of the plant that is not digested—is an important part of a child's diet. There are two types of fibre, and each has a specific role. Insoluble fibre, found mainly in wheat bran, vegetables, and the peels of fruits and vegetables, promotes regular bowel movements and may reduce the incidence of some cancers. Soluble fibre, found mainly in fruit, oat products, and beans, helps to regulate blood sugar levels and bowel movements. A general rule for the number of grams of fibre your child needs daily is her age plus five. Children who eat according to Canada's Food Guide will get the fibre they need, but to ensure your meals include enough fibre, choose whole grain breads, pasta, and rice over their white equivalents, buy cereals with 4 to 6 grams of fibre per serving, and serve fruits and vegetables with their skins on, after washing them thoroughly.

What to drink

When your child is thirsty, the best thing you can offer her is water. Despite its perennial popularity, children don't need to drink juice—which should come as a relief on laundry day. If you do offer her juice, however, only give her 100 per cent fruit juice, and limit it to no more than 125 to 175 millilitres (4 to 6 ounces) a day. Avoid fruit cocktails or drinks that contain added sugar and water but little or no real juice. Never give her pop, coffee, or energy drinks.

Your school-age child needs 500 millilitres (16 ounces) of milk a day to meet her vitamin D requirements. Be careful not to exceed 625 to 750 millilitres (20 to 24 ounces) of milk daily, as too much milk can fill up her small stomach and prevent her from eating other nutritious foods. She also needs 800 milligrams of calcium every day, which she can get from three servings of dairy products.

Dealing with a Picky Eater

Many children go through stages when they refuse to eat certain foods, are easily distracted at mealtimes, or eat very little. If your child refuses certain foods or entire meals, let him make the choice, but don't get roped into making a snack 15 minutes after lunch. Stick to the rule that the kitchen doesn't reopen until it's time for the next snack or meal. You may have to deal with some crankiness, but don't give in or worry that you're neglecting your child. He'll be more than ready to eat when the next meal comes around.

MAKE A NOTE, MAKE AN APPOINTMENT, OR GO TO THE HOSPITAL?

If your child is refusing most foods, **make a note** to mention it to his doctor at his next appointment.

You can encourage a reluctant child to eat by including at least one thing on the table that he is sure to enjoy, like his favourite vegetable. He will also be more likely to eat if he helped make the meal, so get him to do something simple like tear up lettuce for salad. Make food more intriguing by cutting it into interesting shapes (heart-shaped sandwiches, perhaps), or serving raw (or cooked, if that's his current foible) fruits or vegetables with yogurt dip. Eliminate distractions by turning off the television and banning toys at the table. You should also watch how you talk about food in front of him. If he hears you discuss your aversions or your dieting habits, he'll pick up on the fact that it's normal for adults to dislike certain foods and not eat healthy meals—which, of course, it is, but he doesn't need to know that yet.

Pica

Children often put strange things in their mouths, but when they eat non-food materials like paper or dirt on a regular basis, it's a condition called pica. Though pica is not well understood, it may indicate that some nutrient is lacking in a child's diet, or that the child is craving attention. Consumption of some materials may not be harmful, but the tendency itself often reflects an underlying problem, such as iron deficiency anemia.

MAKE A NOTE, MAKE AN APPOINTMENT, OR GO TO THE HOSPITAL?

If your child has regularly been eating a non-food substance for a month, **make an appointment** with his doctor to assess his behaviour. The doctor may order some blood tests.

Food Safety Issues

Food poisoning is a common affliction for both adults and children, but is especially dangerous for young children, and can sometimes lead to complications. Bacteria thrive in moist, warm mediums, and can double in number every 15 minutes when food is between 4°C and 60°C (40°F and 140°F). To avoid serving food contaminated by bacteria, you only need to take a few simple precautions.

Only buy food that complies with government and local health regulations, which means that you should not buy home-canned food like homemade jams and pickles, or unpasteurized juice, milk, or cheese. Purchasing safe food is only part of the solution, however. How you store and prepare it is also vital. Don't pack your refrigerator full to bursting; store food so that air can circulate around shelves and walls. Keep the temperature at or below 4°C (40°F), heed best-before dates, and follow guidelines about the length of time a food can be safely stored. In the pantry, keep the temperature cool, at about 18°C (64°F). Store food in clean metal, glass, or hard plastic containers that are rodent- and insect-proof. Avoid containers and bottles that are made with bisphenol A, also known as BPA. (For information on BPA, see "Product Safety" in Resources for the Health Canada website.) Keep track of when you buy foods, and use the "FIFO" system: first in, first out. Keep the cupboards dry, and repair any holes or cracks.

When you prepare meals, wash raw fruit and vegetables well before serving, and wash the tops of cans before opening. Thaw frozen foods in the refrigerator or microwave rather than at room temperature. Cook hamburger meat and chicken until they are no longer pink, and cook eggs until both yolks and whites are firm. Serve perishable foods immediately after preparing them or refrigerate them until mealtime. Cover and refrigerate leftovers immediately following the meal, and use them within three days.

Using a microwave

A microwave oven can be a lifesaver when you have a hungry child. However, because microwaves heat unevenly, they can cause dangerous hot spots in food, so use the low to medium setting for short intervals. Stir and test any reheated food thoroughly before offering it to your child, and if you are heating more than one kind of food, test the temperature of each separately. Only heat food in containers and wraps labelled as microwave safe—disposable plastic or polystyrene containers can release toxic substances into food. Remember that food may be hot even though its container feels cool, so check it carefully. Wipe up food spills in the microwave immediately to prevent microbial growth.

INJURY PREVENTION

Your child is becoming increasingly strong and agile—a wonderful thing to experience, but a whole new challenge when it comes to child-proofing your home. She's able to open drawers and cupboards she could never reach before, and childproof caps and latches may no longer be infallible. Now's the time to check your home again, making extra sure that chemicals, medicines, and hazardous objects are well out of reach, and that the phone number for Poison Control is next to every phone in your home. It's also a good time to teach your child some key safety lessons. Make sure that she knows her full name, her address, and her phone number, and teach her how to dial 911 in an emergency. If she takes a bus to school, teach her how to get on and off safely. She should stand five big steps back from where the bus will stop, and should watch for traffic before she leaves the curb or the bus. Remind her that she must sit still in her seat while the bus is moving.

Of course, her improved agility doesn't mean that she won't take a tumble now and then. In fact, her ability to do more will encourage her to push her limits, which makes this the prime time for playground injuries like cuts, scrapes, bruises, and bumps. It also means she'll be playing in the water and taking part in sports that require safety equipment. Creating a safe environment for living and playing means giving your child an environment where she is free to explore without getting hurt, and where she is encouraged to grow into her own unique person. Knowing how to prepare her for risks great and small and how to soothe her bumps and scrapes will help you feel confident when you send her out the door to play.

Changing to a Booster Seat

Sometime between four and five years of age, and when she weighs at least 18 kilograms (40 pounds), your child will be ready to move from a forward-facing car seat to a booster seat. Booster seats come in both high-back and backless styles, and they must be used until your child is at least eight years old and 1.45 metres (4 feet 9 inches) tall. A booster seat keeps the seat belt in the correct place over your child's body: the shoulder strap flat against her chest (and not touching her neck) and the lap belt low and snug against her hips.

Read the instruction manual to make sure you install your seat properly and you're using the correct seat belt system. Your local police department, fire department, or public health unit may also be able to check that it's installed properly. You can either make an appointment or attend a car seat check event, which are sometimes held at malls and community centres. When you put your child in the seat, use the booster seat's belt-positioning clips, located on the sides of a high-back booster or attached to a special strap on a backless model, to ensure that the shoulder straps sit correctly on your child's torso. Never put the shoulder belt behind her back or under her arm, and never let the lap belt ride up over her stomach, as both positions could cause serious injury in a collision.

Strap your child into her booster seat every time she travels in the car, even for very short trips. Even when your booster seat is empty, keep it buckled up so it doesn't move around. If your vehicle is in a crash, replace the booster seat, even if there was no one in it at the time. It's also ready to be replaced when it reaches its expiry date or, if there is no expiry date, when the seat is 10 years old.

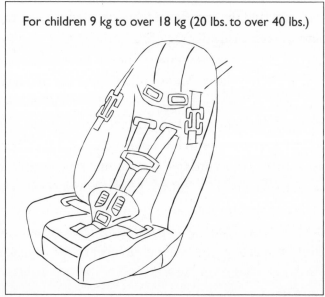

For children 9 kg to over 18 kg (20 lbs. to over 40 lbs.)

Figure 5.1: Combination child/ booster seat

Source: *Child Safety Seats*, Alberta Infrastructure and Transportation. Revised May 2003.

Air bags can expand at 322 kilometres (200 miles) an hour, so they can be deadly to children, who have weaker back, neck, and stomach muscles than adults. Their heads are also bigger in relation to their bodies, so it's more difficult for them to remain upright in a collision, putting them in danger of taking the blunt force of the air bag. According to the law, your child must ride in the back seat until the age of 12 years, and preferably in the middle of the seat, which is the safest place in the car because it is well away from air bags.

Teaching Traffic Safety

Your child deserves as many opportunities to play outside in the fresh air as he can get, but being outside usually means being close to traffic. Parents often think their children can handle traffic safely by themselves before they are actually ready, but children don't have the skills to be safe pedestrians until about age 10. As well as being hindered by physical limitations such as a slower reaction time and a reduced field of vision (one-third narrower than that of adults), children lack the mental maturity and the experience to judge a dangerous situation. They are impetuous and easily distracted, and they aren't able to accurately determine where a sound is coming from or how far away a vehicle is and how fast it is travelling. Many children assume that if they can see a vehicle, the driver can see them, which may be unlikely since they're small and easily hidden by parked cars and street furniture.

To protect your child until he is old enough to handle traffic on his own, have him play in traffic-free areas as much as possible, and closely supervise him when he's around any kind of traffic until he's at least 10 years old. Traffic doesn't just include roads and streets; he should also be watched while around footpaths, parking lots, driveways, and unfenced yards. The best way to protect your child near traffic is to hold his hand securely. If your hands are full, have him hold on to a stroller, your bag, or your clothing. Try not to relate holding your hand with punishment, which can be a challenge if you often need to rein in a rambunctious child. Make up for any negative associations by encouraging and praising him whenever he holds your hand.

As much as you may want him to avoid traffic until he is mature enough to handle it, getting lots of experience will help keep your child safe. Go for frequent walks together and practise crossing the street. Spend some time walking a bit behind him so he can experience being a pedestrian on his own. Talk to him about pedestrian safety whenever you're in traffic, even if you're in the car. Ask him what the traffic lights and signs mean, and why pedestrians must stop at the curb and watch for the walk light or look both ways before crossing the street. Listen critically to his responses, though. Just because he can repeat the rules doesn't mean he understands how to put them into practice.

One of the most important ways you can teach your child to be safe in traffic is to set a good example. Your child will imitate you, especially your bad behaviour, so never jaywalk, even on a deserted street. He should also be aware of how traffic works when he is in a vehicle, so watch for pedestrians at crosswalks and corners when you are driving, and obey all traffic rules when you ride a bike...while wearing your seat belt or helmet, of course.

Dr. Sacks Says

How often have you seen a mom crossing a busy street in the middle of the block with a child in tow? Is the minute saved really worth teaching your child a terribly dangerous lesson?

Helmets

One of the most thrilling events of childhood is the day you learn to ride a bike. As quintessential as that moment is, however, precariously balancing on two wheels still involves its share of spills. According to Safe Kids Canada, head injuries are the cause of most serious injuries and fatalities to children playing on wheeled vehicles, but a helmet significantly reduces the risk of serious head injury while biking. When your child is riding a bike or taking part in any number of other sports, like in-line skating, skateboarding, riding a scooter, ice skating, skiing, snowboarding, or horseback riding, the single most important safety precaution you can take is to make sure she wears a helmet. The best way to encourage your child to wear a helmet is to wear one yourself when you're riding, skating, or skiing with her.

Dr. Sacks Says

Make it a rule: no helmet, no wheels.

Different helmets are designed for different sports, but your child will probably only need two helmets: a bike helmet and a hockey helmet. A bike helmet is also appropriate for in-line skating and scooters. Bike helmets are single-impact helmets, which means that once they've been in a hard fall, they must be replaced. Hockey helmets should be used for ice skating, and can also protect your child when she is tobogganing. They are multi-impact helmets designed to last through several falls. Your child's helmet wardrobe can get complicated if she wants to try skateboarding, skiing, and snowboarding. Sports that involve more backwards falls require helmets that protect the back of the head, but these helmets may not be appropriate for biking, which involves more forward falls. Multi-sport helmets are designed to meet the standards of more than one activity, but they may not cover all your needs, so read the label. (See "Injury Prevention" in Resources for up-to-date information on helmet use from Safe Kids Canada.)

Figure 5.2: CSA International certification mark

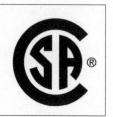

Any helmet you buy should have a certification mark from CSA International, CPSC (Consumer Product Safety Commission), ASTM (American Society for Testing and Materials), or Snell. In Canada, hockey helmets must have a CSA mark. When you buy a helmet, take your child to the store so she can try on different ones. For maximum protection, a helmet must fit properly, and it should be lightweight so your child's head and neck can support it. It should sit comfortably around her head (not on top of it) without falling over her ears and eyes—the distance between the front of her helmet and her eyebrows should be two of her finger widths. The straps should go in front of and behind her ears, and should fasten snugly under her chin. Never use a second-hand helmet unless you know its history, as it may have been in a crash, and you may not be able to tell how old it is. Replace helmets when they're older than five years, as the plastic becomes brittle with age.

Pool Safety

Children love water, so a backyard pool is an irresistible attraction in summer. Water is extremely dangerous for children, though, so if you have a backyard pool, you must take precautions to ensure the enclosure is secure, and be extra diligent about childproofing your yard and supervising your child. Your pool should be surrounded by a four-sided fence (do not use your house as one side of the fence) that is at least 1.25 metres (4 feet) high, with gaps no wider than 7.5 centimetres (3 inches). A rigid, motorized pool cover can add another measure of safety, but keep water from collecting on the top of the cover, as even a small puddle can pose a danger to young children. If you have an above-ground pool, remove and lock up the ladder when the pool is not in use.

Inside the house, all windows and doors that lead outside should be latched. Many drownings happen when children wander out of an unlocked door while parents are distracted. You can also purchase a pool alarm (the kind that detects underwater movement is best) and child safety wristbands, which sound an alarm when they get wet. If your house has an alarm, set it to beep every time a door is opened.

The Canadian Paediatric Society recommends that children be at least four years old before taking formal swimming lessons, so now is a good time to take an adult/child swim class, where you both can learn about water safety. However, even if your child has taken swimming lessons, and may even be able to swim, she still needs to be constantly supervised when she's in or around water. Until she's six, an adult must stay right beside her at all times when she is in the water. (In fact, there's no age when swimming alone is safe—even adults should have someone else nearby.) For extra protection, put a life jacket on your child. Most important, never let your guard down when it comes to pool safety. Alarms, fences, and life jackets are essential, but they must be combined with your vigilance.

Play Injuries

There's no way around it: no matter where it occurs or how closely it's supervised, playtime will inevitably result in the occasional cut, scrape, bruise, or bump. Most of these injuries will be superficial, and your child will often be back in the game in a minute or two, so try not to react immediately. If he isn't crying or seriously hurt, a flurry of hugs and hysterical questions will only upset him. A few simple guidelines are all you need to deal with minor injuries.

Cuts and scrapes

When your child has a scrape or cut that needs obvious attention, wash your hands well and examine it. If it's bleeding, apply direct pressure with a clean towel or bandage for 10 minutes. After the bleeding stops, check for glass, stones, or any other debris in the cut, and wash it out with cool running water or use tweezers to extract the foreign matter. Wash the wound well with soap and warm water, pat it dry, and apply a little bit of antibacterial ointment, which may help reduce the risk of infection and will help prevent bandages from sticking to the wound.

Small cuts and scrapes may heal better when left unbandaged, so leave it open to the air unless it's in an area that is used constantly, like the palm of the hand. Deep cuts should be bandaged, and the bandage should be changed daily or whenever it gets wet, until the cut is no longer raw or open. If your child is in pain, you can give him ibuprofen or acetaminophen (but never aspirin).

MAKE A NOTE, MAKE AN APPOINTMENT, OR GO TO THE HOSPITAL?

If your child's cut bleeds continuosly and significantly for more than a few minutes, even if it's a minor cut, or if his wound is red, swollen, or has pus, or if the area is warm to the touch, it could be infected, so **make an appointment** to see his doctor.

Take your child to the hospital immediately if

▷ the bleeding doesn't stop after 10 minutes of direct pressure;
▷ the wound contains debris that you can't (or don't think you should try to) remove;

> ▷ you think the wound might need stitches (see "Does my child need stitches?" below);
> ▷ your child has been bitten by an animal or other child, and the skin is broken; or
> ▷ the wound is on his face, as even small facial wounds can cause scarring.

Does my child need stitches?

A wound that is stitched or glued properly leaves much less visible scarring. For best results, stitches should be administered within eight hours of the injury. Your child may need stitches if his cut is open or has jagged edges, it is in an area that stretches with movement, like the palm of the hand, or it is deep or more than half an inch long, as there may be some damage to underlying muscles, nerves, or tendons.

MAKE A NOTE, MAKE AN APPOINTMENT, OR GO TO THE HOSPITAL?

If you think your child needs stitches, if you are not sure about the severity of his cut, or if he won't let you examine it, **take him to the hospital.**

Bruises

Bruises start when small blood vessels near the skin's surface get bumped and rupture. Blood seeps into the skin, turning it black and blue. As the bruise heals, the body starts to reabsorb the blood, and the skin turns green or yellow. Some children are more prone to bruising than others, and bruises show up more visibly on children with fair skin, but almost all children will get the occasional bruise. To treat the initial pain, you can ice the area for 15-minute periods a few times during the first 48 hours, and give your child ibuprofen or acetaminophen according to package directions if it is needed.

MAKE A NOTE, MAKE AN APPOINTMENT, OR GO TO THE HOSPITAL?

Most bruises heal on their own within a couple of weeks, but you should **make an appointment** to see your child's doctor if

▷ the bruise is on a large joint, such as the knee or elbow, and your child is having difficulty using the limb or refuses to use it;

▷ the bruise was the result of a serious fall (from a bike, for example) or another traumatic event, which may have caused other less obvious injuries;

▷ significant pain continues for more than 24 hours;

▷ the bruise doesn't fade within 14 days;

▷ your child bruises very frequently, and his bruises are accompanied by nosebleeds or bleeding gums, which may indicate a medical problem; or

▷ he has unexplained bruising on an area of his body other than his limbs. If you have any concerns about his safety while at daycare or anywhere else, talk to his doctor.

Black eyes

Although it may look frightening, a black eye is just a type of bruise, and should be treated the same way as all bruises: with ice and, if necessary, pain relief. Forehead bumps often turn into black eyes, so treat them immediately with ice to reduce the swelling that may appear around the eye the next day.

MAKE A NOTE, MAKE AN APPOINTMENT, OR GO TO THE HOSPITAL?

It's important to rule out an eye injury, so if your child has impaired vision, if he is unable to move his eye in all directions, or if there is blood in the white of his eye, **take him to the hospital immediately.**

Make an appointment to see his doctor if his black eye has not faded within two weeks.

Head injuries

When children play, they fall, and when they fall, they often hit their heads. Most of the time your child will probably stand up, cry for a minute or two and rub her head, then be right back on the jungle gym. In most cases, head lumps without any other symptoms can just be watched to ensure they heal. Applying ice for a few 15-minute intervals and giving her ibuprofen or acetaminophen can help with the pain.

MAKE A NOTE, MAKE AN APPOINTMENT, OR GO TO THE HOSPITAL?

Make an appointment to see your child's doctor if, within a day or two of a fall, she has a lingering headache or is light headed.

Take her to the hospital immediately if she

▷ is unconscious for any length of time;
▷ vomits after a fall;
▷ has blood or pinkish fluid draining from her ears or nose;

> ◦ is unusually sleepy;
> ◦ has a severe headache;
> ◦ has slurred speech or blurred vision;
> ◦ won't stop crying or screaming;
> ◦ has weakness or coordination problems; or
> ◦ has convulsions.

Concussions

A concussion is a brain injury that affects memory and thought processes for a short time. It can be caused by a blow to the head or neck, like a hit from a ball or puck, or by anything that suddenly jars her head, like a fall. Your child doesn't need to lose consciousness after the injury to have a concussion. The symptoms may include headaches, dizziness, ringing in the ears, blurred or lost vision, sleepiness, and nausea. Someone who has had a concussion will also be confused, and may not know what day it is, where she is, or what happened before the injury. Signs to look for if you think your child has had a concussion are poor coordination or balance, a blank stare, crossed eyes or pupils of unequal size, persistent vomiting, excessive sleepiness, slurred speech, and delayed response when you ask her questions.

MAKE A NOTE, MAKE AN APPOINTMENT, OR GO TO THE HOSPITAL?

If you think your child has a concussion, **take her to the hospital** as soon as possible, or if she's unconscious, call an ambulance and do not move her or remove her sports equipment, such as a helmet.

After your child has had a concussion, she should not be left alone. Follow the instructions given to you by the hospital, and check on her during the night, as problems caused by a head injury can get worse later in the day and at night. If you are concerned about how she's breathing or sleeping, wake her up.

MAKE A NOTE, MAKE AN APPOINTMENT, OR GO TO THE HOSPITAL?

If your child has been diagnosed with a concussion and is recuperating, **take her to the hospital immediately** if you can't wake her up, if she has a seizure, or if her symptoms recur, don't improve, or get worse.

The signs and symptoms of concussion usually last for 7 to 10 days, but they may last much longer, especially if your child has had a concussion before. The most important treatment for a concussion is rest. If your child resumes her normal activities before she is completely better, she is more likely to get worse and to have symptoms longer. Once she is completely better at rest, she can gradually increase her activity level, but see her doctor first to ensure that she is healed.

ooooo

Parenting is all about letting go, and this is never more obvious than when she goes off to "big school." Even though she'll be spending a great deal of time away from you, she will benefit from the understanding you've given her of what makes her safe, healthy, and happy. The lessons you've learned and passed on to your child in her first five years will continue to apply for the next fifteen, and as always, most of the teaching you provide throughout her life will be done by setting a good example for her. Parenting is a lifetime job, and sometimes one of the most challenging, but the rewards of helping a child develop into a happy, unique individual cannot be put into words.

Common Illnesses

Your child will experience numerous and varied illnesses throughout her childhood as a result of being out in the world, exposed to other children, but she'll likely get through them unscathed. Immunization will help protect her from many serious illnesses (see page 95 in Chapter Two for information on immunization). However, some minor illnesses, like colds and pinkeye, run rampant through daycare and school on a regular basis, and there's little you can do to prevent them. Fortunately, there's also little to be concerned about when they do strike, so all you really need to know is how to recognize them, what to do to keep your child as comfortable as possible when she is ill, and when you should seek help. For the latest information on common illnesses, check the Canadian Paediatric Society's Caring for Kids website, www.caringforkids. cps.ca, and see "Health" in Resources for other reliable sources. For more information on serious illnesses and conditions, see "Cerebral Palsy," "Diseases and Conditions," and "Special Needs" in Resources.

INCLUDED IN THIS CHAPTER

WHAT TO WATCH FOR

You know your child well, so you'll probably be able to tell when something isn't quite right. However, it helps to be alert for certain signs so that you can tackle illnesses and infections early. Knowing your child's usual activity level, eating patterns, and behaviour will help you sense when all is not right.

SIGNS AND SYMPTOMS OF INFECTION

‣ Unusual behaviour (lethargy, sleepiness, loss of appetite, irritability, persistent crying)

‣ A runny nose

‣ Coughing

‣ Difficulty breathing

‣ Vomiting

‣ Diarrhea

‣ Change in skin colour (paleness, jaundice)

‣ Rash

‣ Fever

Fever

One of the most common symptoms of infection is fever. It is also the symptom that most frequently causes parents to overreact, but a fever alone is rarely cause for concern, and it will usually go away after 48 hours as the infection subsides. A fever in itself will not hurt your child, but it may be symptomatic of something serious, so you should carefully observe your child and watch for other symptoms she may have along with a fever. The exception is babies younger than six months—they should see a doctor when they have a fever. The height of a fever does not tell you how serious her illness is—her behaviour is usually a better indication. If she has an appetite and is relatively active, it's unlikely that the illness is serious.

FEVER TEMPERATURES

Your child has a fever when her body temperature is higher than normal, but "normal" varies for each part of the body. Fever is defined as a temperature above

- 38.0°C (100.4°F) by rectum or ear;
- 37.3°C (99.1°F) by armpit; and
- 37.5°C (99.5°F) by mouth.

Take your child's temperature if she seems ill or is complaining of pain. If you do need to talk to a doctor, this information will help the doctor discuss the illness with you. The most accurate way to take a child's temperature is by the rectum, but for some not-so-mysterious reason many children aren't keen to have their temperature taken this way. (Would you?) Although taking a temperature under the armpit or by ear isn't as precise, it should at least let you know whether your child has a fever. Don't take your child's temperature by mouth until she is over five years old because it's too hard for her to hold the thermometer under her tongue for the requisite minute. Never use a mercury thermometer, in case it breaks. Instead, use a digital thermometer made of non-breakable plastic, and wash it with cool, soapy water before and after each use. Fever strips are very inaccurate, so they are not recommended.

Temperature-taking methods

Rectum

To take a rectal temperature with a digital thermometer, first clean the thermometer with cool, soapy water and rinse. Cover the silver tip with plenty of petroleum jelly. Place your child on her back with her knees bent. Gently insert the thermometer in the rectum to about 2.5 centimetres (1 inch), holding it in place with your fingers. After about one minute, you will hear a beep. Remove the thermometer and read the temperature. A normal rectal temperature is between 36.6°C and 38.0°C (97.9°F to 100.4°F). Clean the thermometer thoroughly when you're done.

Armpit (Axillary)

Use either a rectal or an oral thermometer to take an axillary temperature. Clean the thermometer, and place the tip in the centre of your child's armpit. Make sure her arm is tucked snugly against her body. Leave the thermometer in place for about one minute, until you hear a beep. Remove the thermometer and read the temperature. A normal axillary temperature is between 34.7°C and 37.3°C (94.5°F and 99.1°F).

Ear (Tympanic)

Though quick to use, the tympanic method can produce temperature readings that are too low, even when you follow the thermometer manufacturer's directions, not to mention that the thermometers are expensive. The tympanic method should not be used under two years of age.

To take a tympanic temperature, after cleaning the thermometer, gently pull your child's ear back to straighten the ear canal. Insert the thermometer until the canal is fully sealed off. Hold the button down for one second, then remove the thermometer and read the temperature. A normal tympanic temperature is between 35.8°C and 38.0°C (96.4°F and 100.4°F).

Treating a fever

Children over six months old can be treated for fever at home. Keep your child comfortable and give her plenty of fluids. Remove extra blankets and clothing so heat can leave her body, helping to lower her body temperature. Be careful not to take off too much clothing, though; you want her to be cool, not cold. Do not sponge your child with lukewarm water or give her an alcohol bath or a rub, as these do not effectively lower body temperature.

NEVER GIVE ASPIRIN (ACETYLSALICYLIC ACID OR ASA) TO A CHILD OR TEENAGER WITH A FEVER.

If the fever is due to chickenpox, influenza, or certain other viral infections, aspirin can increase the risk of Reye's syndrome, a serious condition that damages the brain and liver.

You don't always need to give your child medication for a fever, as it only reduces her temperature for a couple of hours at a time, but it may make her more comfortable. Acetaminophen and ibuprofen are the best medications for lowering a fever. Unless your doctor says otherwise, give the dose recommended on the package until your child's temperature comes down. Only give your child ibuprofen if she is over six months old. Do not give your child acetaminophen and ibuprofen at the same time.

MAKE A NOTE, MAKE AN APPOINTMENT, OR GO TO THE HOSPITAL?

A fever *rarely* warrants a trip to the hospital. **Make an appointment** to see your child's doctor if your child

▹ has a fever higher than 39°C (102°F) and is acting ill;

▹ has had a fever for more than 72 hours;

▹ is excessively cranky, fussy, or irritable; or

▹ is persistently wheezing or coughing.

If your child is younger than six months old and has a fever, **take her to the hospital immediately.**

If she is older than six months, **take her to the hospital** if she

▹ is feeding weakly or not at all;

▹ is dehydrated;

▹ is excessively sleepy, lethargic, or unresponsive;

▹ loses consciousness;

▹ has a stiff neck;

▹ has a quickly spreading purple or dark red rash; or

▹ cries inconsolably or very weakly.

Febrile seizures

If your child has a very high fever (over 39.0°C/102.0°F), it can occasionally cause a seizure—an episode in which she may twitch, drool, roll her eyes, and stiffen her limbs. The seizure can last anywhere from a few seconds to several minutes. While they are terrifying to watch, febrile seizures are almost always harmless and do no damage to a child. They are surprisingly common, though. Between the ages of six months and five years, 2 to 5 per cent of children will have a febrile seizure, and a third of those will have more than one. Most will outgrow this response to fever by six years of age.

Febrile seizures are often the first sign of fever, so they really can't be prevented. If your child has a seizure, simply place her on her side (in case she vomits) and allow the seizure to run its course. Try to keep track of how long the seizure lasts by counting the seconds out loud so you can tell the doctor afterward.

MAKE A NOTE, MAKE AN APPOINTMENT, OR GO TO THE HOSPITAL?

If a seizure lasts longer than five minutes or if your child turns blue or has difficulty breathing, **call 911** immediately. No matter how long the seizure, **make an appointment** to take your child to the doctor afterward just to make sure the seizure wasn't caused by an infection or some other problem.

COMMON GASTROINTESTINAL ILLNESSES

Illness	Symptoms	How it spreads	What you can do
Constipation	· Infrequent, painful bowel movements · Stomach cramps · Hard, dry stool, sometimes with blood on the surface	· It is not contagious	· Increase the amount of dietary fibre your child eats by serving more raw fruits and vegetables, whole grains, and legumes. · If necessary, give a mild children's laxative. · Your child can keep going to daycare or school.
Stomach flu (gastroenteritis)	· Diarrhea and/or vomiting · Fever · Loss of appetite · Stomach cramps · Blood/mucus in bowel movements	· Direct contact · Indirect contact with germs on hands, toys, or other objects	· Give acetaminophen or ibuprofen for fever. · Give frequent small feeds. · Use an oral rehydration solution to prevent dehydration. · Keep your child home from daycare or school until her diarrhea stops.
Pinworms	· Itchiness around the anus and vagina, especially at night	· Direct contact · Indirect contact with toys, toilet seats, clothes, or bedding	· Make an appointment with your child's doctor. · The doctor will give you a test kit. · Wash pyjamas, underwear, and bedding in hot water. · Your child can keep going to daycare or school.

Source: Adapted from www.caringforkids.cps.ca.

Constipation

Babies often appear to have difficult bowel movements, but straining and struggling is normal when they are learning about their reflexes and how to control their developing muscles. A baby is constipated only if he has hard, dry stool. When a young child is constipated, his bowel movements are infrequent and painful, he may have stomach cramps, and his stool will be hard and dry, sometimes with bright red blood on the surface.

Some drugs may cause constipation, but it is usually the result of either dietary problems or withheld bowel movements. If your child drinks a lot of milk or juice, he will feel too full to eat foods that help his bowels work well. A diet with not enough roughage like whole grains, fruits, and vegetables can cause constipation, as can a diet with too much dairy. A child may withhold bowel movements when he is toilet learning and is afraid to use the potty, or he may withhold if he has a painful tear (fissure) around the anus. Exercise helps the bowels function, so a child can also become constipated if he doesn't get enough physical activity.

To keep your child's bowels functioning normally, make sure he drinks plenty of fluids, especially water. Instead of giving him fruit juice, give him whole fruit, which has fibre. Other foods that are high in fibre are vegetables, whole-grain breads and cereals, and legumes (split peas, soy, and lentils). He should be drinking milk and eating dairy products in amounts appropriate for his age. Children who depend on the bottle for their nutritional needs without getting any solids often become constipated. After 12 months of age, he shouldn't have more than 3 cups (750 millilitres/24 ounces) of dairy products per day. Children between two and eight years need only 2 cups (500 millilitres/16 ounces) of milk per day.

Another important way to avoid constipation is to try to keep toilet learning a stress-free experience. Don't pressure him into toilet learning—let him set the pace. If he's worried about using the potty, he may hold back bowel movements. He may also avoid eating, which will only make the problem worse, and may eventually lead to chronic constipation. Try to get your child used to a regular daily toilet routine, and make sure he has firm support for his feet to make it easier to push.

Because there's such a wide range of normal, it's important that you check your child's diaper, taking note of the frequency and consistency of his bowel movements, to get a sense of what is normal for him. If you notice a change early, you can deal with constipation before it becomes a problem. Do what you can with diet, and make sure he is able to go to the toilet comfortably. You can give him a mild children's laxative if necessary, but if you find the problem hasn't been resolved after a few doses, talk to your child's doctor.

MAKE A NOTE, MAKE AN APPOINTMENT, OR GO TO THE HOSPITAL?

Make an appointment to see your child's doctor if

▷ you find that you need to give your child a laxative more than a few times to treat his constipation;

▷ your child has stool leakage or staining in his underwear or diaper, as this may be a sign of severe constipation (the doctor will prescribe stronger laxatives to clear the excess buildup); or

▷ there is blood spotting when you wipe him, as he may have an anal fissure. The doctor may prescribe stool softener or an ointment, as well as an increase in fibre in his diet.

Make a note to mention it to your child's doctor at his next appointment if your child has regular bowel movements but his stool is hard. Ask the doctor for dietary advice.

Diarrhea

Diarrhea is a very common problem in childhood. It's usually mild and brief, but it can sometimes have severe consequences, especially for infants. A child has diarrhea if he has more bowel movements than usual, and if stools are less formed and more watery than usual. Acute diarrhea, usually caused by gastroenteritis (or "stomach flu"), lasts less than one week. During this time, you can treat your child by keeping him well hydrated. Giving him an oral rehydration solution (ORS) can help him stay hydrated. Because diapers are so absorbent now, you may not be able to tell if he has urinated, so check the amount of moisture in his mouth and look for tears in his eyes. Watch to see that he is not listless. Do not give your child an over-the-counter medication unless instructed by the doctor.

There are many possible causes of diarrhea. Usually, it's caused by a virus, but less often it is caused by bacteria. The most common causes are viruses such as rotavirus, which can't be treated with antibiotics; parasites like giardia; bacteria such as campylobacter, salmonella, shigella, and E. coli; and food poisoning. Some bacterial diarrhea can be treated with antibiotics, but children will often get better on their own before the bacteria are identified.

Diarrhea germs are easily spread from person to person, and especially from child to child. They spread readily among children who have not learned how to properly use the toilet. The spread of the infection can be reduced if adults and children wash their hands carefully after every diaper change and going to the toilet, and before preparing and eating food (see "Washing Hands" on page 362 for proper techniques). Safe food handling is another important factor in preventing diarrhea (see page 310 in Chapter Five).

MYTH BUSTERS

Myth: The flu shot prevents the stomach flu.

Fact: The flu shot prevents influenza, which is a respiratory infection. It does not prevent stomach flu.

—Dr. Krista Baerg, MD, FRCPC

Rotavirus

Rotavirus is the most common cause of acute diarrhea in babies and young children. It usually affects children between the ages of six months and two years. Rotavirus illness starts between 12 hours and four days after being exposed to the germ. The first signs are usually a high fever (39°C/102°F) and vomiting. Within 12 to 24 hours, children start to pass large amounts of watery diarrhea. The illness usually lasts three to seven days.

When children have rotavirus, their stool contains large numbers of the germs. Rotavirus can spread directly (for example, by handling a contaminated diaper and not washing your hands properly) or indirectly (by handling a toy that has germs on it). Outbreaks of rotavirus in Canada usually happen in the winter and spring, between December and May. A vaccine to prevent rotavirus is available in Canada.

Giardia

Giardia is a parasite that is common in daycare centres, especially where children are in diapers. It affects children differently; some may have no symptoms, while others will. Symptoms include diarrhea, stomach cramps, gas, loss of appetite, and even weight loss. It is spread when someone comes in contact with the infected stool and touches other objects that children then place in their mouths. It can be prevented by thoroughly washing hands after changing a diaper or helping a child go to the toilet (or going to the toilet yourself, of course).

A child may have the giardia parasite in his stool and not have any symptoms; if so, no treatment is necessary. If your child is sick, however, his doctor will prescribe a drug to treat the infection, of which your child must take the full course to prevent the infection from recurring. The doctor may need to take stool samples from different days to confirm that your child has giardia. As with all diarrheal illness, small, frequent feedings of something easily digestible, like oral rehydration solution (ORS), is the most important treatment. He should stay home from daycare while his diarrhea persists.

Dehydration

When sick children have diarrhea or vomit, they can lose large amounts of bodily fluids, which are made up of water and salts, and become dehydrated very quickly. Dehydration can be very dangerous, especially for babies. Infants and children can die if they are not treated. To avoid dehydration, a child with diarrhea should continue to drink an appropriate quantity of appropriate fluids—not water, soup, or homemade concoctions, but oral rehydration solutions (ORS) found in the pharmacy.

MAKE A NOTE, MAKE AN APPOINTMENT, OR GO TO THE HOSPITAL?

Take your child to the hospital immediately if he has any of the following signs of dehydration.

▷ He is very listless.
▷ He has fewer than four wet diapers in 24 hours.
▷ He is thirstier than normal.
▷ He has no tears when he cries.

> ▸ He has dry skin and a dry mouth and tongue.
> ▸ He has sunken eyes.
> ▸ His skin is greyish in colour.
> ▸ He has a sunken fontanel (the soft spot on his forehead, if he is younger than 18 months).
> ▸ He has persistent vomiting and cannot hold even a small amount of fluids down after four to six hours.

If you are breastfeeding, keep feeding as usual. If your child is eating solid foods, offer him the foods he usually eats. If you are formula feeding, try giving your baby an ORS and withholding formula and food for 24 hours or so. If he refuses the ORS and is not vomiting, continue formula feeding (you don't need to dilute the formula), and offer him the food he normally eats.

Oral rehydration solutions

Oral rehydration solutions can help keep children well hydrated when their diarrhea is serious, and replenish fluids when they show signs of mild dehydration. They are precise mixtures of water, salt, and sugar that can be absorbed by the body even when a child is vomiting. They are available at pharmacies in ready-to-serve preparations, frozen pops, and powders. Although powders are cheaper and more convenient to store, they have to be mixed very carefully to work properly, so it's best to buy an ORS that has already been mixed.

If your baby is not breastfeeding or formula feeding well, give him small amounts of ORS often, gradually increasing the amount until he can drink normally. The amount and frequency depends on his age and weight, but the following table gives a good guideline for the first four hours.

Amount of oral rehydration solution to give your child

Age	Amount to give per hour
6 months and under	30 to 90 millilitres (1 to 3 ounces)
Between 6 months and 24 months	90 to 125 millilitres (3 to 4 ounces)
Over 24 months	125 to 250 millilitres (4 to 8 ounces)

If your child refuses ORS by cup or bottle, give the solution using a medicine dropper, a small teaspoon, or a frozen pop. If your child vomits, you may need to stop giving him food and drink, but continue to give ORS using a spoon. Give 15 millilitres (1 tablespoon) every 10 to 15 minutes until vomiting stops, then increase the amounts gradually until your child is able to drink the regular amounts.

MAKE A NOTE, MAKE AN APPOINTMENT, OR GO TO THE HOSPITAL?

If your child is still vomiting after four to six hours, **take him to the hospital.**

After four hours and up to 24 hours (the recovery stage), keep giving your child ORS according to package directions until his diarrhea is less frequent. When vomiting decreases, start him breastfeeding or drinking formula as usual, or eating regular food in small, frequent feedings. After one or two days, he can resume his normal diet. The number of stools may increase at first (one or two more than usual each day), and it may take a week or more for stools to become completely formed, but this is part of the normal healing process.

Foods to avoid

If your child is sick and has frequent diarrhea, do not give him plain water. Drinking only water may lead to low blood sugar or low sodium levels in your child's blood. Do not make your own ORS or give your child sugary drinks such as fruit juice, sweetened fruit drinks, carbonated drinks, sweetened tea, broth, or rice water. These have the wrong amounts of water, salt, and sugar, and they can actually make his diarrhea worse. Too much fruit juice can also cause diarrhea—known as "toddler's diarrhea"—so if you do give your child juice (although you really don't need to), limit it to 125 to 175 millilitres (4 to 6 ounces) a day.

MAKE A NOTE, MAKE AN APPOINTMENT, OR GO TO THE HOSPITAL?

Make an appointment to see your child's doctor if your child is younger than six months and has diarrhea, or if he

▷ has diarrhea for more than a week;
▷ has a fever with diarrhea; or
▷ continues to refuse his normal diet after the diarrhea subsides.

Take your child to the hospital immediately if he is listless, has bloody or black stools, or has signs of dehydration (see the "Make a Note, Make an Appointment, or Go to the Hospital?" box" on page 339).

Pinworms

Pinworms are whitish-grey, threadlike worms that cause itching and irritation around the anus, and in girls they can irritate the vulva and the vagina, often causing a lot of pain during the night. For information on treatment and prevention, see page 303 in Chapter Five.

COMMON RESPIRATORY ILLNESSES

Illness	Symptoms	How it spreads	What you can do
Common cold	· Runny nose · Sneezing · Coughing · Sore throat · Headache · Sometimes fever, but it usually isn't very high	· Direct contact · Indirect contact with germs from the nose or mouth (on hands, toys, tissues, etc.) · Droplet transmission (when a child coughs or sneezes and droplets reach other children who are close by)	· Offer fluids and plenty of rest. · Give acetaminophen or ibuprofen for fever. · To clear nasal congestion, try a bulb syringe and saline nose drops. · Use a cool mist humidifier. · Gargling with salt water will help ease a sore throat.
Croup	· Hoarse voice and barking cough · Rapid, laboured, or noisy breathing · Fever		· If symptoms continue or worsen, make an appointment with your child's doctor. · If your child has a cold, he can keep going to daycare or school if he feels well enough to take part in activities.
Influenza	· Fever · Chills · Cough · Headache · Muscle pain		· If your child has the flu or croup, keep him home from daycare or school until the fever is gone and he feels well enough to take part in activities. If he has laboured breathing, take him to the hospital.
Strep throat	· Fever · Sore throat · Swollen, tender neck glands		· Make an appointment with your child's doctor to get a throat swab. · Strep throat is treated with an antibiotic. · Keep your child home from daycare or school until she has taken the antibiotic for at least one full day.

(continued)

(continued)

Illness	Symptoms	How it spreads	What you can do
Ear infection	· Crankiness or fussiness · Trouble sleeping · Tugging at ears · Fluid draining from the ear	· May be caused by a respiratory infection, but is not contagious	· Make an appointment with your child's doctor. · An antibiotic may be needed. · Your child can keep going to daycare or school.
Pinkeye (conjunctivitis)	· Scratchy feeling or pain in the eyes · Watery or pussy discharge from the eyes · Whites of the eyes are pink or red	· Direct contact · Indirect contact with germs on hands, tissues, washcloths, etc.	· Keep eyes clean, and wipe from inside out. Use a clean cloth each time. · Make an appointment with your child's doctor. · If your child's eyes have pussy discharge, he should stay home from daycare or school until he's been treated with warm-water compresses and antibiotics for 24 hours.

Source: Adapted from www.caringforkids.cps.ca.

Colds

Your child will get many, many colds, sometimes as many as 8 to 10 each year, especially if she's in daycare. Come the winter, it may seem like she always has a cold. Colds tend to be more common in fall and winter because your child spends more time indoors and in closer contact with others, and because the cold outdoor air and dry indoor heating dry out her mucus membranes and make her more susceptible to viruses. Young children have more colds than older children and adults because they haven't built up immunity to the more than 100 different cold viruses that are around. Once you've had a cold virus, you become immune to that virus, and that's why children get fewer colds as they get older. By the time they start school, children who attended daycare will have fewer colds than other children.

Cold viruses are found in the nose and throat. Because children often touch their noses, eyes, and mouths, put things in their mouths, and touch each other during play, cold germs spread easily when they touch their runny noses or mouths or when they cough or sneeze, and then touch other objects or people. The typical symptoms are a runny nose, nasal congestion, sneezing, coughing, and a mild sore throat. Some children may not want to eat, they may have a headache, or they may be more tired than usual. Colds can sometimes cause fever, but the fever usually isn't very high. Colds usually last about a week, but can last for as long as two weeks.

MYTH BUSTERS

Myth: You can catch a cold if you get chilled or wet.

Fact: Researchers actually had volunteers sit on ice to test this theory, but it turned out to be false. Colds are actually caused by viruses that infect the nose, throat, and sinuses.

—*Dr. Krista Baerg, MD, FRCPC*

Since there's no cure for the cold, keep your child comfortable for the week or two it will take her to get over it—and get her ready for the next one. Over-the-counter cough and cold medicines aren't effective and should not be given to children under six years of age. Besides, coughing helps clear mucus from the chest, so it may be annoying, but it serves a purpose. Colds cannot be treated with antibiotics; antibiotics are used only when children develop complications, such as an ear infection or pneumonia. (See the Caring for Kids website at www.caringforkids.cps.ca for up-to-date information on antibiotics from the Canadian Paediatric Society.)

Make sure your child stays hydrated and gets plenty of rest. If she doesn't want to eat, offer her plenty of fluids and small, nutritious meals. Monitor her temperature—it's fine to give her acetaminophen or ibuprofen (but not aspirin) to lower her fever if she's uncomfortable. If she is having trouble feeding because of a stuffed nose, saline nose drops or spray (not medicated drops) can help, but do not use them more than three or four times in a day. A rubber suction bulb can also clear mucus from the nose. A cool mist humidifier may make a child with a stuffy nose more comfortable, although a hot-water vaporizer shouldn't be used because of the risk of burns. (Clean and dry the humidifier regularly to prevent mould from growing.) Your child can continue her normal activities if she feels well enough to do so, and can even continue to play outside in winter. If she has a fever or complications such as an ear infection, she may need a few days of rest at home.

The best way to reduce the spread of colds is to wash hands, both yours and your child's. If you can, keep babies under three months old away from people with colds. Avoid sharing toys that children place in their mouths until the toys have been cleaned. Teach your child to avoid spreading a cold by covering her nose and mouth with tissues or her sleeve when she sneezes or coughs, by throwing out tissues right away, and by washing her hands after wiping her nose or handling tissues.

Make sure your child has received all of the recommended immunizations (see page 95 in Chapter Two for information on immunization). While they won't prevent colds, they will help prevent some of the complications, such as bacterial infections of the ears or lungs. Influenza vaccine protects against the flu but not against other viruses.

Dr. Sacks Says

Taking your child to the doctor for a cold may only increase her risk of catching one there!

Cold, allergies, flu, or more serious?

Not sure what the runny nose, sneezing, and congestion really mean? Colds are most likely to occur between November and April, but allergies tend to show up in the spring, summer, and early fall. A child with allergies will likely have itchy, watery eyes and a runny nose, but the mucus coming out of her nose will continue to run clear, instead of thickening and turning yellow or green as it tends to in children with colds.

The influenza (flu) virus strikes more quickly than a cold, may be accompanied by vomiting or diarrhea, and causes high fever, coughs, and body aches. While children with colds usually have energy to play and keep up their daily routines, children with the flu feel sicker and usually stay in bed.

Some respiratory viruses that cause colds in older children and adults may cause illnesses that are more serious when they infect infants and young toddlers. This is because young children can become dehydrated more quickly than older children can if they aren't taking in enough fluids, and because very young immune systems have trouble containing infections. Some illnesses, including croup (hoarseness, noisy breathing, barking cough) and bronchiolitis (wheezing, difficulty breathing), can resemble a cold at the start, but are caused by specific viruses and may require treatment.

If a child gets many colds, it's not a sign that she has a weak immune system; it just means she's exposed to many viruses. The only reason to have a child's immune system tested is if her colds frequently lead to more serious problems, like frequent pneumonia.

Croup

Croup is a viral infection of the throat and vocal cords, or larynx. It often begins like a cold, but then fever, cough, and difficulty breathing develop. For information on treatment, see page 251 in Chapter Four.

MAKE A NOTE, MAKE AN APPOINTMENT, OR GO TO THE HOSPITAL?

Children of all ages should see a doctor if a cold seems to be causing serious problems. **Make an appointment** to see your child's doctor if

▷ your child also has a fever (see "Fever" on page 329);

▷ you think she might have an ear infection (she is cranky, is vomiting, has an earache, has pus draining from her ear, and has a high fever that begins several days after the start of a cold);

▷ she is much sleepier than usual, doesn't want to feed or play, or is very cranky or fussy and cannot be comforted;

▷ she has thick or discoloured (yellow or green) discharge from her nose for more than 10 to 14 days;

▷ she wakes in the morning with one or both eyes stuck shut with dried yellow pus (although red eyes and watery discharge are common with a cold, pus is a sign of an eye infection and should be treated); or

▷ her cough worsens and she's wheezing. These symptoms could be a sign of pneumonia or respiratory syncytial virus (RSV), a relatively common but potentially serious respiratory illness in babies under 12 months.

Take your child to the hospital immediately if

▷ she is having trouble breathing, or is breathing very rapidly and seems to be working hard to breathe;

▷ her lips look blue;

▷ she is coughing so badly that she is choking or vomiting;

▷ she is refusing to drink, or has been vomiting for more than four to six hours;

▷ she is listless; or

▷ she is wheezing severely

▷ she is gasping

Ear Infections

Most children will have had an ear infection by the age of three. The most common childhood ear infections affect the middle ear. Fluid and bacteria normally drain away from that area through the Eustachian tube, which connects the middle ear to the back of the nose and throat. If the Eustachian tube becomes blocked when your child has a cold or allergies, the fluid stays trapped in the middle ear. Bacteria multiply there and cause swelling around the eardrum, which in turn causes pain. Doctors diagnose ear infections by checking the eardrum for redness and swelling and for decreased movement of the tympanic membrane.

Babies are susceptible to ear infections because their Eustachian tubes are short (only about half an inch long) and horizontal, so when they have a cold or the sniffles, the fluid is unable to drain properly. As they get older, the tubes lengthen and become more vertical, making ear infections much less common.

A middle ear infection often occurs after another illness, such as a cold. Along with the usual symptoms of a cold, a child with an ear infection will often (but not always) have earaches, be cranky or fussy, have trouble sleeping, and tug or pull at her ear, and she may not respond to quiet sounds. Other less common symptoms are fluid draining from her ear, loss of balance, and a fever after a few days of a cold.

Middle ear infections in children younger than two years of age are usually treated with antibiotics. However, new research suggests that for many ear infections, "watchful waiting" is all you need to do. Most ear infections are not serious and will heal well. When antibiotics are prescribed to treat bacterial ear infections, your doctor will choose one that is specific for the type of bacteria causing the infection. Sometimes antibiotic ear drops can clear an external ear canal infection, and some specific types can even alleviate a middle ear infection. Most children feel better within the first two or three days after starting an antibiotic, but to cure the infection, they must take all the medication prescribed. Your child may need to return for another examination so that the doctor can see whether the infection has cleared.

Sometimes fluid may stay in the middle ear for up to six weeks after the infection has cleared, causing temporary hearing loss. Usually, the fluid drains on its own and hearing improves without additional medical treatment. In the meantime, your child could develop another ear infection and require further treatment. In children younger than three years of age, speech and language development could be delayed if fluid remains in their ear for more than several months and causes hearing loss. Children with this problem, or who have chronic ear infections, may be candidates for a tympanostomy, a procedure in which a tube is inserted through the eardrum and into the middle ear to drain the fluid. This operation is the most common surgical procedure in North America on children under four years of age. The decision to operate needs to be carefully considered by the parents, the child's doctor, and an ear, nose and throat specialist who sees many children with recurrent ear infections.

Although most ear infections are caused by colds, other factors can make them more frequent, such as allergies, exposure to cigarette smoke, attending daycare, using a pacifier too frequently, and bottle-feeding while lying down. The risk factors you can control—smoking, excessive pacifier use, and bottle-feeding while lying down—should be eliminated as soon as possible. One way to reduce the chance of ear infections is to vaccinate your child against pneumococcus, one of the most common bacteria that can cause ear infections. The vaccination is actually for pneumococcal meningitis, but it also appears to reduce the incidence of pneumococcal ear infections. However, the vaccine will not prevent all ear infections.

MAKE A NOTE, MAKE AN APPOINTMENT, OR GO TO THE HOSPITAL?

If your child is taking antibiotics for an ear infection, **make an appointment** to see her doctor if she

▷ still has an earache after two or three days of treatment;

▷ has a fever over 39°C (102°F), or has a fever that lasts more than three days;

▷ is very sleepy;

▷ is still fussy or cranky; or

▷ isn't hearing well.

Take your child to the hospital immediately if she is listless, breathing quickly, or having trouble breathing.

Influenza

In young children, the symptoms of the flu aren't very different from those for the cold, although there's a greater chance of high fevers in babies. The virus spreads quickly from person to person in crowded places, like daycare and school. The virus is found in the nose and throat, so it usually spreads when children touch their noses, mouths, or eyes and then touch something else, or through sneezing or coughing. Babies may only have a high fever, while young children may have stomach pain, earaches, croup, and even febrile seizures. In school-age children, the flu begins with a sudden fever, chills, head and muscle aches, fatigue, loss of appetite, a cough, and a sore throat.

Influenza outbreaks are most common between November and April, but you can lessen your child's chance of getting the flu by having her immunized. For information on the influenza vaccine, see page 103 in Chapter Two. If your child gets the flu, keep her home from daycare or school until her fever is gone and she is back to her normal activity level, make sure she's comfortable, and let her rest. Give her plenty of fluids so that she stays hydrated, and offer her small, nutritious meals. If she has a fever, you can give her acetaminophen or ibuprofen to control the temperature. The flu should not be treated with antibiotics.

MYTH BUSTERS

Myth: If you get a flu shot, you will get the flu.

Fact: The flu shot will protect your child from the viruses it is designed to treat. It does not protect her from the hundreds of other less dangerous viruses she comes in contact with that may make her mildly ill.

—*Dr. Diane Sacks, MD, FRCPC*

Pinkeye

Pinkeye, also known as conjunctivitis, is an infection that covers the white of the eye and the inside of the eyelid. It starts out feeling scratchy or painful, often with lots of tears. The whites of the eyes are pink or red, and the eyelids can be stuck together in the morning with discharge. There are two kinds: non-purulent pinkeye (most likely caused by a virus), which has clear discharge and little pain, is the most common, and is just allowed to run its course. Purulent pinkeye (caused by bacteria), which has white or yellow discharge, matted or red eyelids, and eye pain, is treated with antibiotic drops or ointment.

Pinkeye is easily spread when infected people touch their eyes and then touch objects or other people, who then touch their own eyes. If the person with pinkeye also has a cold, she can spread it by sneezing or coughing. Sometimes an eye can become pink due to factors other than a virus or bacteria, such as allergies or exposure to irritants like smoke or chemicals.

If your child has purulent pinkeye, she should stay home from daycare or school to avoid infecting others. Her doctor will prescribe antibiotic eye drops or ointment, and after 24 hours of being on antibiotics, she can return to school. Warm compresses, such as a warm, damp cloth placed over the eyes, will help ease the discomfort of both forms of pinkeye. When you wipe discharge from your child's eye, wipe from the inside out, and use a clean part of the cloth each time. Make sure you and your child wash your hands thoroughly every time you touch her eyes. Proper hand-washing is also the key to avoiding pinkeye if someone else has it.

MAKE A NOTE, MAKE AN APPOINTMENT, OR GO TO THE HOSPITAL?

Make an appointment to see your child's doctor if the whites of your child's eyes are pink or red, if she has white or yellow discharge in her eyes, and if she complains that her eyes hurt or feel scratchy. It's not always easy to tell the difference between purulent and non-purulent pinkeye, so if you have any doubt, the doctor should see your child and determine whether she will need antibiotic treatment.

Strep Throat

Strep throat is a bacterial infection that is fairly common in children. It is characterized by a very sore throat, a fever, and swollen, tender neck glands. Your child may also have a headache, stomach ache, nausea, or vomiting. Strep throat is passed by either direct contact with someone's saliva, runny nose, or open sore, or indirect contact when someone sneezes or coughs.

Dr. Sacks Says

Even the most experienced doctor can't always identify strep throat by looking, so make sure your child gets a positive throat swab before being subjected to 10 days of antibiotics.

Strep throat is really hard to diagnose, so your child's doctor should take a throat swab for testing if strep throat is suspected. If it turns out to be strep throat, the doctor will prescribe antibiotics. You will need to keep your child home from school or daycare for 24 hours after she starts the antibiotics, but after that she can return to normal activity if she is feeling well enough. You can ease her sore throat by having her gargle with warm salt water (if she's old enough to know how to gargle). Check that she gets plenty of rest and fluids, and treat her fever with acetaminophen or ibuprofen (not aspirin) if she's uncomfortable.

The best way to prevent the spread of strep throat is to wash your hands and your child's hands thoroughly and regularly. Teach you child to sneeze and cough into a tissue or her sleeve, and to throw out tissues right away.

MAKE A NOTE, MAKE AN APPOINTMENT, OR GO TO THE HOSPITAL?

Make an appointment with your child's doctor if your child has a sore throat, a fever, and a tender neck.

COMMON RASHES AND SKIN INFECTIONS

Illness	Symptoms	How it spreads	What you can do
Cold sore	• Blisters on the lips or in the mouth • May also have a sore throat	• Direct contact with the sore • Indirect contact with infected person's towel, cup, utensils, etc.	• Usually clears up on its own. • Apply ice to the sore or give acetaminophen or ibuprofen to ease discomfort. • Your child can keep going to daycare or school.
Fifth disease	• Red rash on the cheeks spreads over the rest of the body after a couple of days • Child does not feel very ill	• Direct contact • Indirect contact with germs in saliva, on hands, tissues • It's not contagious once the rash appears	• Usually clears up on its own. • Your child can keep going to daycare or school if she feels well enough to take part in activities.
Hand, foot, and mouth disease	• A skin rash that looks like red spots, often with small blisters on top, on the hands and feet (and sometimes other places) • Small, painful ulcers in the mouth • Fever, headache, and sore throat • Loss of appetite • Lack of energy	• Direct contact • Indirect contact with infected person's saliva	• Will clear up on its own. • Make sure your child drinks lots of water. • Your child can keep going to daycare or school if he feels well enough to take part in activities.

(continued)

(continued)

Illness	Symptoms	How it spreads	What you can do
Impetigo	· Red bumps, blisters · Oozing or honey-coloured crusty lesions around the mouth, nose, or exposed skin of the face	· Direct contact with skin of infected person · Indirect contact with germs on clothing, towels, etc.	· Gently wash the infected skin with clean gauze and soap. · Make an appointment with your child's doctor. · Keep your child home from daycare or school until she has taken the antibiotic for at least one full day.
Ringworm	· Ring-shaped rash with a raised edge; is itchy and flaky · If it is on the scalp, there may be bald patches	· Direct contact · Indirect contact with clothing, combs, etc.	· Make an appointment with your child's doctor. · Keep your child home from daycare or school until after he has started treatment.
Roseola	· Initial fever · When fever disappears, a rash appears · Crankiness or fussiness · Rash with small red spots for 1 to 2 days, mainly on the face and body	· Direct contact with saliva of infected person · Not very contagious	· Give acetaminophen or ibuprofen for fever. · Fluids and plenty of rest. · Will clear up on its own. · Your child can keep going to daycare or school if she feels well enough to take part in activities.
Scabies	· A rash that is very itchy and red, especially at night · Rash between the fingers or toes, in the groin area, or around wrists or elbows · In children younger than two, the rash can appear on the head, face, neck, chest, abdomen, and back as white, curvy, threadlike lines, tiny red bumps, or scratch marks	· Direct contact · Indirect contact with clothes or personal items of infected person	· Make an appointment with your child's doctor. · Everyone in your home must be treated. · Wash bedding, clothing, and towels in hot water and dry at the hottest dryer setting. · Store things that can't be washed in an airtight plastic bag for 1 week. · Keep your child home from daycare or school until after he has started treatment.

Source: Adapted from www.caringforkids.cps.ca.

Cold Sores

Cold sores, which are caused by the herpes simplex virus, are small, fluid-filled blisters that appear on or near the lips. A child can contract the virus by sharing a towel, cup, or utensil with an infected person, or by kissing an infected person. Besides blisters, symptoms can also include a sore throat or mouth. The symptoms may cause your child discomfort, or they may be so mild that he barely notices them. They disappear within a week or two, but the virus may remain in his body and reactivate in the future. The blisters can flare up periodically when your child is under stress, has a fever, or is spending a lot of time in the sun, but the other initial symptoms probably won't come back.

Cold sores aren't usually dangerous, but your child can become dehydrated if he refuses to drink because of the pain, and cold sores can cause a serious infection if they spread to his eyes. They can also be dangerous if they spread to a newborn or an immuno-compromised person. If your child has a cold sore, try to keep him from touching his eyes, and make sure he washes his hands regularly with soap and warm water. The cold sore should go away on its own, but in the meantime you can apply ice to it or give your child ibuprofen or acetaminophen (not aspirin) to ease the discomfort. There are medicines on the market that can treat cold sores, but they should only be used on children who get severe outbreaks, and they must be taken in the very early stages of an outbreak.

Fifth Disease

Fifth disease is an infection of the respiratory system that is caused by a virus called parvovirus B19. It is most commonly seen in preschool and school-age children, and spreads the same way as a cold does: on the hands of someone who has the infection, on something that has been touched by someone who has the infection, or in the air after an infected person has sneezed. At least 50 per cent of children will get fifth disease, but once they've had it they won't get it again.

Fifth disease is also known as "slapped cheeks syndrome" because the infection starts as a very red rash on the cheeks, making the face look like it has been slapped. One to four days later, a red, lace-like rash appears, first on the arms, and then on the rest of the body. The rash may last from one to three weeks and may be accompanied by fever. The illness is often very mild in children, and they may not even feel sick. Adults usually get a more severe case, with fever and painful joints.

The infection is highly contagious, but most children are no longer contagious by the time the rash appears, so your child may continue attending daycare or school if he feels well enough to take part in the activities. The disease is not dangerous, but pregnant women and people with certain types of anemia need closer supervision.

There is no vaccine to prevent the infection and no medication to treat it, and since it's a viral illness, antibiotics will not help. Much like a cold, you just need to let the virus run its course. Fluids, lots of rest, and acetaminophen or ibuprofen (not aspirin) for fever or discomfort are all the treatment that is necessary.

Hand, Foot, and Mouth Disease

Hand, foot, and mouth disease (HFMD) is a viral infection that usually occurs in the summer and fall. It can affect people at any age, but is most likely to affect young children. HFMD is usually not a severe illness, and children recover in a week to 10 days without treatment, but the mouth sores are often quite painful. It may be a full-time job getting your child to drink enough to stay hydrated. Symptoms of HFMD include fever, headache, sore throat, loss of appetite, lack of energy, a rash, and small, painful ulcers in the mouth. The rash consists of red spots, often topped by small blisters. It usually appears on the hands and feet, but can affect other parts of the body as well.

The virus that causes the infection is found in saliva and spreads like a cold, from person to person through the air or by touch. Your child can have the virus in his body for about 10 to 14 days before getting sick, and he may be contagious for one or two weeks after. There is no treatment for the infection, and because it's a virus, antibiotics won't help.

If someone in your child's class or daycare has HFMD, watch your child for symptoms. Make sure everyone in your home washes their hands before preparing food and after wiping their noses, changing a diaper, and using the toilet. If symptoms appear, just make sure your child is comfortable, drinking lots of fluids, and eating normally. Avoid spicy or acidic foods if he has ulcers in his mouth. If he feels well enough, he can still go to daycare or school.

MAKE A NOTE, MAKE AN APPOINTMENT, OR GO TO THE HOSPITAL?

Make an appointment to see your child's doctor if your child has HFMD and refuses to drink enough to be well hydrated.

Impetigo

Impetigo is a highly contagious bacterial infection that is very common among children, and occurs when bacteria enters the skin through a cut or scrape. It causes blisters that can appear as red clusters filled with fluid, or larger ulcer-like sores. For information on treatment, see page 301 in Chapter Five.

Ringworm

Ringworm, or tinea, is a skin infection caused by a fungus. The infection causes an itchy, flaky rash that may have a ring-shape with a raised edge, and may cause an area of baldness if it's on the scalp. For information on treatment, see page 301 in Chapter Five.

Roseola

Roseola is a common infection in young children: most often in children between 6 and 24 months old, and rarely in children under 4 months or over four years. Children with roseola have a high fever, but are otherwise more cranky than ill for the first three to five days. Because of the high fever, some children who are prone to febrile seizures may have one with this infection (see "Febrile Seizures" on page 333). When the fever clears, a rash of small red spots on the face and body will take its place. The rash lasts anywhere from a few hours to two days. However, roseola is contagious before the rash appears, and spreads through close contact with saliva, either by sneezing, coughing, or touching, so make sure everyone in your home is washing their hands regularly and thoroughly.

Dr. Sacks Says

The very worst part of roseola is the irritability that accompanies the virus.

There is no treatment for roseola; all you need to do is let it play out. Give your child acetaminophen or ibuprofen (not aspirin) to lower his fever. If he feels well enough to continue normal activities, he can still attend daycare.

> ## MAKE A NOTE, MAKE AN APPOINTMENT, OR GO TO THE HOSPITAL?
>
> **Make an appointment** to see your child's doctor if your child has had a febrile seizure, if he has had a fever for more than 72 hours, or if he is younger than six months old and has a fever.

Scabies

Scabies is caused by mites that burrow under the skin—a nasty thought and a very, very itchy condition, but not particularly harmful. Mites do not carry disease, nor do they mean that your child is dirty. However, they cause a rash that is extremely itchy and red, especially at night. The rash usually appears between fingers and toes, in the groin area, and around wrists or elbows, although it can appear in other places too. In children under two years of age, it appears as white, threadlike lines, tiny red bumps, or scratch marks.

Scabies is passed when you touch someone who has it, or you touch their clothes or other personal items after they have touched them, as the mites can live for three days off of people. If one person has scabies, everyone else in your home may need to be treated at the same time. You will also have to wash your child's bed linens, towels, and clothing in hot water and dry them in a dryer at the hottest setting to kill the mites. Anything that can't be washed can be stored in an airtight plastic bag for a week.

The doctor will prescribe a cream or lotion, and you may have to do two treatments, one week apart. After you have applied the first treatment, your child can return to school. He may be itchy for a few weeks after being treated, but that doesn't mean the mites have come back.

MAKE A NOTE, MAKE AN APPOINTMENT, OR GO TO THE HOSPITAL?

Make an appointment to see your child's doctor if you think your child has scabies.

PREVENTING AND CONTROLLING INFECTION

Good hygiene—especially proper hand-washing—is the key to controlling the spread of germs. Of course you and your child are going to get the occasional cold, but you can minimize the chance that it will decimate everyone in the family, office, and daycare if you wash your hands properly, especially after diapering and helping your child use the toilet, and clean up a bit around your home.

Washing Hands

Proper hand-washing is the most important and most effective thing you can do to prevent infection and stop it from spreading. The moment you finish washing your hands you start to collect germs again by opening doors, wiping faces, playing with toys, and changing diapers. You cannot avoid collecting germs, but you can reduce the chance of infecting others by knowing when to wash.

Whether they are visibly dirty or not, wash your hands before cooking, eating, feeding your child (including breastfeeding), and giving medication. Wash your hands after changing a diaper, helping your child to use the toilet, using the toilet yourself, taking care of a sick child, handling pets or animals, cleaning pet cages or litter boxes, wiping or blowing your own or your child's nose, and preparing food. Teach your child to wash her hands before eating and drinking, before and after playing in the water, after playing outside or with clay or sand, after touching animals, after she has her diaper changed or she uses the potty, and after sneezing, coughing, or wiping her nose. Also, teach her to sneeze into her sleeve when she doesn't have a tissue. Although there is no specific evidence, using a small amount of hand sanitizer when away from home should be useful in a pinch.

You've been doing it for decades, but have you been doing it correctly? To properly wash your hands, you don't need hot water. Friction is what really gets your hands clean. Turn on the taps and get your hands wet from wrist to finger tips. Use a mild liquid soap; not an antibacterial soap, which kills good bacteria as well as bad, or a bar soap, which can carry germs from other users. Lather well for 10 to 15 seconds, rubbing your hands together and making sure to wash the backs of your hands and between your fingers. Rinse your hands under running water for 5 to 10 seconds. If you are in a public washroom and can't turn off the taps with your elbows, use a paper towel. Dry your hands, and use hand lotion if your hands are dry, as cracks in your skin can trap germs.

How to wash your hands

Step 1	Wet your hands under running water.
Step 2	Scrub your hands with soap for 10 to 15 seconds.
Step 3	Rinse your hands under running water for 5 to 10 seconds.
Step 4	Dry your hands with a clean towel.

While your child is too young to use the sink, wash her hands with a wet cloth and soap. Rinse them, and dry them with a towel. Toddlers can be taught to wash their own hands, but try to make it fun and relaxed. Hands should be washed for 15 to 30 seconds, so sing the alphabet with your child while she washes her hands.

How to wash your child's hands

Step 1	With a warm, damp, soapy cloth, wipe your child's hands, scrubbing gently.
Step 2	Using another warm, wet cloth, wipe the soap off your child's hands.
Step 3	Dry your child's hands with a clean towel.

When water and soap are not available, use premoistened hand wipes or alcohol-based hand rubs. To use a hand rub, put about half a teaspoon in your hand and rub your hands together, making sure you cover the backs of your hands, between your fingers, and down to your wrists. Rub for about 10 to 15 seconds, until your hands are dry. If your hands are visibly dirty, use a paper towel or hand wipe to remove as much dirt as you can first, use the rub, and then remove any residue with another paper towel or hand wipe. When using rubs on your child's hands, put the rub in your own palm and rub it on her hands between yours. Keep hand rubs out of the reach of children because they may be harmful if swallowed. They are also flammable, so make sure to thoroughly dry your child's hands and your own when done.

Dr. Sacks Says

Children love to mimic the adults around them using hand sanitizer.

Diaper and Toilet Routines

When you are changing your child's diaper or helping her go to the toilet, follow practices that will keep germs from spreading. Never change your child's diaper or put her potty in an area where food is prepared. However, you may find that diapering "on the run" becomes a common pitfall, so try to only diaper your child on a dedicated diapering surface and well away from the kitchen and dining room. Wash your hands and your child's hands thoroughly after every diaper change or trip to the potty.

Before you change your baby's diaper, have all the supplies you'll need handy. Remove the diaper, fold it closed, and place it well out of her reach. Clean her bottom from front to back with a warm, damp cloth, and only use soap if you need it to wash off stool. Dry her well by patting instead of rubbing. Only use diaper cream or a paste of petroleum jelly and cornstarch if she has redness or a diaper rash. Keep one hand on her at all times as you put on a new diaper so she doesn't fall. Wash your hands and your child's hands, then move your baby to a safe place. Dispose of the dirty diaper right away in a sealed container, and wash your hands again. It's a good idea to disinfect the diaper-changing surface every once in a while with a mild bleach solution (1 part bleach to 100 parts water), rinse the surface well, and then allow it to air dry.

Dr. Sacks Says

Diapering a young child must qualify parents for the cattle-roping competition in the rodeo.

When you help your child use the toilet, remove her diaper first and sit her on the potty or toilet. Wipe her from front to back, and if using the toilet, flush it. Diaper her and help her to dress, then wash your hands and hers as well. If using a potty, carefully empty it into the toilet without splashing, then rinse the potty and carefully empty the rinse water into the toilet. Wipe the potty clean with toilet paper and flush the paper down the toilet. And, of course, wash your hands again. Once again, disinfect the potty from time to time with a mild bleach solution, rinse, and let it air dry.

Cleaning

Keeping a clean home may seem impossible when you're chasing a toddler around all day, but it can minimize the spread of germs, helping everyone in the home to stay healthy. Kitchens and bathrooms should be cleaned regularly and even disinfected. Cleaning means removing all the visible dirt with a household cleaner and a cloth. Friction removes most germs, so wipe or scrub surfaces, then disinfect with a mild bleach solution (1 part bleach to 100 parts water), leaving it on the surface for two minutes. Wear rubber gloves when disinfecting, and store all cleaning products in a locked cupboard well out of your child's reach.

Toys will get very dirty and germy in the course of play, so it helps to buy toys that are easily washable in hot, soapy water, the dishwasher, or the laundry. If you have a wading pool, empty, clean, and disinfect it after each use. Sandboxes are irresistible to children, but they're also irresistible to animals and bacteria. When your sandbox is not in use, keep toys inside your home, and cover the box with screening or mesh, which will keep animals out but allow air to circulate and sun to kill the bacteria. Rake the sand every once in a while to aerate it and help the process. If an animal does get into the sandbox (or your child doesn't make it to the toilet in time), empty the sandbox, throw the sand out, clean and disinfect the sandbox, and allow it to air dry before filling it with new sand. If there's only urine in the sand, rake the sand to aerate it, and leave it in the sunlight for a couple of days before letting your child use it again.

Because children spend a lot of time on the floor, whether they're crawling and exploring or just playing, it's important to keep the floors clean. Minimize the amount of dirt that comes into your home by making everyone remove their shoes at the door (or at least trying). Sweep, vacuum, and mop floors regularly, and don't forget to dust too!

GIVING MEDICATION TO YOUR SICK CHILD

Using medications safely means knowing when they're necessary and when they're not. Babies under three months of age should never be given medication unless recommended by a doctor. Do not give over-the-counter medication to babies and young children without first talking to a doctor. Many are ineffective, and they may even be harmful. The only exceptions are acetaminophen and ibuprofen for treating fever in children over six months of age. In many cases, non-medicinal treatments take care of the problem. Saline drops clear a stuffy nose, a cool-mist humidifier or vaporizer may also help to loosen congestion, and plenty of clear fluids, like oral rehydration solutions, can help avoid dehydration.

GETTING THE MOST FROM YOUR PHARMACY

If your child's doctor says that medicine is necessary, know how to administer it properly. Ask your doctor or pharmacist the questions below.

- How much, how often, and for how long should the medication be taken?
- How should it be stored?
- Are there any special instructions, like whether it should be taken with food?
- What are the common side effects or reactions?
- Does it interfere with other medications?
- What happens if your child misses a dose?

Your pharmacist is a valuable part of your healthcare team. Stick with the same pharmacy so that all the records of the medications your child has taken will be in one place.

There are various ways to measure and give medication. For babies, a calibrated syringe or a plastic dropper is usually easiest. A regular spoon is not the same as a measuring spoon, so don't use it to measure medication. If the prescribed dose is different from the unit on your syringe or measuring spoon, don't try to convert it. Buy a syringe or measuring spoon with the proper units instead.

Know your measurement abbreviations

Abbreviation		Measurement
tbsp	=	tablespoon
tsp	=	teaspoon
oz	=	ounce
ml (or mL)	=	millilitre
mg	=	milligram

Getting Children to Take Medication

Getting a child to open wide and take his medicine can sometimes be a monumental accomplishment. There are some tricks you can use, though, and none of them involve a spoonful of sugar. Before you give your child medication, let him know a few minutes in advance so he can finish whatever he's doing. Give him his medication somewhere quiet and comfortable, away from distraction. Be honest and matter-of-fact about what will happen. Tell him what you're going to do just before you do it, be straightforward if he asks why he's taking it, and explain to him how it might taste or feel. Don't tell him it's candy, as he may be tempted to find it on his own and accidentally overdose—just say that it might have a fruit flavour (but only if it's true). If he takes his medicine, be sure to praise him; if not, wait 15 minutes and try again.

When you're giving medication, have everything you'll need—measurement container, medication, glass of water, tissues—in place before you start, and wash your hands first. Read the label to check the correct dose, and measure the dose with the right container. When you've given the medication, wash the measuring container and your hands.

If using a syringe, try squirting the medication into the inside of your child's cheek; there are no bitter taste buds there, as there are on the back of the tongue. Be careful storing them, as some syringes have a small plastic cap on the end that can be a choking hazard. Always store medication syringes with the medication, and out of reach of your child. For babies, you can also get medication dispensers that look like pacifiers. You put the medication into a small measuring cup attached to a pacifier and give it to your baby to suck. The medicine slips past his taste buds, making it more palatable.

Some pharmacists can add flavourings like chocolate, fruit, or bubble gum, along with a sweetener, to make medicines like antibiotics and cough syrup more appealing to children. Only a small amount of flavouring is needed to disguise the taste. While a better taste may be an incentive for a child who has to take medication regularly, some experts say the chemicals in the flavouring may diminish the effectiveness of the drug. Some children may also be sensitive to certain dyes or sweeteners. Ask your doctor or pharmacist for more information about the safety of mixing the medication with a flavouring.

Some medications taste better chilled, or you can try mixing liquid medication with a small amount of soft food, like yogurt or applesauce, or put it in a bottle or sippy cup with a bit of juice. Use only a very small bit of food or liquid because your child may not receive his full dose if he doesn't finish the food or juice. Check with your pharmacist to see if chilling your child's medicine is safe, or to make sure that the medication's effectiveness will not be altered by mixing it with food or liquid.

MAKE A NOTE, MAKE AN APPOINTMENT, OR GO TO THE HOSPITAL?

Make an appointment to see your child's doctor if he has any of the following reactions after taking a medication:

> rash

> hives

> severe pain anywhere in the body

> vomiting or diarrhea

Take your child to the hospital immediately if his face or lips swell, he has trouble breathing, or he starts to wheeze. This may be the sign of an anaphylactic reaction to medication. If his breathing is very laboured, **call 911.**

Safe Medication Use

Most medications are given on an as-needed basis, like when your child needs pain relief. Other medications need to be given exactly as his doctor has prescribed, even if he is feeling better before they are finished. For example, you need to finish all doses of prescribed antibiotics, even after symptoms disappear, to kill bacteria in the body. The infection can return if the antibiotic is stopped too early.

Aspirin given to a child can cause Reye's syndrome, a potentially life-threatening disease that can put a child into a coma. Always read labels because some over-the-counter medications contain aspirin but may call it by other names such as salicylate, acetylsalicylate, or ASA. Aspirin and medications containing salicylates are not appropriate for children except in very specific cases and when supervised by a doctor.

DISPOSING OF MEDICATION

It's important to dispose of unused medication properly so it doesn't end up in curious hands or contaminate the environment. Check if your pharmacy will take back unused or expired medication. Some do and some don't, so call before you go. Your local hazardous-waste facility—the same one that disposes of old paint, batteries, and antifreeze—may also take medications. Again, call and ask. If neither of these options is available, secure the childproof cap, put tape around the bottle or put it into a tightly closed bag, and put it into a garbage can that is not accessible to your children.

Sometimes pharmacists dispense more medication than is necessary in case some spills, is measured incorrectly, or your child spits it out. If you have medication left over after the course of treatment is completed, throw it out, and keep an eye on the expiration dates of any medicine in your cabinet. Never give your child medication that is prescribed for someone else. Even if he has the same condition as the person for whom the medicine was prescribed, he may require a different drug or different dosage.

Both prescription and over-the-counter medications come with a printed sheet of information and instructions. Before administering your child's medication, read all the instructions carefully. If you're not sure about something, don't hesitate to ask a doctor or pharmacist. No question is ever silly when it comes to your child's health.

7

Keeping Your Child Safe

Your child is curious and adventurous by nature. It's how he learns about his world and his place in it, and it's all a part of normal, healthy development. The bumps and bruises that often come with exploration may seem inevitable, but you can keep them minor. Really, there is no such thing as an accident—almost any injury can be prevented. Although this chapter at times may seem to contain a long list of rules and hazards, the main message is that you have control over your child's safety. By taking some basic measures to prevent injuries, you can provide your child with a safer environment in which to play and explore.

Childproofing can go a long way to keeping your child safe, but there's so much you can do to protect your child that it's often hard to know where to start. This chapter gives guidelines for purchasing and using common baby gear and toys, as well as a comprehensive list of childproofing measures. However, childproofing is not infallible, so supervising your child, teaching him about safety, and knowing how to avoid common injuries are also important factors in keeping him safe. For those times when he may hurt himself, your best strategy is to be prepared with a first-aid kit and knowledge of the basic steps you'll need to take to help him, which are also provided here. For additional preparation and confidence, the Canadian Paediatric Society recommends taking courses in first aid and CPR before you your child is born, then taking regular refresher courses to maintain your skills. (See "Injury Prevention" in Resources.)

INCLUDED IN THIS CHAPTER

Dr. Sacks Says

"If only I'd..." is the most unfortunate phrase a parent can say.

TAKING CONTROL OF YOUR CHILD'S SAFETY

When it comes to your child's safety, always keep these three important ideas in mind: anticipate, supervise, and childproof.

1. **Anticipate.** Your child will develop at his own pace, but you must be at least one step ahead of his milestones. Often developments like crawling or grabbing are surprisingly sudden—one minute your child is only able to kick and squirm when he's lying on the carpet, the next he's halfway across the room and headed for the stairs. Cover electrical plugs and install safety gates long before he can crawl, remove breakable or dangerous objects out of reach before he can grab them, and anchor heavy furniture to the wall before he can stand and climb.

   Another thing you can anticipate is *when* your child is most likely to injure himself. Children are most prone to injury late in the afternoon or early in the evening, when they're excited, hungry, or tired, or when they're off their regular routine. Knowing this, you can try to schedule quiet play for the times your child is most injury-prone.

2. **Supervise.** Supervising a young child doesn't mean occasionally glancing up from your book. When your child is active, he can get into trouble in a matter of seconds, so keep an eye on him at all times. You can always read when he's sleeping in his crib (if you're not napping too, of course!). If you have to do something that will take your attention away from him, make sure he's safely in his crib or playpen. A few minutes in a safe, confined place while you make a phone call or use the bathroom can be lifesaving.

3. Childproof. Your child needs to explore and experiment in order to develop, but in a home full of sharp corners and unlocked cupboards, exploration and experimentation can be fraught with peril. Let your child develop freely and fully by giving him a safer environment to play in. Childproofing means taking a look at your home from your child's eye level and anticipating all the trouble he can get into. For a comprehensive list of things you can do to childproof your home, see "Childproofing Checklist" on page 420.

Dr. Sacks Says

Even before your child is born, check each room in the places he will live and play, and redecorate with safety in mind. Style may have to wait.

Teaching Your Child

Children will learn a lot about safety from you, so make sure you model safe behaviour. That means no more jaywalking, no riding a bike without a helmet, and no tossing caution to the wind and going outside without a hat, sunglasses, and sunscreen. Start teaching your child basic rules for staying safe when she's a toddler. Young children love to "remember the rules"—and they're more than happy to point out when you've forgotten them. (Sadly, this enthusiasm for rules won't last.) Remember to praise her when she gets them right.

When she's a preschooler, teach her simple, concrete rules that are easy to follow, and show her some of the specific hazards in her environment. Gradually teach her rules for playing so that she doesn't get the impression you're out to ruin her fun. She doesn't need to know them all at once—and in any case, there's no way she'll remember them all.

Here are some basic rules you can teach your toddler.

- When a caregiver calls your name, immediately stop, look, and listen—stop whatever you're doing, look at the adult, and listen to what the adult tells you.
- After playing with toys, pick them up off the floor so no one trips on them. (Helping her clean up always makes it more fun.)
- If a toy is broken or dirty, bring it to an adult.
- Use the handrail when climbing or going down stairs. (When you're childproofing, check that the handrail is stable.)
- Learn which tap is hot and which tap is cold, and always turn the cold one on first.
- Stay away from things that have hazard symbols on them (corrosive, flammable, explosive, and poison).

Figure 7.1: Hazard symbols

 Corrosive   Flammable   Explosive   Poison

MORE BASIC RULES FOR PLAY

- Always take off your helmet in the playground. A helmet strap can catch on playground equipment.
- Keep your shoes on when playing outside.
- Don't push or shove around play equipment. Wait your turn.

Swings

- Keep away from moving swings.
- Sit in the middle of the swing seat, and hold on with both hands. Don't stand or kneel on the seat.
- Don't jump off a moving swing.

‣ Only one person is allowed on a swing at a time.

‣ Don't push empty swings.

Slides

‣ Don't wear a scarf or any clothing with strings on it when you use the slide.

‣ Wait your turn at the foot of the ladder.

‣ Slide feet first.

‣ Don't slide lying down.

‣ Leave the slide quickly once you reach the bottom.

Climbing structures

‣ Only one person is allowed on one rung or bar at a time.

‣ Use both hands to climb, and grip with your fingers and thumb.

‣ Drop with your knees bent, landing on both feet.

‣ Stay off the climbing structure when it's wet.

Seesaws

‣ Only go on the seesaw if you're four years of age or older.

‣ Sit up straight and face your partner.

‣ Hold on tight with both hands.

‣ Keep your feet out from under the seesaw.

‣ Tell your partner when you want to get off, and get off carefully.

Ride-on toys

‣ Always wear your helmet.

‣ Never go on the road.

‣ Get off the toy before you go down a step or curb.

‣ Keep your hands and feet away from the wheels.

Water play

‣ Never swim without an adult.

‣ Don't run or push others around the water.

‣ No ride-on toys are allowed around the pool.

Winter play

‣ Don't build snow tunnels.

‣ Don't play on roadside snowbanks.

‣ Don't touch metal objects with your mouth in cold weather.

‣ And finally, everyone's favourite: Don't eat yellow snow!

When you begin to teach your preschooler more specific rules, make sure the rules are clear, and try to make them positive and not frightening. Instead of saying "Don't take your skipping rope on the slide, you'll trip over it and hurt yourself," say "Toys stay on the ground when we climb." Enforce rules consistently, and adapt them to your child's developmental stage. Young children can't remember very many rules, so when you have to remind her over and over again, be patient. Praise her when she follows a rule without you having to remind her; if she picks up her toys unprompted, thank her and remind her that now no one will trip on them. When she doesn't follow a rule after you've reminded her, make sure there are consequences—give her a time-out, or have her clean up a mess she's made.

SAFE PLAY

In addition to some small toys and countless books, your child will probably also have one or two large toys. When he's a baby, you may get him an activity centre or bouncy chair to keep him occupied or to soothe him. As he grows, toys such as swing sets and tricycles will be a valuable outlet for his boundless energy and a wonderful incentive to get him to play outside. As always, safety should be your first consideration when you're purchasing and using these toys.

Activity Centres

Stationary activity centres have replaced baby walkers, which are now banned in Canada. An activity centre has a seat that is surrounded by a tray, and often objects such as spinners, mirrors, buttons that play music, and bouncing toys are attached to the tray within reach of the baby. The baby can turn in his seat, bounce, and rock, but the centre stays in one place. Even though your baby can't move the centre, that doesn't mean you should leave him unattended in it, however. Keep the activity centre well away from stairs, plants, bookshelves, curtain cords, and hot surfaces. Don't leave your baby in the centre for more than half an hour, and when he's done, clean the centre and check that the toys aren't broken or loose.

Don't use an activity centre until your baby is four months of age or older, as his neck isn't strong enough yet to control his head. Follow the activity centre's weight and height guidelines, since a baby who is too big for a centre can tip it over and injure his head. **If he can move the centre, he's too big for it**—and that will happen sooner than you think.

Baby Swings and Bouncy Chairs

Baby swings and bouncy chairs are popular because they're an easy, hands-free way to calm down a fussy baby. Your undivided attention is always the best tool for calming your baby, but it doesn't hurt to have a little help. When you buy a swing or chair, make sure it has a strong, stable base and that you follow the age and weight guidelines. Don't buy a swing that has a carrier or bed, as a baby can slide forward against the side of the carrier and suffocate. Put the swing or chair on the floor away from high-activity areas and cords or things he can grab and pull on top of him. Never put a baby swing or bouncy chair on a raised surface such as a table, as the motion can move it over the edge, or other children can push it off.

When you put your baby in the swing or chair, always use the seat belt and crotch strap (unless the swing has a crotch pillar), and secure the harness snugly to keep him in place. In a swing, prop him up so that his head doesn't roll forward and get trapped between the backrest and the bars the seat hangs from. Let it rock or bounce gently, and not too quickly. Don't leave him unattended, and don't leave him in the swing or bouncer for more than 20 minutes. If he falls asleep, take him out of the swing and put him into his crib to sleep.

Ride-on Toys

To be fun and safe, a ride-on toy must be the right size for your child. If it is too small, it can be unstable; if it's too big, it can be hard to control. Children under 12 months of age are too young for all ride-on toys. If your child can walk with some steadiness, he may be able to straddle a ride-on toy and push with his feet, but he is still too young to pedal or steer.

Some ride-on toys tip easily, so test a toy's stability by placing your weight directly on the handlebars or rear of the ride-on toy to see if it flips forward or backward. Toys are more stable if the seat is close to the ground and they have a long wheelbase. Ride-on toys for children aged 12 to 18 months should have four or more recessed wheels, and should be pushed by foot. Straddle toys are easier to steer than ones a child sits inside.

Your child will be ready to learn to pedal when he's around two years old, but he probably won't be able to steer yet. That becomes easier when he's three. When he can steer and pedal, he's ready for a tricycle. A good tricycle should have a low centre of gravity, widely spaced rear wheels with rubber tires, padded handlebars, non-slip pedals and handgrips, and hubcap wheel covers instead of spokes. Keep your child's tricycle inside so it doesn't rust, and check it regularly for loose, missing, or damaged parts.

When your child is using a ride-on toy, follow age, weight, and height specifications. Make sure he can put both feet flat on the ground when sitting in the seat. A child on a wheeled toy can move very quickly, so keep him away from stairways, decks, porches, and swimming pools, and off the driveway or street. Teach him that if he wants to ride his tricycle, he must wear a helmet.

Dr. Sacks Says

It's a real shame that many parents jump over this wonderful tricycle stage and go straight to a bicycle with training wheels. Try a trike! Hold the bike!

Swing Sets

Backyard swing sets and outdoor play centres can be great fun if you're lucky enough to have a spacious backyard. The first precaution you should take is to check that you do have enough room in your yard for the equipment. Buy equipment that is age-appropriate for your child, and always follow the manufacturer's instructions for assembling it. Modifying it can make it less safe. Anchor it securely to the ground, but make sure that pegs are easy to see so that no one trips over them. Tighten all nuts and bolts securely, cover any bolt that extends beyond a nut with an acorn nut or plastic cap, and file down any sharp points or edges. You can buy plastic covers for the swing chains so that your child doesn't pinch his fingers in the chain loops, a minor but ubiquitous swing injury. Adjust the heights of the swings so your child can get on and off safely but can swing his legs under him when he's sitting in the seat. If the equipment doesn't seem stable, it isn't, so don't hesitate to call the customer service number and ask for help.

Maintaining play equipment is as important as putting it together properly, since plastic can become brittle when it's exposed to sun, rain, and cold. Every once in a while, check any parts that hold a child's weight. You can usually buy replacement parts, such as swing seats and ladder rungs, from the retailer or the manufacturer.

COMMON INJURIES

Minor injuries like bumps, scrapes, and bruises are a part of childhood, and are the consequence of your child exploring her environment and being out in the world. If you anticipate, supervise, and childproof, her injuries will stay minor. If you take a first-aid course and have a first-aid kit on hand, you can easily treat her minor injuries. Chapters Two through Five cover many age-specific hazards, so this section addresses the hazards that are most common to all age groups: falls, scalds and burns, near-drowning, and poisoning and choking.

Falls

More kids visit the hospital because of a fall than for any other reason. Falls from diaper-changing tables, staircases, playground equipment, and cribs are still all too common. Crawling, cruising, walking, and running are accomplishments we all celebrate, but they're accompanied by safety hazards you'll need to consider.

Tips for prevention

Birth to 12 months

Your baby can wriggle enough to fall off of something before she is able to crawl or even turn over, so keep a hand on her at all times when you're changing her diaper. Your change table should have a guardrail and be easily accessible storage for supplies. Have everything you'll need assembled before you start so you don't have to go looking for something, and don't even think about answering the phone. That's what voicemail is for.

Never lay your child down anyplace she could fall off of if she rolled over, like the couch. She should always sleep in her crib. Bassinets and cradles are not safe because babies outgrow them quickly and can tip them once they are too big and strong, often by three months. Keep stuffed toys, comforters, and pillows out of your baby's crib and playpen, because once she is able to pull herself up on her feet, she may be able to climb on top of them and fall out. All she really needs in her crib is a light blanket.

A crawling baby can move faster than you think, so keep an eye on her at all times and put gates across all stairways. If your baby uses a stationary activity centre, check the label to make sure it's the right size for her. If she's too big for it, she could move it or tip it over. Keep activity centres, baby swings, bouncy chairs, and infant carriers on the floor, never on a raised surface, and away from high-traffic areas and stairs.

A baby in a swing, infant chair, or car seat should **never** be placed on a raised surface like a tabletop or car trunk. The movement of the swing or chair, or of your squirming baby, can shift it off the surface, or another child or a pet can knock them off. Baby swings and bouncy chairs are meant to be used on the floor. When your baby is in any kind of chair, including high chairs, strap her in securely with the harness provided. Make sure her high chair is sturdy and has a wide and stable base so it won't tip. Keep the high chair away from counters or tables—anything that she could push or pull on and tip the chair over. Never let your child climb or stand up in the high chair. If she's big enough to try to climb out, it's time to switch to a safe booster chair.

Stroller-related injuries usually happen when a child isn't strapped in properly or is left unattended, so always use the safety harness and crotch strap, and never leave a child unattended in a stroller. Never prop the stroller handles against something, such as a chair, to create a sleeping space, and never park a stroller on a sloping surface, such as a driveway or hill. Do not hang bags or other items from a stroller or allow other children to play on it as the extra weight can cause it to tip over. Always remove your baby from the stroller before carrying it up or down stairs and when using an escalator.

12 to 24 months

When your baby is learning to walk, she often can't control her movements very well, and she has a hard time stopping. You might not be able to stop her from bumping into walls or tripping over the cat, but you can pad sharp corners on furniture and fireplace hearths and keep things tidy so there are fewer sharp things for her to fall into or obstacles for her to trip over. Time to put that beautiful glass coffee table into storage.

Make sure that stair safety gates are secure. They should be mounted into the wall at the top and bottom of all staircases, and have vertical bars so your baby can't climb them. Pressure-mounted gates are good between rooms, but should never be used on staircases as they are not as strong as hardware-mounted gates.

Keep all windows and doors locked even when you're home. If you need to have an open window, make sure it opens no more than 10 centimetres (4 inches), or install a guard so that your child won't fall out, even if there's a window screen. Screens do not prevent falls from windows. Move furniture away from windows and railings so your talented climber isn't tempted to use her new skills at the window or on the balcony.

When your baby is in her crib, always raise and lock the crib rail in its highest position. Keep large toys and blankets out of the crib and playpen, and set the crib mattress at its lowest level so she can't climb out. If she's big enough to try, or is 89 centimetres (35 inches) tall, it's time to consider moving her to a toddler bed. A good way to transition into a bed is to have her sleep on her mattress on the floor first.

Two to three years

Once your child is in a toddler bed, there's a chance she can fall out. Buy a bed that's low to the ground and has permanent side rails rather than portable ones. The spaces between the vertical bars of the rails should be no wider than 6 centimetres (2⅜ inches). Children younger than six years should never sleep in the top bunk of a bunk bed. In fact, it's not a good idea to have a bunk bed at all if you have young children in the home since they'll be tempted to climb the ladder.

Falls from playground equipment become more likely once your child is fully mobile. You can help minimize the risk of injury by taking her to playgrounds that have equipment designed for preschoolers, making sure the playground surface is safe (sand, wood chips, pea gravel, or shredded rubber) and that the equipment is in good shape, and watching her at all times when she's playing. You should also stay within arm's reach, as even if the equipment suits your toddler, she may have a hard time going from a standing to a sitting position without losing her balance. Never help her climb to unsafe heights.

Inside the home, put non-slip backing on rugs and mats so they don't trip your running toddler, and clean up any spills right away. Wearing shoes or slippers with non-slip soles, rather than socks alone, can also help prevent a fall. Teach your child to put her toys away when she's done with them so no one trips on them.

Ride-on toys can be falling hazards for toddlers if the toys are too large or too small, or if they tip easily. Make sure the height and weight guidelines are appropriate for your child, and that the ride-ons don't tip when you put your weight on any one point. Don't let your child use them near stairs, decks, pools, and roads. If your child has graduated to a tricycle, make sure it's the right size for her and that she wears a helmet whenever she rides.

Bicycles can be falling hazards even when a parent is at the handlebars. If you want to get a bike carrier for your child, discuss it with a reliable supplier first. Be aware that her weight will make the bike more unstable, so ride carefully. Never put her in the carrier without doing up the harness, and never leave her in the carrier with the bike resting on its kickstand.

Bike trailers are another option for taking your child along on a bike ride, but they can be dangerous if she can lean out. Features that can help avoid injuries in bike trailers include a rotating hitch that will allow the trailer to stay upright even if the bike falls over, a roll cage that will protect your child if the trailer tips, and an internal harness that will keep her from trying to climb out. It's also a good idea to have someone ride behind you to keep an eye on your child whether she's in a carrier or a trailer.

Shopping carts are yet another of the many wheeled devices your child can fall out of if you're not careful. Check that your store's carts have safety straps; talk to the store's manager if they do not. Never allow your child to stand up in the seat, ride in the basket, or cling to the outside of the cart. If you find it too difficult to pay attention to your child when you're at the grocery store, go when it's less crowded, with fewer distractions, or when someone can watch your child at home.

Four to five years

Once your child is four or five, she's much more agile, so she's less likely to trip or run into things. However, she is also faster, and she's likely to be participating in activities that require more skill, like biking or skating. Appropriate helmets are important for making sure that if she does fall, her head is protected. For more information on helmets, see page 316 in Chapter Five.

Helmets are also important for sledding in the winter. Your child must wear a hockey or ski helmet, not a bicycle helmet, when sledding. Choose a slope that is free of trees, isn't too crowded, and isn't near a road. Teach your child to quickly move from the bottom of the hill after her slide and to walk back up the side. Tell her she must sit or kneel on the sled (not lie down), watch out for others before she goes, and slide down the middle of the hill.

It's important to keep older children's toys away from younger children, but it's also important that those toys be easily accessible for older children. If your child has to climb or pull to get her toys, she's likely to fall or pull them down on top of herself. Climbing might also be an issue in the bathroom. If your child can't reach the sink, get her a stool that's sturdy and has a non-slip surface and base.

Running under the sprinkler in summer is one of the simplest joys of childhood, but water can pool on the lawn, creating slippery spots. You can avoid falls by moving the sprinkler regularly or shutting it off until the water has drained away. Water slides are also falling hazards, so make sure children slide in a sitting position only. Avoid trampolines—they aren't safe for children of any age.

STAY AWAY FROM TRAMPOLINES

Despite efforts to make trampolines safe, trampoline-related injuries have nearly doubled since 1990. Even mini-trampolines that are close to the ground are not safe for young children, as falling off a trampoline is not the only cause of injuries. Since their muscles aren't strong enough for them to land correctly when they bounce, young children can injure themselves simply by bouncing on a trampoline. As a result, the Canadian Paediatric Society recommends that parents do not buy trampolines or allow their children to play on them. For more information on trampolines, visit the Caring for Kids website (www.caringforkids.cps.ca).

What to do in case of injury

Injuries from falls can range from minor bruises to major head injuries. Even minor cuts and scrapes should be washed and kept clean. Here's what you can do to help your child with these injuries.

Bruises

Most bruises are minor and don't need much attention, but if you catch a new bruise right away you can apply a cold compress (ice wrapped in a washcloth, for example) for 10 or 15 minutes to keep it small. **Make an appointment** with your child's doctor if you find any unexplained bruising or if your child has bruises on her back, chest, or stomach. **Take your child to the hospital** if she refuses to use a limb that has been bruised.

Scrapes

To prevent infection, rinse a scrape with lots of room-temperature water to remove dirt and debris. If you still see debris in the wound, dampen some gauze pads and gently sponge the area. Once the scrape is clean, cover it with a sterile non-stick dressing. If you can't remove the debris from the wound, clean it as well as you can, put antibiotic ointment on it, and **take your child to the hospital.**

Cuts

If your child has a cut that is bleeding, first check for debris in the cut. Rinse it out if necessary. Apply direct pressure to the cut with a gauze pad until the bleeding stops, then place a dressing over it with firm pressure and wrap it with tape. **Take your child to the hospital immediately** if she has a wound that is still bleeding freely after it's been compressed for five minutes, or if she has an abdominal injury and vomits blood or passes blood through her rectum.

Dental injuries

If your child has bitten her tongue or lip, apply direct pressure to the area with a clean cloth. Put a cold compress on the area if it is swelling.

If your child knocks a tooth out when she falls, whether it's a baby tooth or a permanent one, try to find the tooth. Don't wash, rub, or scrub the tooth; just put it in a small container, cover the tooth in milk, and put the container on ice to keep it cold. If your child isn't too upset and can produce saliva, ask her to spit into the container a few times instead of using milk. You can also use saline solution to cover the tooth. Never ask your child to hold the tooth in her mouth, as there's a risk that she could swallow or inhale it. **Take her to the dentist or an emergency dental clinic immediately.** Emergency dental clinics are often open on the weekend.

If your child has a broken tooth, use warm water to clean any debris from the injured area, then put a cold compress on her face next to the tooth to minimize swelling. **Take her to the dentist or an emergency dental clinic immediately.**

Fractures

If your child has a very painful, swollen, or deformed limb or body part that she refuses to move after a fall, **take her to the hospital immediately.** If the bone is visible, cover her injury with a clean towel before you go. If you think she may have injured her back or neck, don't move her. **Call 911** and make sure she stays still, with her head supported.

Head injuries

It's not always easy to tell if your child has had a head injury, as the signs may be delayed. If your child has had a mild bump to her head but continues to play normally, keep a close watch on her for the next 24 hours. Even minor head bumps can turn into big goose eggs, but a cold compress on the bump can keep it from getting bigger over the first few hours. For more information on head injuries, see page 322 in Chapter Five. If your child has had a serious head injury and has neck pain, is unable to move her head, or feels numbness or tingling in her arms and legs, **call 911** and make sure she stays in the position she was found in, with her head supported.

Scalds and Burns

Scalds are most often caused by tap water or foods and drinks that are too hot. Foods and liquids heated in the microwave can cause scalding if they aren't stirred before the temperature is tested because they heat unevenly, meaning that some spots will be cool while others are very hot. Burns also come from many sources. Unprotected heaters, fireplaces, stoves, electrical outlets, appliances such as irons and curling irons, and chemicals are all hazards to a mobile child.

Tips for prevention

Birth to 12 months

One of the first things you should do when you childproof your home is install safety covers on all electrical outlets that aren't being used. Put away any leftover safety covers somewhere safe, as they can be a choking hazard. Dangling cords from lamps and electronic equipment are also a hazard, as babies will be far too tempted to chew them or pull on them, so try to keep them behind furniture.

Another extremely important childproofing measure to take as soon as possible is to reset your hot-water heater to 49°C (120°F) so that tap water doesn't burn your child. If you don't know how to reset the temperature on your water heater, call your landlord or utility company.

When you turn taps on, turn the cold tap on first, then the hot, and test the temperature with your whole hand or your elbow, making sure that it's warm but not too warm. When you turn the taps off, turn the hot water off first, then the cold, so that no hot water is left in the pipes for whoever turns the tap on next. You can also buy anti-scald devices for taps at hardware and home improvement stores. If the water cools too much, take your baby out of the bath before adding more hot water, then check the water temperature again before placing him back in.

When heating milk or formula for your baby, **never** heat it in a microwave. Microwaves heat unevenly, creating hot spots, and the container is often a lot cooler than the contents. Instead, warm a bottle up in a pot of hot water. Test the temperature on your wrist, and make sure it's lukewarm. Never, ever carry your baby and your own hot beverage at the same time.

Sunlight can also pose a burning hazard to babies, as their skin is much more sensitive than yours. Sunscreen shouldn't be used on babies under six months of age, so try to keep your baby out of direct sunlight whenever possible, and put a wide-brimmed hat on him (as well as light, loose clothing and sunglasses) whenever he goes outside. A hat that has a flap to protect the back of his neck is ideal. Stay out of direct sun, especially between 10 am and 2 pm. When your baby is in a stroller with a canopy and sides, make sure he doesn't overheat. If your stroller doesn't have a sun canopy, choose a shady route and dress your baby appropriately.

12 to 24 months

Fireplaces, floor heaters, electrical outlets, dangling appliance cords, hot drinks, and unsafe pot handles on the stove present burn hazards for a mobile child. Make absolutely sure all matches, lighters, and electrical cords are well out of reach. Set up play areas away from fireplaces and heaters, or buy a safety barrier for your fireplace, whether it's wood or gas.

When you're in the kitchen, keep your baby behind a safety gate or in a playpen or high chair. When cooking, use the back burners as often as you can, and turn pot handles in toward the stove where your baby can't reach them. Keep hot foods and liquids away from counter and table edges, and don't use tablecloths. If the knobs of your stove are at the front at your child's level, which is common with gas stoves, remove them when you're not using it.

Your toddler can wear sunscreen now when he's out in the sun. Use one with an SPF of at least 30, and reapply it after he's been in the water or after vigorous play. He'll still need to wear a hat and sunglasses. And so will you. Don't forget to lead by example.

Two to three years

Your toddler has many new skills now that he can walk steadily and is more dexterous. He may be able to remove the electrical outlet covers, so it's time to talk to him about the dangers of electricity, and to install tamper-resistant covers. He can turn taps on and off, so install an anti-scald device on all faucets or lower the temperature on the water heater to 49°C (120°F) if you haven't already. He will be able to reach the barbecue, so keep him away from it when it's on, but also when it's off. Barbecues retain heat for a long time, and toddlers can loosen gas or propane fittings.

Four to five years

You can now begin to teach your child about fire safety at home. Tell him what he should do if the smoke alarm goes off and what he can do to prevent fire, and make the lesson positive so you don't frighten him. Teach him about your fire escape plan and how to tell whether it's safe to open a door. Show him how to crawl on his hands and knees to the door if his room is smoky, and how to stop, drop, and roll if he sees fire on his clothes. Tell him that if he finds a lighter or matches, he must bring them straight to an adult. "Child-resistant" lighters are not child-proof, so keep all lighters and matches locked away. Keep any burning candles well out of your child's reach, and keep wicks short so flames aren't high. Loose pyjamas and nightgowns catch fire easily, so dress him in close-fitting pyjamas.

In the bathroom, show your child which are the hot and cold taps, and teach him to turn on the cold tap first. Keep electrical appliances out of reach and away from water, and show him how to unplug them properly by turning them off first, then pulling them out by the plug, not the cord.

If you heat food in the microwave, use low to medium settings, stir well to get rid of any hot spots, and test the temperature carefully before serving the food to your child. If you are heating more than one kind of food at the same time, test each food separately.

When you buy battery-operated toys, check that the battery compartment has to be opened with a screwdriver rather than just a finger. Install the batteries properly yourself, as improperly installed batteries can leak or overheat. If your child swallows a battery, **call the poison control centre.**

What to do in case of injury

Minor burns

If your child has a minor burn without blisters, immerse the burned body part in cold water for 10 minutes, or cover it with cold, wet cloths until the pain stops, for at least 15 minutes, replacing the cloths as they warm up. If he does have blisters or if his burn is as large as his hand, **take him to the hospital.** Do not break the blisters.

Severe burns

If your child has a burn that has many blisters or is over an extensive area, remove him from the source of the burn and **call 911.** If his clothes are on fire, smother the flames with a blanket or coat and make him roll on the floor until the flames are out. Cover him with a clean sheet and a blanket to keep him warm. Do not try to remove his clothing if it is stuck to his skin, and do not dress the wound. Do not apply water, ice, ointments, butter, or any other substance to a severe burn.

Chemical burns

If your child comes into contact with a corrosive chemical, remove any contaminated clothing. If the chemical is dry, like a powder or crystal, brush off as much as you can with a clean cloth. Keep the container and **call the poison control centre,** especially if you think he may have ingested some. Rinse his skin under cool running water for 20 minutes, and make sure the rinse water drains so that it doesn't touch healthy skin after it has touched the contaminated skin.

Electrical shocks

If your child has an electrical shock, disconnect the electrical power if it is safe to do so. Don't touch your child with your bare hands if the power is still on—keep a piece of wool or a thick, dry cloth between your hands and his body, and pull him away from the power source. **Call 911,** then begin CPR if he isn't moving or breathing (see below for more on giving CPR).

GIVING CPR

While you're pregnant and trying to think of all you can do to help your new child, think about taking a first-aid course. Learning first aid will help you be as prepared as possible to take care of your child. (See "Injury Prevention" in Resources for information on first-aid courses.) It's also a first step to becoming trained to give cardiopulmonary resuscitation, or CPR, when you suspect that someone's heartbeat or breathing has stopped. Take a refresher course every few years to make sure your skills are up to date.

If you have taken CPR training recently, here's a quick review.

‣ If a child is not moving or responding, shout for help and ask someone to **call 911.**

‣ Place the child on her back on a firm surface.

‣ Tilt her head and lift her chin to open the airway. Look, listen, and feel to see if she is breathing, but don't take any more than 10 seconds.

‣ If she is breathing and there is no sign of injury, turn her onto her side and wait for help.

‣ If she is not breathing or she only gasps occasionally, give two breaths into her mouth, pinching her nostrils shut. If the child is an infant, cover her nose and mouth with your mouth and give her the breaths. Watch her chest to make sure it rises. If her chest doesn't rise or you think her airway is obstructed, reposition her head and try again.

‣ If she doesn't start breathing on her own, give two rescue breaths, fol-lowed by 30 chest compressions. When you give chest compressions, push down on her breastbone to ⅓ or ½ the depth of her chest. Com-press quickly, at a rate of about 100 times per minute, but allow the chest to recoil fully between compressions.

- **For babies under one year, give chest compressions by placing two fingers just below the inter-nipple line (the imaginary line from one nipple to the other).**

- **For children over one year, give chest compressions by placing the heel of your hand (or use two hands) in the centre of her chest on the inter-nipple line.**

‣ Repeat the cycle of 2 breaths and 30 compressions until help arrives or your child is breathing normally.

‣ If two people are performing CPR, take turns, switching quickly every two minutes or so, in under five seconds.

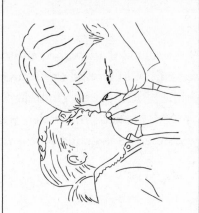

Open airway, check breathing.

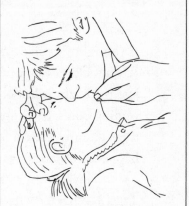

Give 2 breaths, then
30 compressions

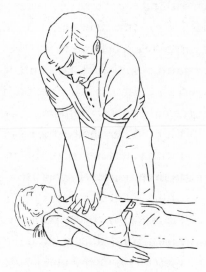

Two-handed chest compressions.

Source: Adapted from *Heartsaver CPR Student Workbook*,
American Heart Association, 2006.

Near-Drowning

A young child can drown in water as shallow as 5 centimetres (2 inches). Always closely supervise your child around any source of water—not just the backyard pool or the beach, but also drainage ditches, creeks, wading pools, bathtubs, toilets, buckets, and coolers with melted ice in them. It only takes a few moments for a child to drown, and it usually happens in silence.

Tips for prevention

Birth to 12 months
When bathing your baby, no matter how little water you're using, you'll need to pay careful attention. Make sure you've placed everything you'll need within reach before you run the bathwater, and do not answer the phone during your baby's bath. Infants can only lift their heads or sit up for a very short time, so they are particularly at risk of drowning if you are distracted or not right there. Only fill the tub with enough water to cover her legs. When she's in the bath, hold her at all times, and support her head with your forearm or the inside of your elbow. Keep her head well away from faucets. **Never** use a bath seat or ring, which actually make bathing more dangerous rather than safer, and don't leave your baby in the care of an older sibling, even for a few seconds. When you're done the bath, immediately drain the bathwater.

12 to 24 months
Buy toilet latches that will keep your child from raising the lid of the toilet. If you or a neighbour have a backyard pool, it must be surrounded on all four sides by a fence that meets or exceeds your municipality's bylaws, is at least 1.2 metres (4 feet) high, can't be climbed, and has a

self-closing, self-latching gate. (The house or patio cannot count as one side of the fence.) It's also a good idea to have an in-pool alarm, which notifies you if anyone is in the pool. Hot tubs should be protected by a hard, locking cover if they're not in an enclosed area that can be locked when not in use. Do not keep standing water, such as buckets, rain barrels, or wading pools, around your home or yard—dump them as soon as you're finished using them.

Two to three years

Toddlers have no sense of how dangerous water is, so you'll have to keep a close watch on your adventurous child, even if she's taken swimming lessons. When she is in the bath, at the beach, or in a pool, always stay within reach of her. For extra protection in pools and at the beach, have her wear a life jacket that's designed for her height and weight, and keep all the straps fastened at all times. All family members should wear life jackets when they're in a boat.

Make sure your child is not left alone around any source of standing water. Put a rubber bath mat or non-slip stickers in the tub so she won't fall getting in and out of the bath, and teach her to stay seated when she's in the tub.

Four to five years

Your child is old enough to begin swimming lessons once she's four. Swimming lessons are available for younger children, but they aren't effective for preventing drowning. If your school-age child has taken swimming lessons, you don't need to stay within reach of her, but you should actively supervise her. Never leave her unattended in or near water, including the bathtub. Don't depend on water wings or inflatable toys to keep her safe; they're not safety devices and should never be used by children who can't swim when they're in water that's higher than their waist.

What to do in case of injury

Near-drowning

If your child is drowning, remove her from the water and **call 911.** Don't try to remove water from her mouth and lungs. If she's not moving or breathing, perform CPR (see "Giving CPR" on page 395) until help arrives.

Hypothermia

If your child falls into cold water and is drowsy, shivering, confused, and stiff, and has slurred speech, discoloured lips, and cold skin, she could have hypothermia. Hypothermia becomes life-threatening when shivering stops or the child loses consciousness. If your child has hypothermia, move her to a warm place and **call 911.** Remove her wet clothing and cover her with blankets or dry clothing until help arrives. Use your own body heat to raise her temperature slowly; do not rub her or use heat pads, hot-water bottles, or electric blankets.

Poisoning and Choking

Children use their mouths to explore their world, so they'll readily stick anything and everything they can in there. If you've done your child-proofing effectively, the only things he'll be able to reach for in your home are harmless toys and household objects he can use as toys, such as pots and pans and plastic containers. Other places may not be as safe, and he may get hold of things that are poisonous, like household cleaners or plants, or that could choke him, like small objects found on the floor or in purses, briefcases, and knapsacks. In your home, post the poison control centre number next to every phone, just in case you need it in a hurry. Make sure everyone who is in your home or who takes care of your child knows where to find the number. (See "Injury Prevention" in Resources for information on poison control centres.)

Any toys your child receives must be appropriate for his age (see "Product Safety" in Resources for information on the *Toy Report*, a buying guide that rates toys by age group). One toy that children can't resist—but that you must keep away from them—is latex balloons. As much as they love them, latex balloons are the second most common cause of death by choking in children (after food) and the most common cause of death by suffocation in children. Children can inhale them while trying to blow them up, or may stick a piece of broken balloon in their mouths. Mylar balloons are safer, but as soon as they deflate, throw them out.

Tips for prevention

Birth to 12 months

Your baby will be crawling before you know it, so even before you come home from the hospital, move cleaning products, chemicals, and alcohol out of reach, out of sight, and in latched cupboards. Go through your home looking for objects and plants that a crawling baby could reach, and move them to a safe place or get rid of them entirely. Vigilantly sweep or vacuum floors every day, and check the floor for small objects like coins, paper clips, and bits of dropped food, like fruit pits.

Toys for children over three years are not safe for babies, so check the labels on your baby's toys to make sure they are age-appropriate. Store older siblings' toys out of reach, and teach them to be careful with their toys around their younger brother or sister. If they're young, don't expect them to remember all the time. You'll still have to supervise. Your baby will put anything he can grab into his mouth, and any object that can fit inside a space the size of a toilet roll is a choking hazard. Check all toys regularly for small, loose, or broken parts.

Your baby's first foods should be ones that don't require too many teeth, like pureed vegetables and baby cereal. Until he has enough teeth to chew with, his food should be soft and not too lumpy.

Babies are at risk of choking if they are given a homemade or poorly designed pacifier, as the nipple can separate from the base. Bottle nipples do not make good pacifiers because they can come apart into two small, chokeable pieces. A pacifier's handle should be hinged so it doesn't get jammed into your baby's mouth if he falls on his face. Pacifiers should have mouthguards so the nipple can only go so far into your baby's mouth, but pacifiers made for newborns are too small for bigger kids' mouths, even with the mouthguard, and can be a choking hazard.

12 to 24 months

Once your child is walking, both his reach and his grasp have improved. Check that small or dangerous items are out of reach and floor-level cupboards are kept latched. Have a safe place to put purses and backpacks so he can't explore them, and keep pet dishes and pet food in an area he can't access.

As your child begins to show interest in the food you're eating, only give him foods that are appropriate in size and consistency for him. Hard or round foods like popcorn, whole grapes, and hot dogs are choking hazards until he is around four years old.

Two to three years

Your toddler has probably figured out how those cupboard latches work by now, and that he can climb on a chair to reach higher cupboards, so move all dangerous household cleaners and other chemicals to a safer place or avoid keeping them in your home at all. Be especially careful outside. Barbecue fluid, antifreeze, and some outdoor plants are poisonous, so lock them up or remove them. See page 423 for a list of poisonous plants. When you use bug spray on your toddler, don't put it on his face and hands, where he can lick it.

Four to five years

Your school-age child might not be as likely to stick things in his mouth, ears, or nose, but he's still curious, so continue to be vigilant about poisonous items and choking hazards. Supervise him when he's playing with art and craft materials, and only give him materials that are non-toxic and approved for use by children. Avoid small beads and buttons, sharp scissors, permanent markers, and instant glue.

By now, most children will be able to eat foods of all textures (whether they will want to is a different matter), but certain behaviour can still lead to choking. Watch *how* your child eats as well as *what* he eats. Teach him to pay attention when he's eating, to chew his food well before swallowing, and to not talk when he has food in his mouth, just like your mother told you. If he's eating any kind of food that's on a stick or skewer, throw the stick out as soon as he's done.

Avoid taking medication (including vitamins) in front of your child, and never refer to it as "candy." You may have removed safety gates because he's grown too big for them (when his chin is level with the top of the gate, or he can climb over it), so you'll need to secure previously off-limits areas in a different way, either by using childproof doorknob covers or latches, or by locking dangerous objects and substances in cupboards.

Dr. Sacks Says

As children seem to be able to open childproof latches more easily than adults, try to eliminate as many poisonous substances from your home as possible.

What to do in case of injury

Poisoning

If you think your child may have ingested something dangerous, **call the poison control centre or 911.** If a hospital trip is necessary, take a sample of what he ingested—for instance, the container, or a piece of the plant—so that you can show it to the paramedics. Never make your child vomit if he has ingested something poisonous.

Mild choking

If your child is choking but can still breathe, cry, cough, or speak, stay with him until he settles down. Encourage him to cough; don't try to remove the object yourself. If his choking becomes worse, **call 911.** Here again is where CPR training becomes invaluable (see "Giving CPR" on page 395).

Severe choking

Your child has a severe obstruction if he is choking and cannot breathe, cry, cough, or talk, and if he is limp, turning blue, losing consciousness, or unconscious. How you respond will depend on how old he is and whether he is conscious.

If he is **under one year of age** and conscious, follow the steps below.

- Place him face-down over your arm so that his head is lower than his body. Rest your forearm on your thigh. If he's a large baby, place him face-down across your lap instead.

- Deliver up to five back blows (slaps), striking high between his shoulder blades.

- If that doesn't clear the blockage, turn him over, cradle him across your lap, and use two fingers to give up to five rapid chest compressions (thrusts) just below the inter-nipple line.

- Repeat the back blows and chest compressions until the blockage is cleared or until medical help arrives.

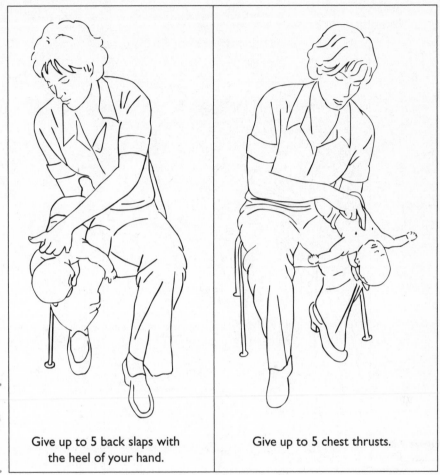

Source: Adapted from *Heartsaver CPR Student Workbook*, American Heart Association, 2006.

Figure 7.2:
How to help
a choking
infant

Give up to 5 back slaps with
the heel of your hand.

Give up to 5 chest thrusts.

If he is **over one year of age** and conscious, perform the Heimlich manoeuvre.

- From behind your child, encircle his abdomen between his navel and breastbone with your arms, and make a fist.
- Press firmly but gently into his abdomen with inward and upward thrusts.
- Repeat until the blockage is cleared or until medical help arrives.

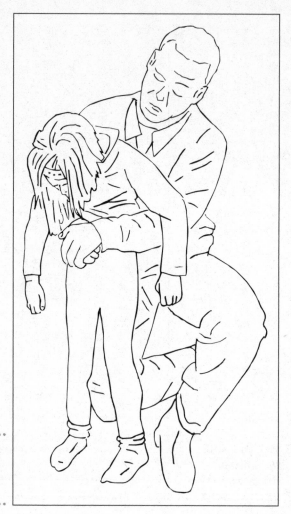

**Figure 7.3:
Heimlich
manoeuvre**

Source: Adapted from *Heartsaver CPR Student Workbook*, American Heart Association 2006.

If your child loses consciousness, **call 911,** then place him on his back on a flat surface, open his mouth and look for anything that might be blocking his airway, and remove the blocking matter with a hooked finger. If you can't see it, don't search for it with your finger—you may push it further down. Perform CPR (see "Giving CPR" on page 395) until the blockage is cleared or medical help arrives.

A WELL-STOCKED FIRST-AID KIT

To be able to help your child in an emergency, keep a well-stocked first-aid kit within easy reach of adults and know how to use it. Keep a small kit in the diaper bag or car as well as in your home, and keep them in securely closed boxes. You can buy pre-packaged kits, but you'll probably need to add some items to them. Your first-aid kits should include the items listed below.

- An assortment of adhesive bandages
- Cotton gauze with non-allergic gauze tape
- Hydrogen peroxide to clean cuts and scrapes
- Antibiotic ointment for burns, cuts, and scrapes
- Calamine lotion
- Tweezers
- Sharp scissors
- A couple of pairs of non-latex or vinyl gloves
- Pain medication (acetaminophen or ibuprofen—**not** aspirin). Carefully check dosage and age requirements, and do not use on a baby younger than three months.
- Antihistamine for allergic reactions
- Saline drops to loosen mucus in a stuffy nose
- Liquid soap or gel hand sanitizer
- Epinephrine device if your child has allergies (in addition to devices you and your child keep with you at all times)
- A small, easy-to-read first-aid manual
- A list of names and phone numbers of emergency contacts. It should be clearly printed or typed, and attached to the inside lid or other visible area of the kit, as well as beside all telephones. Include the following people:

- Your family doctor or paediatrician
- Your local hospital
- Alternate caregivers, such as grandparents or aunts and uncles
- The local or provincial poison control hotline
- Your local police and fire squads
- Two close neighbours (in case you need emergency assistance such as a ride to the hospital or child care for a sibling)
- Your contact information (all numbers) in case of emergency

SAFE PURCHASES

The birth of a child means many things, but one thing it definitely means is that there will be shopping. Whether you're breaking out the credit card, registering for your baby shower, or checking out yard sales and consignment stores for the essentials, you'll have to keep some important safety considerations in mind. Here are some tips on how to wisely buy the most essential items.

Car Seats

A car seat is one of the most important purchases you will ever make for your child. To bring your baby home from the hospital, you'll need a rear-facing infant seat. When she's grown too big for her seat (according to the manufacturer's limits), you'll buy a front-facing seat. And when she's grown too big for that one, it'll be time for a booster seat.

SHOPPING CHECKLIST FOR CAR SEATS

‣ Does the car seat have a National Safety Mark? (See below.)

‣ Is there an instruction booklet?

‣ Is the car seat appropriate for the weight and height of your child?

‣ If the car seat has an expiry date, will the time period cover your needs?

‣ Can the car seat be installed correctly in your vehicle?

‣ Are the harness and tether straps easy to adjust?

Remember to fill out the registration card that comes with your new car seat so the manufacturer can contact you for recalls.

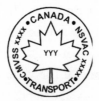

National Safety Mark

Source: Transport Canada, 2000. Reproduced with the permission of the Minister of Public Works and Government Services Canada, 2008.

Choosing a Seat for Each Stage

Birth to 12 months

For at least the first year (and preferably longer), your baby must be in a rear-facing infant car seat every time she travels in the car, from the moment you get in to the moment you're ready to leave the vehicle.

Seats become brittle with age and should never be used after they've been in an accident, so buying a used car seat is not a good idea. Make sure your seat comes with a user manual and is affixed with a label that lists height and weight requirements. Check with Transport Canada (see "Travel" in Resources for information) or your local public health department to ensure the car seat you're using is appropriate for your child's age and weight, and that the seat has not been recalled. Attend a car seat clinic to make sure you've installed your seat properly and are using it correctly. Many police and fire stations can advise you on proper installation, and some hold car seat clinics.

Before installing your first car seat, read and follow the manufacturer's instructions and your vehicle owner's manual carefully. Check that the seat's label indicates the car seat is appropriate for infants, and that it fits in the rear seat of your vehicle. Install the seat in the "kid zone"—the middle of the back seat, away from all air bags. The seat should be positioned at a 45° angle, so if the slope of the vehicle's seat puts the seat at a different angle, use a rolled-up towel or a pool noodle under the seat to adjust the angle. Secure it using the Universal Anchorage System (UAS or LATCH) or the vehicle seat belt. Many lap/shoulder combination seat belts require a special locking clip. Once the seat is installed, make sure you cannot move the seat more than 2.5 centimetres (1 inch) forward or side to side when you pull on it at the anchor point or at the point where the seat belt is routed. Harness straps must be snug and threaded at or just below your baby's shoulders, and the chest clip must be at her armpit level. If you can put more than one finger between the shoulder harness and your baby's collarbone, the harness is too loose.

Dr. Sacks Says

Never let your child scream his way out of his car seat. No car seat means no car ride.

12 months to four years

At 12 months of age, if your toddler has exceeded the rear-facing seat's height or weight requirements, she will be ready to move to a forward-facing car seat. If she doesn't exceed the height or weight requirements, don't rush her into a forward-facing seat—rear-facing seats are safer. When it is time to buy a forward-facing seat, make sure once again that your toddler meets the weight and height requirements, that the seat fits securely in your vehicle, and that you follow both the car seat manufacturer's instructions and your car's manual when you install it. Forward-facing car seats use a tether strap that attaches to an anchor on your vehicle's rear seat. If your vehicle doesn't have an anchor, you'll need to have one installed. Your car dealer will be able to do that.

UAS installation

Car seats manufactured after September 1, 2002, have two UAS connectors that attach to the UAS anchor bars in the rear seats of new vehicles. The UAS symbol marks the location of the anchor bars in the vehicle and the connectors on the car seat.

Figure 7.4: LATCH symbol

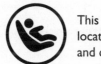

This LATCH symbol marks both the location of anchor bars in your vehicle and connectors on the car seat.

Source: Transport Canada, 2006. Reproduced with the permission of the Minister of Public Works and Government Services Canada, 2009.

Figure 7.5: Sometimes user-ready tether anchors have this symbol.

Source: Transport Canada, 2000. Reproduced with the permission of the Minister of Public Works and Government Services Canada, 2009.

- Attach the two car seat connectors to the vehicle anchor bars and tighten the strap.
- Push down on the child car seat with your knee while you tighten the strap.
- Attach the tether strap to the vehicle's tether anchor and tighten the strap.
- The car seat should not move more than 2.5 centimetres (1 inch) forward or side to side.

Seat belt installation

If your vehicle does not have the UAS or LATCH system, check your vehicle manual's instructions for installing car seats using a seat belt. In some vehicles you will need to use a locking clip with the seat belt to keep the child car seat securely in place.

- Thread the seat belt webbing through the child seat as shown in the instructions.
- Buckle the seat belt and make sure it is tight.
- Push down on the child seat with your knee while you tighten the seat belt.
- Attach the tether strap to the vehicle's tether anchor and tighten the strap.
- The child seat should not move more than 2.5 centimetres (1 inch) forward or side to side.

To secure your toddler in a forward-facing child seat, adjust the harness straps to the slot positions that are at or slightly above her shoulders. She should be in an upright position with her back flat against the back of the car seat. The chest clip should be positioned at her armpit level to hold the harness straps in place. Make sure the harness straps are fastened tightly so that only one finger fits between the straps and your child's chest.

Four years to eight years

When your child reaches 18 kilograms (40 pounds) or exceeds the height requirements of her front-facing seat, which usually happens between the ages of four and five, she can start to use a booster seat. Booster seats come in both high-back and backless styles, and they must be used until your child is at least eight years old and 145 centimetres (4 feet 9 inches) tall. A booster seat keeps the seat belt in the correct place over your child's body: the shoulder strap flat against her chest (and not touching her neck) and the lap belt low and snug against her hips. Buckle the seat belt across the seat even when it's not in use so that it doesn't become a projectile in case of an accident.

If your child is too tall for her forward-facing seat before she reaches 18 kilograms (40 pounds), you can get a combination child/booster seat. With a combination seat, you use a harness until your child reaches 18 kilograms (40 pounds), at which point you remove the harness and use a seat belt instead.

All car seats you use must be labelled with the letters CMVSS (Canadian Motor Vehicle Safety Standard). Mail in the registration card shortly after purchase so that the manufacturer can contact you if there's a recall. Also check the Transport Canada website for recalls and age-specific guidelines (see "Travel" in Resources for information). If you need to replace any parts, only order them from the manufacturer, using the correct model number or name, and don't use any car seat accessories, like trays or cushions, that aren't provided by the manufacturer.

Dr. Sacks Says

This is a product registration card you really should send in. Being notified of car seat recalls can save your child's life.

414 · CARING FOR YOUR CHILD FROM BIRTH TO AGE FIVE

Cribs

A crib is the safest place for your baby when you can't be around to watch him, and it's the safest place for him to sleep. Any crib you use should have a permanent label with the manufacturer's name, the model number or name, the date of manufacture, instructions for assembly, and a warning statement about mattress size and proper crib use. Never use a crib that is missing this label, that is homemade or has been modified, or that was made before 1986, when government safety regulations changed.

Here are some basic safety specifications for cribs.

- Crib bars should be no more than 6 centimetres (2⅜ inches) apart. Make sure that none of the bars are missing or loose.

- The mattress should fit tightly within the crib frame. If there is more than 3 centimetres (1³/₁₆ inches, or two finger widths) between the mattress and crib side when you push the mattress toward the other side, it is too small. A child can become trapped in that space and suffocate.

- Corner posts should be either no higher than 3 millimetres (⅛ inch) above the top of the end panels, or too high to catch on clothing. There should be no cut-out designs in the head or footboards or openings between the corner post and top rail— places where a baby could trap her head or catch her clothing.

- The crib's drop-side latches should be securely in place when the rail is raised. Always raise and lock this rail in its highest position whenever a child is in the crib.

- The mattress support hangers should be secured with the bolts or closed hooks supplied by the manufacturer. These fixtures should all be tight and strong. Don't use a crib where these hooks are Z- or S-shaped.

- Use only the original hardware that came with the crib. If you're missing any hardware, contact the manufacturer.

- The mattress should be firm, flat, and covered with a fitted crib sheet. Never use removable plastic wrapping, dry-cleaning bags, or garbage bags as mattress covers.

- Check the overall condition of a crib regularly, especially if you have moved it.

High Chairs

Even before your baby begins to eat solid food, you may use a high chair to keep him in sight and out from underfoot while you work in the kitchen. However, high chair–related injuries are very common. Whether a high chair is new or second-hand, take precautions.

- Always follow the manufacturer's weight, height, and age guidelines. If the chair does not have a label on it that lists these, you shouldn't use it.

- Make sure your high chair has a wide and stable base.

- If the chair folds, be sure it is securely locked in its upright position when you use it.

- Always use the safety straps so your child doesn't slide out the bottom of the chair.

- Pinching your child's fingers with the tray is a very common injury. Be extra careful when removing or replacing the tray.

Hook-on chairs

A hook-on chair allows your baby to get up close and eat at the table with the family. It works by hooking onto the table surface, and your baby's weight helps to hold it in place. Always use a hook-on chair on a sturdy table that will not tip—if you're outside your home, check the table's stability first. Make sure the chair has locks or clamps that tighten securely, and use the safety straps, including the waist and crotch belt, to keep your baby from sliding forward and out of the chair.

Playpens

A playpen can be a safe place for your baby if you're otherwise occupied for a short time, like while you're making dinner or on the phone. However, you and your baby should be able to see and hear each other when she's in the playpen. A child left unattended in a playpen is not safe.

Here are some basic safety guidelines for playpens.

- Check that the playpen has a permanent label stating that it complies with federal playpen regulations and listing the manufacturer's name, the model number or name, and the date of manufacture. Never use a playpen that does not have this label on it.

- Follow the instructions for assembly, and keep the instruction manual.

- Always comply with the playpen's weight and height limits.

- Check for product advisories and recalls at Health Canada's website (see "Product Safety" in Resources). Never use a playpen that has been recalled.

- Make sure the playpen is stable and sturdy, and that there are no exposed joints or sharp edges that could pinch or scrape.

- The playpen should have sides made of a fine mesh with holes smaller than 6.4 millimetres (¼ inch) across and well-padded surfaces. Don't attach accessories like mobiles or play gyms to the sides.

- Make sure the top rails and sides are locked securely whenever the playpen is set up.

- Check regularly for tears in the vinyl rail covering, the mattress pad, and the mesh. A baby can choke on small pieces of vinyl or be strangled if a button on her clothing catches in a tear.

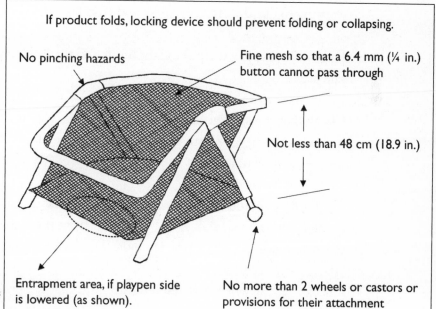

Figure 7.6: Playpen safety specifications

Source: *Information to Dealers of Second-hand Children's Products*, Health Canada, 2003 © Adapted and Reproduced with the permission of the Minister of Public Works and Government Services Canada, 2008.

Strollers

Strollers range in style—and scale—from the collapsible umbrella stroller you can carry on your arm to a two-child stroller with a full dashboard and cup holders. Before you join the stroller set, make sure yours is sturdy and appropriate for the age, height, and weight of your child. Infants younger than four months of age need to recline, so they should only be taken out in a carriage stroller, never an umbrella-style stroller. Some strollers can accommodate a car seat or convert into a carriage, so one stroller may suit all your needs.

Some other stroller-shopping guidelines are outlined below.

- The stroller must have a permanent label with the manufacturer's name, model number or name, date of manufacture, and a warning to use the safety harness and crotch strap.

- Follow the age, height, and weight limits and the instructions for safe use.

- Check that the stroller has a five-point harness system, with belts that come down over both shoulders, two that connect at the waist, and a crotch strap.

- The harness should be solidly attached to the seat or frame of the stroller, and the seat should not pull away from the frame, even when you pull sharply on the lap belt.

- Check that the wheels are fixed tightly, and that the brakes work and are easy to use.

- Make sure there are no sharp edges or tears in the upholstery, pinch points, or sharp corners.

- Safety regulations changed in 1985, so any stroller made before then is not safe.

Before you go out the door, check that brakes, wheels, and handles are in good working order. Do not pad the stroller with pillows or blankets. Always use the brake when putting your child in or taking him out, and always use the harness. Before making any adjustments, such as reversing the handle, make sure your child's hands and feet are clear. If your stroller has a storage basket, check the manufacturer's weight guideline and don't exceed it.

Baby carriers

A front baby carrier, which keeps your baby snuggled close to your chest or stomach, can be used as long as you can put it on and take it off by yourself. Front carriers should have shoulder and head support for your baby and leg openings that are small enough to prevent her from slipping out.

A baby must be at least six months old and have good head control before you can switch to a back carrier. Back carriers should have strong stitching; large, heavy-duty closures to prevent unintended release; and proper safety and anchor straps that fit both mom and baby snugly. The frame should be padded near your baby's face, and the leg openings should be small enough to prevent her from slipping out but large enough to prevent chafing. A back carrier is not safe for a sleeping baby, who should be moved to a crib to sleep as soon as possible.

Dr. Sacks Says

You know that kitchen drawer that's full of stuff you're not sure you need? Now you can use it to store all the manuals, tags, and warranty cards you'll collect from all your baby gear.

CHILDPROOFING CHECKLIST

Childproofing is the key to creating a safe environment for your child. Your home isn't the only place that needs childproofing, though. Don't forget to childproof vacation homes and hotel rooms, and ask grandparents and other caregivers to childproof their homes as well. This list includes the most important things to look for (many of which have been discussed in more detail in this chapter and throughout the book), but you should always assess your child's environment from his point of view for other hazards. Children have their own unique ways of getting into danger, so know your child and his environment.

All Through the Home

- Ensure entryways, hallways, and staircases are well lit and free of clutter.

- Have somewhere safe and out of reach where you and guests can put purses, knapsacks, and briefcases.

- Post a list of emergency numbers next to each phone.

- Use child-resistant doorknob covers to prevent children from accessing stairs, rooms with hazards, and front and back doors.

- Install smoke detectors on every level of your home. There should be one near each sleeping area. Test them monthly, and change the batteries every six months or use a long-life battery, which may last up to 10 years. Replace alarms that are more than 10 years old. In some new homes, smoke alarms may be connected to the wiring of your home.

- Install carbon monoxide detectors on every level of your home.

- Tuck lamp and electronics cords behind furniture, and keep appliance cords out of reach.

- Cover all unused electrical outlets with safety covers, including those on power bars.

- Avoid using extension cords, but if you must, cover unused outlets, and run them behind furniture so your child doesn't trip over them. Do not run them under a rug or carpet.

- Put non-slip backing or double-sided tape on rugs to prevent tripping and sliding.

- Sweep or vacuum your floors daily. Get down on your knees to check under tables, chairs, and beds for small objects.

- Cover sharp corners on tables and fireplace hearths with padding.

- Look for curtain and blind cords that can get caught around a child's neck. Cut them short or secure them to the wall so they are well out of reach.

- Ensure that your windows cannot open more than 10 centimetres (4 inches) by installing window guards. Children can fall out of windows, and screens do not prevent falls.

- Keep furniture away from windows so children can't climb to window height and reach the cords or fall out.

- Keep sharp, breakable, or heavy objects on tabletops and shelves well out of reach. If you can, simply remove them and put them in storage.

- Anchor tall, top-heavy furniture, like bookcases, dressers, televisions, and entertainment units, to the wall with L-shaped brackets or furniture straps to keep them from falling.

- Reset your hot-water heater to 49°C (120°F) or install anti-scald devices on your hot-water faucets. If you have difficulties adjusting the temperature of your hot-water heater, contact your landlord or utility company for help.

- Empty bathtubs, wading pools, buckets, and coolers with melted ice as soon as you're done with them.

- Install safety latches on cupboards and drawers where you keep products that can be dangerous for a baby, such as household cleaners, sharp utensils, and plastic bags.

- Stair and porch railings should not have horizontal bars that allow climbing, and the rungs should be less than 10 centimetres (4 inches) apart.

- At stairway openings, install hardware-mounted safety gates that are fixed securely to the door frame or to studs in the wall. Also use hardware-mounted safety gates to block access to porches, balconies, and other dangerous areas.

- To block access to rooms such as the kitchen, you can use pressure gates. Make sure the pressure bar is on the side away from where your child will be so he doesn't climb on it.

- Put barriers around gas and wood fireplaces and wood stoves to prevent your child from falling against them. Barriers should be at least 56 centimetres (22 inches) high and made of non-combustible materials.

- Choose space heaters that are cool to the touch and have an automatic shut-off. Keep them away from furniture and from fabrics such as bedding and curtains.

- Check paint finishes in older homes for lead content. Paint with lead in it could be hazardous if it's peeling or chipped and your child puts pieces in his mouth. You can buy test kits in paint, hardware, and home improvement stores.

- Keep litter boxes and pet food somewhere where your child can't access them.

- Learn the names of all your houseplants and outdoor plants. Get rid of any that are poisonous or that you are not sure about.

POISONOUS PLANTS

The following are some common plants that are poisonous to humans:

Amaryllis	Boston Ivy
Angel's Trumpet	Caladium
Arrowhead Vine	Calla Lily
Autumn Crocus	Castor Bean
Azalea	Chinese Lantern Plant
Bittersweet	Clematis
Black Locust	Cotoneaster

Croton	Monkshood
Cyclamen	Morning Glory
Daffodil	Mother-in-law's Tongue
Daisy (Chrysanthemum)	Narcissus
Delphinium	Nightshade
Dieffenbachia (Dumb Cane)	Oleander
Elephant's Ear	Peony
English Ivy	Periwinkle (Vinca)
Eucalyptus	Philodendron
Euonymus	Poison Ivy
Foxglove	Poison Oak
Gladiola	Pokeweed
Holly	Potato (all green parts)
Horse Chestnut	Pothos
Hyacinth	Rhododendron
Hydrangea	Rhubarb Leaves
Iris	Rosary Bean
Jack-in-the-Pulpit	Snake Berry
Jequirity Bean	Snow on the Mountain
Jerusalem Cherry	Star of Bethlehem
Jimson Weed	St. John's Wort
Larkspur	Tobacco
Lily-of-the-Valley	Tomato (plant and unripe fruit)
Lobelia	Virginia Creeper
Lupine	Water Hemlock
Marijuana	Wisteria
Milkweed	Yew
Mistletoe	

Source: Ontario Poison Centre, 2008. Adapted from the Hospital for Sick Children's "Plant Safety" brochure.

Your Child's Room

- Keep stuffed toys, comforters, and pillows out of your child's crib and playpen.

- Make sure there are no wall hangings, cords, lamps, or pictures within reach of the crib.

- Hang mobiles well out of reach of your baby, securely fastened to the crib, and remove them once he's able to push himself up on his hands and knees (or when he's four months old).

- Check that cribs, playpens, high chairs, and strollers have manufacturers' labels on them and meet current safety standards.

Toys

- Make sure toys are appropriate for your child's age. If a toy can fit inside a toilet roll, it's too small for children under three years old.

- Follow the height and weight limits of bouncy chairs, baby swings, and activity centres.

- Toys should not have pull strings longer than 15 centimetres (6 inches).

- Throw out broken toys.

- Make sure your child wears a helmet when he's on wheeled toys and when he's skating and sledding.

- Keep older children's toys, which often have small parts, out of reach of babies and young children.

Kitchen

- Keep a fire extinguisher handy in the kitchen and check the test window monthly.

- Keep oven and dishwasher doors closed, and put up a safety gate to keep your child away from the kitchen when they're being used.

- If the knobs on your stove are at the front and at child level, remove them when the stove is not being used.

- When cooking, make sure pot handles don't stick out from the stove. Instead, turn them in toward the stove. Try to cook on the back burners only, whenever possible.

- Push kitchen gadgets and appliances to the back of the counter when you're not using them, and make sure the cords don't dangle.

- Put plastic bags and sharp utensils, skewers, and scissors out of reach in latched drawers or cupboards.

- If you keep any medications in the kitchen, including vitamins, keep them out of sight and out of reach, either in a latched cupboard or in a sealed container in the fridge. You may want to buy a fridge latch so your child can't get into the fridge.

- If your young child needs to be in the kitchen while you're cooking, cleaning, or making hot drinks, place him in a playpen nearby.

- Keep the high chair away from other furniture or appliances that your child could reach.

- Use placemats instead of a tablecloth, which can be pulled, bringing everything on the table down with it.

- Keep garbage cans and compost containers in latched cupboards.

Bathroom

- Keep bathroom doors closed and latched when bathrooms are not being used. Install either child-resistant doorknob covers on the handles or a hook-and-eye latch high up on the outside of the door.

- Give your child a stool for reaching the bathroom sink. It should be sturdy and have a non-slip surface and base.

- Keep all household cleaning products and medications safely capped—locked up, out of reach, *and* out of sight. Never assume that products labelled "childproof" can't be opened.

- Keep the diaper pail in a latched cupboard.

- Unplug appliances such as hair dryers and curling irons when they're not in use, and keep them out of reach. Make sure the cords don't dangle.

- Buy toilet latches so that you can lock toilet lids shut.

Outdoors

- Keep your child away from the barbecue at all times. Even when it is not in use, it can stay hot for a long time, and curious hands can loosen fittings to the gas or propane tank.

- If you have a backyard pool, install a pool alarm. Fencing must completely surround the pool on all four sides (the house or deck does not count as fencing) and must not be climbable. The gate must be able to close by itself and latch securely, and the enclosure must meet or exceed the requirements of your municipality's bylaws.

- Keep dangerous items inaccessible: power tools, lawn mowers and clippers, garden tools, pesticides, insect sprays, barbecue fluid, paint thinner, antifreeze, and other poisonous products.

- Porch and deck railings should be sturdy and kept in good condition, and the rungs should be less than 10 centimetres (4 inches) apart.

- Outdoor play equipment should be sturdy and well maintained. Check for rusting, places that might catch on clothing or pinch fingers, and plastic or metal fatigue.

ooooo

If you've read this chapter from beginning to end, you may be feeling a little overwhelmed by all the things that could possibly go wrong and all that you need to do to keep your child safe. No need to worry. This chapter provides all the information you need to prevent injuries and respond appropriately in the event of an injury, but you can come back to it any time you need it. Use it as a tool when you childproof your home, purchase equipment for your child, supply your first-aid kit, and talk to your child about safety. Use it as a reference guide to quickly find out what to do if your child does become injured.

Keeping your child safe doesn't have to be difficult or daunting. You just have to do a bit of research and preparation at each stage of your child's development, and get used to seeing things in a whole new light. In addition to having an increased awareness of your child's environment, after reading this chapter you should also have a sense of how to look at that environment from her perspective. The more you practise seeing the world through her eyes, the better you'll become at childproofing, supervising, and anticipating her next move, and the safer she'll be.

8

Emotional Health and Well-Being

Your child is unique. She will develop at her own pace, which is determined by genetics, environmental influences, her physical health, and her temperament. This is as true for her emotional health and growth as it is for her physical and intellectual development. Her personality—whether she is a risk-taker or slow to try new things—may play a role in when she accomplishes emotional milestones and how she copes with distress and challenges. Her emotional development is also affected by her attachment to her parents. By creating a strong emotional attachment to your child, you give her a sense of security that will help her grow into an emotionally strong adult. Attachment also forges the kind of relationship that allows you to teach her how to behave appropriately, manage her moods, and become resilient.

Although infants and very young children are rarely diagnosed with mental health disorders, one in five children will be diagnosed with a mental health disorder before adulthood. Anxiety disorders, attention deficit hyperactivity disorder, autistic spectrum disorders, and some other behavioural disorders can often be identified in young children. As with physical conditions, early identification can decrease the impact these disorders can have on a child's life. If you have a family history of mental health disorders, or if your family is going through divorce or dealing with alcoholism, chronic illness, or any other traumatic event, discuss it with your child's doctor.

INCLUDED IN THIS CHAPTER

EMOTIONAL DEVELOPMENTAL MILESTONES

Reaching the following emotional developmental milestones allow your child to grow into a trusting, independent child who feels secure in himself and others. The normal range for many milestones is quite large, but if his behaviour interferes with his health or his relationships with family, friends, caregivers, and teachers, he should see a doctor. If you feel there is "something missing," or if interactions with him are more frustrating than fun, don't be embarrassed to ask. You are not alone, and a little bit of guidance can make a big difference.

2 to 7 Months

This is a special time to learn about your baby's temperament. Newborns are able to receive and react to stimuli such as touch, smell, taste, and movement, and communicate with caregivers by crying or wiggling. Does your infant thrive on noise and activity, or does he become overwhelmed by too much touching and movement? Gradually you will learn just what your baby's cries and movements mean, and how to tell when he is overstimulated and needs quiet time.

What to expect
- He has an increasing sense of himself and of others.
- He recognizes his caregivers more and more.
- He begins to realize that he can make things happen; for instance, he knows you will respond when he cries.
- He may begin focusing on his parents' eyes.

7 to 15 Months

The first 15 months are a critical time for developing a special, trusting attachment with your baby. Your baby will begin to respond to the behaviour, and even the feelings, of other people. With his increased mobility, you'll learn more about his personality: Is he a fearless explorer, or a cautious observer? It's also important to be aware of your own response as your baby starts to go out into the world.

What to expect

- He has increased emotional control, although he often requires comforting.

- He is beginning to be aware of feelings other than distress, such as happiness or excitement.

- He has an increasing sense of himself as separate from others. The amount of distress he shows when you leave or a stranger appears gives good insight into your baby's temperament.

- He is becoming increasingly attached to his parents, and often has a special greeting by 12 months.

- He is becoming more interested in exploring, including shaking, banging, and mouthing everything he can get his hands on, but he often checks to make sure you're still there.

- He has increasing separation distress, which will peak at about 18 months of age.

15 to 30 Months

Helping your child be independent and positive about the world becomes more difficult now, as the need to set limits interferes with his desire to see and do for himself. Tantrums become common as his excitement meets up with devastating disappointment (see page 224 in Chapter Four for more on tantrums). If you have worked at forming a healthy attachment with your child, you will know when to intervene and when to sit back and let him experiment and explore (see page 437 for more on attachment). As independent as he wants to be, a securely attached toddler will still rely on his parents for reassurance and help.

What to expect
- He is starting to identify himself (me, I, mine).
- He enjoys pretend play more and more.
- He is learning to feel satisfied with his accomplishments.
- He has increased problem-solving ability.
- He is beginning to assert himself without being aggressive.
- He is able to accept discipline without a strong fear of losing his parents' love.
- He is beginning to show empathy.

30 Months to Five Years

During his preschool years, your child's emotional extremes should decrease significantly. He should be able to use words to deal with his emotions and express his fears, and it's normal for him to have some specific fears, such as lightning or dogs. By age three, most children can separate from their parents for a short period without much crying or clinging, although some need more help preparing for change.

What to expect

- He has less separation and stranger anxiety.
- He is increasingly able to play with other children.
- He can control his emotions, to some extent.
- He has a firm understanding of himself and his family.

MAKE A NOTE, MAKE AN APPOINTMENT, OR GO TO THE HOSPITAL?

Make a note to mention to your child's doctor at your next scheduled appointment if he doesn't reach these milestones.

2 to 7 months

- ▷ He often can't be comforted.
- ▷ He doesn't develop a general smile (when something makes him happy) or a social smile (when someone smiles at him or when he recognizes someone).
- ▷ He doesn't develop a specific social smile by seven months.

7 to 15 months

- ▷ He shows persistent signs of distress (crying, irritability).
- ▷ He doesn't respond when primary caregivers arrive or leave.
- ▷ He is very difficult to feed, and as a result is not meeting growth milestones.

> He isn't interested in exploring objects.
> He doesn't show interest in other people.

15 to 30 months

> He is increasingly and consistently defiant.
> He is often aggressive.
> He is often frustrated and angry, but will not turn to or respond to his parents when he's upset.
> When people try to hug him, he rejects them.

30 months to five years

> He rarely plays with other children.
> He continues to have tantrums.
> He is constantly frustrated.
> He cries or clings persistently when a parent leaves, even for short periods or in familiar places, and cannot be soothed.
> He has persistent and severe sleeping difficulties.

ATTACHMENT

In the beginning, your child's healthy emotional development is all about attachment: the deep emotional bond that a baby forms with a person who cares for her. A secure attachment forms when a parent or caregiver responds to her needs consistently in warm and sensitive ways. Holding, rocking, or talking softly to her all help promote attachment. You know you have a secure attachment with your child when you can easily soothe her, she wants to be near you, and she responds to you even from a distance.

A consistent, sensitive, and warm response to your baby's needs appears to set the stage for healthy emotional development. Consistency is important, but that rare meltdown—which all new parents have—does not affect the strong bond you are forming through the rocking and soothing you give her most of the time. Attachment helps provide a solid base from which a baby can explore the world. It makes her feel safe and secure, and helps her learn to trust others.

The rewards of this strong attachment are significant. In the first two months of life, even though infants show little observable preference for a particular caregiver, warm, sensitive, and dependable responses set the stage for attachment. By four weeks, your baby will respond to your smile. By three months, she'll be smiling right back at you, and at four months her smile will turn into laughter. By four to six months of age, she begins to expect your response when she's distressed. From two to seven months, babies tend to interact differently with caregivers than with strangers, but in general they still do not show strong preferences.

With continued appropriate responses to your baby's needs, by the end of the first seven or eight months (or even earlier in some babies), she will have a special smile and response for you. Her increasing attachment may also bring about distress with strangers—unfortunately, even with grandma, although by 12 months she should show preferences for a small number of caregivers. Amazingly, by seven or eight months your baby might be able to read your emotions, and she will begin to respond to your stress, anger, or sadness.

From 12 to 18 months, with the advent of crawling and walking, babies use their attachment figure as a secure base from which to venture out and explore the world, and as a safe haven to return to when they are frightened or distressed. From 18 months to about four years of age, healthy attachment leads to tolerance of separation, learning to cooperate, and signs of self-control. But she's not ready to fly solo yet—if you have a strong attachment with your child, she will continue to show you that she needs your love and protection.

Dr. Sacks Says

Parenting is really the art of letting go at the right time. In order to let go, though, you must be properly attached to your child to begin with.

MAKE A NOTE, MAKE AN APPOINTMENT, OR GO TO THE HOSPITAL?

Insecure attachment can jeopardize a baby's healthy emotional and social development. If you feel you cannot give your baby the attention she needs, it is important that you **make an appointment** to talk to a doctor. Your own physical or mental health may need attention that, when treated, will allow you to confidently care for your child.

A strong attachment also depends on your child's ability and willingness to look at faces and receive responses back, as well as her ability to make eye contact. If your child doesn't show interest in people or make eye contact with them, **make an appointment** with her doctor.

MANAGING MOODS

Newborns are very aware of how they feel, and even at that age, they tolerate stress differently. Although you may be learning plenty about your own moods in the early days, this is also a great time to learn about your baby's temperament. Knowing what upsets him (such as loud noise or rough play) and how much he can take before he is distressed will allow you to respond appropriately to him and to avoid certain situations, if necessary. As children grow, they begin to understand that not everyone feels the same, and they learn that they have feelings about other people. By age two, your child can start to see that the characters in his favourite book feel differently from time to time. Eventually he will learn that feelings do not remain the same, and that he has a role in changing his own feelings.

All of these little lessons will help your child deal with his moods. He should also learn how his moods affect his behaviour. You can show him how to deal with moods by using words to describe your own feelings and how they relate to your behaviour: "I was angry because I burned dinner, so I yelled at the dog." It is one thing to tell your young child to use words, and another to do it yourself, however. We are used to acting on our feelings rather then talking about them, and you'll be surprised to find how hard it is to describe your feelings. You may find you react to situations with a default feeling that may or may not be appropriate—you may get angry when you are actually sad, or sad when you are just really tired. Even if your child grows up to not be a particularly verbal person (think of most teenage boys!), if he can learn to recognize his own moods, he can learn to act on them appropriately.

Dr. Sacks Says

Finding out how people feel about a problem gets you a whole lot closer to the truth than asking them what happened, even when it's just toddlers fighting over a toy.

DISCIPLINE

Disciplining a child is one of the most important roles you have as a parent—and perhaps one of the most difficult. Healthy discipline is part of a comfortable, secure family environment, and it helps your child fit into the real world. To be effective, discipline must be about teaching your child, not just forcing her to obey, while at the same time letting her know you love and support her. There are no shortcuts in discipline; teaching about limits and acceptable behaviour takes time and a great deal of energy, and can be frustrating. Especially when you realize you're starting to sound like your parents.

Discipline is most effective when it is given by an adult who has a strong bond with your child, and it must be supported by any other adults that happen to be around. Each parent should develop his or her own style. Two people will rarely approach child discipline in the same way, so it is important that you discuss your approaches and support each other in most situations. Don't have these discussions in front of your child, though. If you argue about discipline in front of her, you'll only confuse her.

Discipline should be applied with mutual respect in a firm, reasonable, and consistent way. The foundation of effective discipline is respect. Since the goal is to teach her, teaching is always most effective when the student and teacher respect each other. Your child should always understand you are directing the discipline at her behaviour, not at her personally. Harsh discipline, such as humiliation in the form of verbal abuse, shouting, or name-calling, will make it hard for her to hear the lesson you're trying to teach. She'll also be less likely to listen to you even when you're not shouting, as she won't be able to trust you.

Firm discipline doesn't mean always saying "no." Use different words with varying intensity, and use "no" sparingly—and watch that you're not saying "no" simply out of habit. Reasonable discipline involves adjusting your expectations, so set just enough rules to get her safely through the day, and add more as she is able to handle them. Inconsistently applied rules show her your rules are weak and don't have to be followed, so make sure you discipline her each time she disobeys.

Effective discipline has many positive outcomes. It fosters appropriate behaviour, it protects your child from danger, and it helps her grow into an emotionally mature adult by teaching her to develop self-discipline, a healthy conscience, and a sense of responsibility. The boundaries discipline draws create a safe environment and are the basis for developing self-discipline many years later. A disciplined person is able to postpone pleasure, is considerate of the needs of others, is assertive without being aggressive or hostile, and can tolerate discomfort when necessary. Learning these lessons prepares your child for all that life can, and will, present to her.

Your discipline should always be appropriate to your child's level of development. Much has been said about age-appropriate discipline throughout this book, but the following are some guidelines for appropriate discipline at different age levels. For more on age-specific discipline strategies, see the Growth and Development sections of Chapters Two through Five.

Infants (Birth to 12 Months)

Your infant needs a routine in order to regulate her body's functions, but also to have a sense of security. Base a schedule for eating, sleeping, and playing on her cues, but don't respond to her so quickly that she never gets upset, as she needs to develop some tolerance of frustration and the ability to calm herself. Discipline before the age of one year shouldn't involve time-outs or consequences yet. Even the youngest crawling baby will understand and respond to a firm "no." It is important to remember that physically harming or spanking your child is not an appropriate disciplinary measure at any age.

Early Toddlers (One to Two Years)

Your one- and two-year-old will experiment with her control of the physical world and with her ability to exercise her own will. Since this is how she learns and grows, you need to be tolerant of her exploration, so use discipline only when needed to keep her safe, limit aggression, and prevent harmful behaviour (for more on toddler aggression, see page 153 in Chapter Three). Try removing her from a situation or a forbidden object from her hands with a firm "no" or a very brief explanation, then redirect her to another activity. Stay with her for a bit to make sure she doesn't do it again and to reassure her that you still love her. Early toddlers are very susceptible to fears of abandonment, so don't use solitary time-outs yet. Also, your child can't fully understand directions or explanations, and she's not mature enough to respond to them, so keep your words simple and brief.

Late Toddlers (Two to Three Years)

Your child continues to struggle for independence and control, and the frustration that often results from her setbacks and thwarted attempts can lead to the dreaded temper tantrum (for more on tantrums, see page 224 in Chapter Four). Equally frustrated parents are most likely to resort to spanking or yelling at this age. You should continue to supervise your child and set rules and routines, but also be realistic about her ability to understand and follow rules. If you know her pattern of reaction, you can interrupt or prevent situations that make her especially frustrated. Develop a strategy to stop her before the tantrums start. At this age, toddlers can't control their behaviour based on explanations or directions alone, but they do respond to time-outs (for more on time-outs, see page 222 in Chapter Four). Think, plan, and practise to master the skill of effective discipline…and it is a skill. If she does have a tantrum, give her a simple explanation and reassurance once she's settled down, then redirect her to some other activity, preferably away from the scene of the tantrum.

Preschoolers and Kindergartners (Three to Five Years)

Sometime between three and five years of age, your child will learn what her limitations are, she'll learn how adults expect her to act, and she'll no longer need to rely on others for her immediate needs. She's able to follow instructions and understand explanations now, but she doesn't always remember the rules—especially the ones she doesn't like—and she still needs to be supervised. Approval and praise, not lectures, are the most powerful motivators for good behaviour. Good role models (that's you!) are also important. To keep situations from getting out of hand, you can use time-outs and redirection. You can also use minor consequences as a way to teach her the cost of her actions. The consequence must immediately follow the incident, and it must be related to what she's done wrong. For instance, if she throws something and makes a mess, have her help you clean it up before she moves on to the next activity.

OPINIONS ON DISCIPLINE

There is a great deal of controversy about the appropriate way to discipline children. Both medical and popular literature are replete with diverse opinions about the short- and long-term effects of various disciplinary methods, especially the use of spanking. The Canadian Paediatric Society strongly discourages the use of spanking or any other form of physical punishment. See "Discipline" in Resources for a list of helpful books on the topic, and the Caring for Kids website (www.caringforkids.cps.ca) for more information.

RESILIENCE

What can we do to help prepare any child—whether he's shy or outgoing, brainy or average, athletic or clumsy—to reach his potential and to face life's challenges? As a parent, you are in a unique position to help your child learn to cope with difficult situations, and learn how those situations can make him stronger. Helping your child become more resilient is one of the most important things you can teach. The factors that make a child resilient are having a significant person in his life, developing positive self-esteem, being able to solve problems, and cultivating compassionate relationships with other people.

A Significant Other

Research and clinical experience have shown over and over again that a significant person who is consistently present in a child's life plays a crucial role in helping him develop resilience. A significant person is someone your child spends a lot of time with and knows he can turn to when he needs help. This can be a family member, such as a grandparent or an aunt, or it can be a teacher, coach, or neighbour. Of course, this significant other can also be you, since parents are the primary role models for children.

Self-Esteem

Your child's self-esteem affects his ability to function in the outside world, and the foundation of self-esteem is a positive attachment with his parents. You can help him feel good about himself by really understanding and respecting his strengths and limitations. The truth is that children are average at most things they do. They'll probably excel at a few activities—and may be quite bad at some. It's important that you accept this and adjust your responses. If you over-praise every accomplishment, it will only detract from the things he actually succeeds at that took him real effort. This also means that you can't decide in advance what your child should be good at, and ignore his attempts or successes at other activities. Your child is his own person—he won't be the next Gretzky just because that's what you want for him. If you give him support and genuine praise, he'll be successful at the things he's actually good at.

Dr. Sacks Says

Remember that cousin who was pretty bad at most things but good at breaking everything he touched? He probably runs a successful wrecking company now!

Now that few of us have large families, with a variety of people and a long memory of how different children are when they're growing, we compare our children's strengths and limitations to those of our neighbours' children. Parents often decide what activities a child will participate in according to what they or the other parents in their community consider important. However, you know your child best, and you should be aware of her abilities and her personality. These will change as she grows, of course, but by knowing and supporting who she really is, you will raise a self-confident individual.

Problem Solving

You probably solve dozens of problems every day in order to successfully navigate your way through life. We all solve problems in a very specific way, usually without knowing it, and it's important to pass that knowledge on to your child if you want her to be confident and capable.

THE PASTE SYSTEM

Successful problem solving uses the PASTE system:

P— First, clearly define the **problem.**

A—Think of all the possible **alternative** solutions, even some that may seem improbable. For each of these solutions, think of all the pros and cons, and the consequences of each choice. (If one alternative was perfect, there wouldn't be a problem!)

S—**Select** one of the solutions.

T—**Try** it out.

And here is the most important part:

E—**Evaluate** the result. Did the solution work out? If not, go and try one of the others.

Source: Hoffman, A. *Assessment and Management of Health Risk Behaviors* (Hanley and Belfus, 1990).

It's pretty easy to tell when your child has a problem—depending on the age, there's usually crying, screaming, sulking, or toy-throwing involved. Once you've calmed her down, use these opportunities to teach her how to solve problems. First, help her figure out what her problem is. If she can't find the words to describe it or she doesn't really know why she's upset, suggest some ideas of what you think it could be. You may be wrong, but talking about it will get your child thinking about her feelings and the situation. If she isn't able to talk yet, try showing her what you think made her upset. Then offer a few solutions, and try one to see if it works.

You can practise problem solving with her in everyday situations, not just in the wake of a temper tantrum. A trip to the supermarket is an opportunity to teach your child the importance of choosing a solution, evaluating the result, and making mistakes. Talk about choices, discuss the pros and cons of each, and decide what you would do if your choice didn't work out. We learn more from our mistakes than from situations that go smoothly, often because we don't realize what we did to make something work out.

Dr. Sacks Says

Making mistakes is the most human of endeavours, and your child is nothing if not human. Making mistakes is how we learn. Of course, making the same "mistake" over and over is how we manipulate, and your child will learn that skill pretty quickly.

Compassionate Relationships

As adults, we know how important strong relationships with family and friends are for getting through difficult times. At some point we learned that to be able to rely on people when we need them, we also need to be there for others and help them when they're in trouble. Teaching your child the value of cooperation and compassion, and the rewards of helping someone when they are distressed, will enrich his life immeasurably. Just as important, it will allow him to build support networks in his various environments—family, school, and eventually work—that will help him through his own challenges.

When he can recognize that people have feelings different from his own, often by three or four years, you can begin to explain that you sometimes feel sad, scared, or tired, just like the characters in his books.

Explain to him how you would help a character in trouble, or ask him what he would do. Let him know that everyone in the family deserves time to play, and that if he helps you with the chores, you'll have more time to play with him. Helping with chores also teaches your child that everyone in a relationship needs to contribute. Make him part of the team, and let him know that what he does to help around the home benefits the whole family. The idea of chores seems to have disappeared with the dinosaurs, but they teach cooperation like nothing else can.

MENTAL HEALTH CONCERNS

Although the vast majority of children will be physically and mentally healthy, mental health concerns are a reality for many parents. There is a lot of evidence that suggests that addressing these concerns early in a child's life can diminish the serious effects of mental health disorders. Great strides have been made in helping young children with conditions such as anxiety disorders, autistic spectrum disorders, and attention deficit hyperactivity disorder (ADHD), and all involve helping parents attend to their children's special needs.

Ignoring emotional and mental problems is the wrong thing to do. They do not go away on their own, and they can significantly limit your child's healthy development if they're not dealt with. It's important to recognize the symptoms that occur during these very early years. It's not unusual for parents who are watching their children struggle with certain emotional issues to recognize issues that they need to address in themselves.

As with all of the advice in this book, one of the goals of this section is to help you know when you should consult the doctor. A discussion of your child's behavioural development and emotional health issues should be part of every well-child visit. If you have concerns about your child's emotional and mental health, mention them to the doctor, who may want to schedule another appointment to talk about these issues in more depth. Most paediatricians are very knowledgeable about normal emotional developmental milestones. Your child's doctor may recommend some books for you to read. He may also refer your child to one of the many specialists who deal with these issues, such as a psychologist, psychiatrist, neurologist, or developmental paediatrician, if he feels that your child requires further assessment.

Anxiety and Fear

Your newborn comes equipped with a neurobiological system that is programmed to respond to signs of danger, such as noise, quick movement, or loss of physical support. While she soothes quickly when reassured by just about anyone in the early months, by five or six months, or sometimes even earlier, she saves her best smiles for her most important caregivers. Soon strangers will cause her to cry, and she will only be soothed by those she recognizes. This reaction peaks at eight or nine months, although strangers may cause her distress on and off throughout her first two years.

Some children, however, are slow to warm to people, or fear new situations or trying new things. These fears are usually temporary, and may go away in a reasonable period of time. If her fears stop her from achieving developmental milestones—for instance, if she's not able to fall asleep by herself at 12 months or settle into a new childcare situation after a few weeks when she's three years old—you'll need to help her gradually work up to being able to do some tasks. See pages 226 to 229 in Chapter Four for information on helping your child deal with fears and phobias.

Anxiety in babies is usually characterized by extreme separation distress or feeding problems. An anxious baby will scream for an extended period of time every time you leave her or ask her to try a new food. Don't indulge her fears by sleeping with her or letting her eat only what she likes. Instead, tell her that you know she can do it, and reward her honest attempts.

Toddlers can develop phobias if they have been through a traumatic event, such as choking or near-drowning. Phobias go beyond the normal, manageable fears most children have, and they can prevent your child from following her daily routine. If your child is consistently afraid of the same thing and is inconsolable, often even at the thought of her fear, she may have a phobia, and she should see a doctor.

By age three, your child should be able to separate from you with little clinging or crying, and even the most fearful three-year-old should adapt to a new situation within a few weeks. Specific fears such as storms, dogs, or doctors may still upset her, but as long as she can get through her daily routine, she should be fine. However, if she always refuses to sleep alone, if she can't go out when it's raining, or if she still refuses to play with other children, mention it to her doctor. Children often sense stress in the home, such as divorce or illness, and it can make them fearful. Your child's doctor may be able to guide you in helping her cope with upheaval in the home. There are also many books that can help you understand your anxious child and that suggest approaches for helping her (see "Anxiety" in Resources for recommendations).

If your child tends to be fearful, make sure you set a good example and show her how to be confident. Any sign that you may be worried about a situation can send a fearful child into a panic. She will also need more explanation, preparation, and reassurance before she tackles anything new or scary. Introduce her to fearful situations in a slow but deliberate manner. Show her pictures of what is going to happen, or take her to the place (such as school or the dentist's office) on a quiet day before she needs to go there. If she is afraid of group play, have her play with one child she knows well, such as a cousin. Once she's comfortable with that idea, have her play with a neighbour for a little while. Ask her teacher to suggest a classmate she should play with next, and eventually you can introduce her to playing with more than one child. Reward her each time she tries a new situation, even if she's not successful. If she's really distressed or uncomfortable, let her know that you understand but that she must at least try. You should also make sure her childcare situation suits her. Just being in an active, noisy daycare centre may upset a child who enjoys quiet.

When you're helping your child become less anxious about meeting new people or new situations, you're bound to get a lot of unsolicited advice. You don't need to listen to it, though—you know your child best, so trust your instincts. Often people will try to pressure your child before she is ready, but this may only make her more fearful. All you can do with people who don't understand your child's fear is explain that although the situation is challenging for your child, she is working on change—as long as it's the truth. Make sure you really are helping your child to face her fears, not helping her avoid them.

MAKE A NOTE, MAKE AN APPOINTMENT, OR GO TO THE HOSPITAL?

Make a note to mention it to your child's doctor if she

> is very difficult to feed;
> has persistent and severe sleeping difficulties;
> doesn't adjust to a new childcare situation after a few weeks;
> has a fear that interferes with her normal routine; or
> after three years of age, cries or clings persistently when a parent leaves, even for short periods or in familiar places, and cannot be soothed.

Autistic Spectrum Disorders

Young children are extremely social. Your baby is programmed to smile at four in the morning when he wakens you to feed, even though you probably won't be smiling at that particular time of day. During the first year and over the following two or three years, his emotional development will include being afraid of strangers, experiencing separation distress, learning to mimic you, being curious, and being interested when you point something out. It will also include that wonderful imaginary play that lets him be a superhero whenever he wants. His ability to communicate progresses from crying and smiling to pointing, waving, using more diverse facial expressions, babbling, saying words, and eventually putting them together into sentences. The amount of exploring your baby does may depend on his temperament and how adventurous he is, but he should show some interest in a new toy or situation. You should also notice that he is interested in your own reactions.

As is normal in all aspects of your child's development, the timing of these accomplishments depends on his personality, his health, and what is going on in his environment, and the range of normal is pretty wide. However, if your child doesn't seem to relate to others, especially his parents; if he fails to develop social gestures like smiling and waving; and if he doesn't babble, point, or talk at appropriate times, a discussion with his doctor is in order. People with autistic spectrum disorders have difficulty relating to others and communicating, although as the name suggests, the degree to which a person is affected can range from mild to severe. They can also have intense reactions to noise or changes in their environment, and can have repetitive behaviours.

Autistic spectrum disorders are related to the nervous system, and are sometimes seen with other congenital or genetic disorders. We do not yet know exactly what causes autistic spectrum disorders, but we do know a lot about what doesn't cause them: they are not caused by vaccinations.

Because they are often diagnosed at the same age as vaccinations are given, however, people have erroneously connected them. To date, study after study has shown they are not related. The risk of not immunizing your child far outweighs any medical risk of vaccination.

What we do know about autistic spectrum disorders is that they are more common in males, they seem to recur in some families, they run very different courses in different children, and they can be helped by early diagnosis and intervention. Doctors use screening tools that can make an early diagnosis so that a child with an autistic spectrum disorder has access to the most current therapies. Screening tools certainly help, but because your doctor only sees your child for a short time, it's up to you to bring up any concerns. The most effective therapies for autistic spectrum disorders are now thought to be individualized ones that address the specific needs of each child. Behaviour therapy is used to work on specific skills, such as using a fork, while other therapies deal with social skills. For the most current information on autistic spectrum disorders, see "Emotional and Mental Health" in Resources.

MAKE A NOTE, MAKE AN APPOINTMENT, OR GO TO THE HOSPITAL?

Make an appointment with your child's doctor if he doesn't smile in response to another person's smile by 4 to 6 months, or if by 18 months

- he doesn't babble or talk;
- he doesn't respond when his parents arrive or leave;
- he isn't interested in other people;
- he isn't interested in exploring;
- he doesn't look when you point things out to him; and
- he doesn't respond to affection.

Attention Deficit Hyperactivity Disorder

We hear so much about attention deficit hyperactivity disorder (ADHD) that you would be a rare parent indeed if you weren't convinced that your perpetually moving, doing-without-thinking 18-month-old isn't affected by it, especially after a day of trying to keep up with him and rescue him from disaster. Children have different activity levels, often depending on the situation (for instance, a home full of guests may find a normally docile child jumping around), and parents have equally different tolerance levels. By the age of three or four, however, your child should be able to spend some quiet time with you.

If, as he matures, he fidgets chronically, is easily distractible, has trouble playing quietly, and runs around in inappropriate situations, you should bring this to his doctor's attention. Earlier signs of ADHD are significant problems with playing and sharing with playmates or sitting to listen to a short story, and very frequent falls or bumps due to recklessness. There are three types of ADHD: hyperactive-impulsive, inattentive, and a combination of both. Girls are more likely to have inattentive ADHD—they may not be constantly moving, but they won't be able to pay attention to something for very long. Because they don't cause as much havoc as children with hyperactive-impulsive or combination ADHD do, the disorder is often missed in those with inattentive ADHD. A child may have inattentive ADHD if she daydreams a lot, is easily distractible, is disorganized, has poor problem-solving skills, and finds that she can't follow along in class.

ADHD is a real neurobiological condition that may get in the way of your child's ability to learn and interact with his classmates, so it needs to be addressed. A full assessment must be done before any diagnosis is made. Hyperactivity in a single setting may say more about the setting than about your child, so his doctor will make a diagnosis based on how he behaves in a number of settings. ADHD is one of the most inherited conditions known, so a family history of the disorder is also significant in making the diagnosis. Your observations of your child in a variety of situations are crucial for an accurate diagnosis, so it's important to learn as much as you can. See "Emotional and Mental Health" in Resources for some sources of information on ADHD.

A Parent's Role

As difficult as it may be to admit that a child has an emotional or mental health disorder, it should be addressed as soon as it becomes a concern and before it interferes in any way with her life. Recent knowledge has led to approaches—often non-pharmaceutical for children this age—that may change how these disorders affect children and can help them develop coping skills for life. Always keep in mind that your child's emotional and mental health is the important issue. Fear of what people will say should never keep you from asking questions and seeking help. By doing so, you will keep her moving forward through a healthy childhood and adolescence, and toward a productive adulthood.

Dr. Sacks Says

There are many approaches to helping your child achieve good mental health. Hiding your concerns from healthcare providers is not one of them.

One of the most remarkable experiences of raising a child is watching her unique personality develop as she goes from a smiling, drooling infant to a thinking, talking student. She will always be her own person, but you can encourage her to become a resilient and compassionate person by forming a strong attachment with her when she is a baby and by teaching her to practise self-discipline, solve problems effectively, and recognize her feelings and act on them appropriately. These skills will help her become an emotionally healthy adult who can deal with adversity and develop valuable relationships. Your attention and approval make all the difference in her emotional health, so spend time with your incredible child. Read, play, and sing with her, listen to her, hug her often, and value her for the remarkable individual she is.

Enjoy!

Appendix

YOUR CHILD'S DEVELOPMENT

At the end of 3 months, most infants can . . .			
Gross Motor	**Fine Motor**	**Social/Language**	**Cognitive**
· roll from front to back · control head and neck movement when sitting · raise their head and chest when lying on their stomach · stretch out and kick their legs when lying on their stomach or back · push down with their legs when feet are on a firm surface	· bring their hands together · open and shut their hands · bring their hands to their mouth · take swipes at a hanging object	· smile when you smile and on their own · be expressive and communicate with their face and body · copy some body movements and facial expressions	· watch faces closely · follow moving objects · recognize objects and people they know

At the end of 8 months, most babies can . . .			
Gross Motor	**Fine Motor**	**Social/Language**	**Cognitive**
· roll both ways (front to back, back to front) · sit on their own · support their whole weight on their legs · control their upper body and arms	· hold and shake a hand toy · move an object from hand to hand · use their hands to explore an object	· reach for a person they know · smile at themselves in a mirror · respond when other people express emotion · copy speech sounds	· track a moving object, and find one that is partially hidden · explore with hands and mouth · struggle to get objects that are out of reach · look from one object to another · watch a falling object

(continued)

(continued)

At 12 to 14 months, most babies can ...			
Gross Motor	**Fine Motor**	**Social/Language**	**Cognitive**
· reach a sitting position without help · crawl on hands and knees, or scoot around on their bums · get from a sitting to a crawling or prone (on their stomach) position · pull up to a standing position · cruise, holding onto furniture · stand briefly without support · walk holding an adult's hand, and maybe take 2 or 3 steps on their own · start to climb stairs with help	· finger-feed using thumb and forefinger · put objects into a container (and take them out again) · release objects voluntarily · poke with an index finger · push a toy · begin to drink from a cup · scribble with a crayon · begin to use a spoon	· be shy or anxious with strangers · copy during play · have favourite toys and people · test limits to actions and behaviours · put out an arm or leg to help when being dressed · take off socks · come when called (respond to name) · say "mama" or "dada" with at least one other word with meaning · communicate a need without crying · stop an action if you say "no"	· explore objects in different ways (shaking, banging, throwing, dropping) · know the names of familiar objects · respond to music · begin to explore cause and effect

At 18 months, most babies can ...			
Gross Motor	**Fine Motor**	**Social/Language**	**Cognitive**
· climb into chairs · walk without help · climb stairs one at a time with help	· build a 3-block tower · use a spoon well · turn a few board-book pages at a time · turn over a container to pour out the contents · drink easily from a cup	· say 5 to 10 words · follow a simple instruction · remove some clothing on their own · point to a named body part · point to familiar objects when asked · help with simple tasks	· use objects as tools · fit related objects together (e.g., in a shape sorter)

At 24 months, most toddlers can ...			
Gross Motor	**Fine Motor**	**Social/Language**	**Cognitive**
· pull a toy while walking · carry a large toy or more than one toy while walking · begin to run	· build a tower of 4 blocks or more · complete a simple shape-matching puzzle · turn board-book pages easily, one at a time	· start to put 2 words together · copy the behaviour of adults and other children	· begin "make-believe" play

- kick or throw a ball
- climb into and get down from chairs without help
- walk up and down stairs with help

- get excited about being with other children
- play alongside other children
- show increasing independence
- show defiant behaviour

At three years, most toddlers can . . .

Gross Motor	Fine Motor	Social/Language	Cognitive
· walk up and down stairs, alternating feet (one foot per stair) · run easily · jump in place · throw a ball overhead	· make up-and-down, side-to-side, and circular lines with a pencil or crayon · build a tower of more than 6 blocks · hold a pencil in a writing position · screw and unscrew jar lids or big nuts and bolts · string big beads · work latches and hooks · snip with children's scissors	· show spontaneous affection for playmates they know · begin to take turns · understand the concept of "mine" vs. "someone else's" · object to changes in routine · anticipate daily activities · speak in sentences and ask a lot of questions · put toys away · ask for help · know their full name	· match an object in their hand or the room to a picture in a book · include animals, dolls and people in make-believe play · sort easily by shape and colour · complete a puzzle with 3 or 4 pieces · understand the difference between 1 and 2 · name body parts and colours

At four years, most children can . . .

Gross Motor	Fine Motor	Social/Language	Cognitive
· hop and stand on one foot for up to 4 seconds · kick a ball forward · catch a bounced ball	· draw a person with 2 to 4 body parts · use children's scissors · draw circles and squares · twiddle thumbs · do a finger-to-thumb sequence (e.g., Itsy-Bitsy Spider)	· look forward to new experiences · cooperate with other children · play "mom" or "dad" · be very inventive · dress and undress · imagine monsters · negotiate solutions to conflicts	· understand counting · follow a 3-part instruction · recall parts of a story · make up and tell simple stories · understand "same" and "different" · enjoy rich fantasy play · know their address

Source: *Well Beings: A Guide to Health in Child Care*, 3rd Edition. Canadian Paediatric Society, 2008.

RESOURCES

For up-to-date and in-depth information on many topics, visit the websites of the Canadian Paediatric Society, www.cps.ca and www.caringforkids.cps.ca. You can also consult the following organizations and resources, which have been selected by the Canadian Paediatric Society.

General Information

Canadian Association of Family Resource Programs
www.parentsmatter.ca
Tools and resources for parents from FRP Canada.

Centers for Disease Control and Prevention (U.S.)
www.cdc.gov
In addition to comprehensive information on specific diseases, the CDC website has a wealth of information on healthy lifestyles, injury prevention, development, and immunization, among other topics.

Invest in Kids
www.investinkids.ca
Information on development by stage, as well as tips on positive parenting.

Multiple Births Canada
www.multiplebirthscanada.org
Everything you need to know if you're expecting more than one.

Adoption

Books on adoption:

The Family of Adoption by Joyce Maguire Pavao (Beacon, 2005)

Making Sense of Adoption: A Parent's Guide by Lois Melina (HarperCollins, 1989)

Why? Children's Questions, What They Mean and How to Answer Them by Ruth Gurian and Anita Formanek (Houghton Mifflin, 1983)

Allergies

Allergy Safe Communities
www.allergysafecommunities.ca
This website has an anaphylaxis emergency plan that you can fill out and give to your child's school or care provider.

Anaphylaxis Canada
www.anaphylaxis.ca
www.safe4kids.ca
An organization that helps people who have deadly allergies, with a website dedicated to children.

Anxiety

Books on anxiety:

Freeing Your Child from Anxiety: Powerful, Practical Solutions to Overcome Your Child's Fears, Worries, and Phobias by Tamar E. Chansky (Broadway, 2004)

Help for Worried Kids: How Your Child Can Conquer Anxiety and Fear by Cynthia G. Last (Guilford Publications, 2005)

Helping Your Anxious Child: A Step-by-Step Guide for Parents by Ronald Rapee (New Harbinger Publications, 2008)

Keys to Parenting Your Anxious Child by Katharina Manassis (Barron's, 2008)

Your Anxious Child: How Parents and Teachers Can Relieve Anxiety in Children by John S. Dacey and Lisa B. Fiore (Wiley, 2002)

Asthma

Allergy/Asthma Information Association
www.aaia.ca
A charity devoted to creating safe environments for people with asthma and allergies.

Asthma Society of Canada

www.asthma.ca

www.asthmakids.ca

Information and support for people with asthma, and a dedicated site for children.

Children's Asthma Education Centre

www.asthma-education.com

A program of the Children's Hospital of Winnipeg, its website has lots of information and answers for parents.

Lung Association of Canada

www.lung.ca

Information on asthma, as well as other lung diseases.

Breastfeeding

La Leche League Canada

www.lalecheleaguecanada.ca

Information and support for breastfeeding mothers. For their Breastfeeding Referral Service, call 1-800-665-4324.

Motherisk

www.motherisk.org

Canada's expert on the safety of medications, infections, chemicals, and more, during pregnancy and breastfeeding.

Bullying

L'Arche Canada
www.larchecanada.org/resources/parentsguide.htm
An excellent guide for helping parents deal with bullying.

Cerebral Palsy

Provincial cerebral palsy organizations:

Cerebral Palsy Association of BC
www.bccerebralpalsy.com

Ontario Federation for Cerebral Palsy
www.ofcp.on.ca

Quebec Cerebral Palsy Association
www.paralysiecerebrale.com

Contact information for associations in other provinces is available on the Ontario Federation for Cerebral Palsy website. Select "CP Organizations" from the "Resource Centre" menu to access the list.

Scope
www.scope.org.uk
Scope is a UK-based organization that helps people with cerebral palsy. The "Early Years" section has information for parents of young children with cerebral palsy.

United Cerebral Palsy Association
www.ucp.org
The website of this American organization includes information for
parents and families.

Child Care

Canadian Child Care Federation
www.cccf-fcsge.ca
Information on childcare options in Canada and learning tools.

Dental Health

Canadian Academy of Pediatric Dentistry
www.capd-acdp.org
Search for a paediatric dentist in your area.

Discipline

Books on discipline:

The Difficult Child by Stanley Turecki (Bantam, 2000)

How to Behave So Your Children Will, Too! by Sal Severe
(Penguin, 2003)

Kids are Worth It! Giving Your Child the Gift of Inner Discipline
by Barbara Coloroso (Penguin, 2003)

No More Misbehavin': 38 Difficult Behaviors and How to Stop Them
by Michele Borba (Wiley, 2003)

Raising Your Spirited Child by Mary Kurcinka (HarperCollins, 2006)

Your Defiant Child: 8 Steps to Better Behavior Russel A. Barkley
and Christine M. Benton (Guilford Publications, 1998)

Diseases and Conditions

See also "Allergies," "Asthma," and "Cerebral Palsy."

Canadian Celiac Association
www.celiac.ca
Information about celiac disease, including gluten-free diet resources.

Canadian Cystic Fibrosis Foundation
www.cysticfibrosis.ca
Resources for helping families live with cystic fibrosis and find local
chapters of the foundation.

Canadian Down Syndrome Society
www.cdss.ca
Information and resources for parents with children who have Down
syndrome, provided by Canadian professionals.

Canadian Hemophilia Society
www.hemophilia.ca
Look under "CHS Programs" for "Step by Step," a program for
families of children with bleeding disorders.

Epilepsy Canada
www.epilepsy.ca
The "Kidz Korner" provides information on epilepsy specifically directed to children.

Heart and Stroke Foundation of Canada
www.heartandstroke.com
Provincial websites provide information on congenital heart disease, including resources for children and parents.

Juvenile Diabetes Research Foundation
www.jdrf.ca
Resources for parents on helping their children live with diabetes.

Variety Children's Health Centre
www.vchc.ca
Information and resources for parents of children with congenital heart defects.

Emotional and Mental Health

See also "Anxiety" and "Discipline."

Autism Society Canada
www.autismsocietycanada.ca
A resource for learning about autistic spectrum disorder, treatment, and support, and for keeping up with the latest research.

Canadian ADHD Resource Alliance
www.caddra.ca
Information on ADHD provided by Canadian doctors.

Children and Adults with Attention Deficit Hyperactivity Disorder
www.chadd.org
Provides a lot of information for families dealing with ADHD.

Growth

Centers for Disease Control and Prevention (U.S.)
www.cdc.gov
To view the CDC's growth charts, select "Growth Charts" from under the "Life Stages and Populations" menu.

World Health Organization
www.who.int/childgrowth/en
For WHO's child growth standards, select "Child Growth Standards" from under the "Programmes and Projects" menu.

Health

College of Family Physicians of Canada
www.cfpc.ca
Look under "For Patients" for information on many different health topics.

Children's hospitals:

Alberta Children's Hospital
www.calgaryhealthregion.ca

BC Children's Hospital
www.bcchildrens.ca

Centre hospitalier affilié universitaire de Québec
www.cha.quebec.qc.ca

Centre hospitalier universitaire de Sherbrooke
www.chus.qc.ca

Children's Hospital at London Health Sciences Centre
www.lhsc.on.ca/about_us/childrens_hospital

Children's Hospital of Eastern Ontario
www.cheo.on.ca

CHU Sainte-Justine (Montreal)
www.chu-sainte-justine.org

IWK Health Centre (Halifax)
www.iwk.nshealth.ca

Janeway Children's Health and Rehabilitation Centre (St. John's)
www.easternhealth.ca

Kingston General Hospital
www.kgh.on.ca

McMaster Children's Hospital (Hamilton)
www.mcmasterchildrenshospital.ca

Montreal Children's Hospital
www.thechildren.com

Royal University Hospital (Saskatoon)
www.saskatoonhealthregion.ca

Stollery Children's Hospital (Edmonton)
www.capitalhealth.ca/hospitalsandhealthfacilities/hospitals/stollery-childrenshospital

Toronto Hospital for Sick Children
www.aboutkidshealth.ca

Winnipeg Children's Hospital
www.hsc.mb.ca

Immunization

Canadian Coalition for Immunization Awareness and Promotion
www.immunize.cpha.ca
Information for parents on recommended vaccines and vaccine safety.

Canadian Paediatric Society
Your Child's Best Shot: A Parent's Guide to Vaccination
 by the Canadian Paediatric Society (2006)
www.cps.ca
www.caringforkids.cps.ca
Complete information on vaccinations in Canada.

Every Child By Two
www.vaccinateyourbaby.org
Information on vaccine safety and immunization schedules.

Public Health Agency of Canada
www.phac-aspc.gc.ca

For up-to-date information on the immunization schedule in your province or territory, select "Immunization & Vaccines" under the Health & Safety menu, then select "Immunization Schedules," and then "Routine Schedule for Infants and Children" under "Provincial/Territorial Immunization Programs."

Injury Prevention

Canadian Association of Poison Control Centres

www.capcc.ca
To find the poison control centre closest to you.

Children's Hospital of Eastern Ontario

www.plan-itsafe.com
The Plan-it Safe website has lots of great information on injury prevention.

Is Your Family Prepared?

www.getprepared.ca
This Government of Canada website offers information on how to prepare an emergency kit for your home and what to do during an emergency.

Red Cross

www.redcross.ca
Information on first aid and water safety, and first-aid and CPR training for parents and caregivers.

Safe Kids Canada

www.safekidscanada.ca
Tips for keeping kids safe around water, playgrounds, and wheeled toys, as well as safety information on lots of other topics.

St. John Ambulance
www.sja.ca
First-aid courses, including courses specifically for new parents and caregivers.

Newborns

Best Start
www.beststart.org
Ontario's maternal, newborn, and early child development resource centre supports people across Ontario who work with expecting and new parents, but many of the resources provided on the website are also useful for parents.

Prevent SBS British Columbia
www.dontshake.ca
Valuable information on dealing with a crying baby and preventing shaken baby syndrome.

Nutrition

Books on feeding children:

The Baby's Table: Over 100 Easy, Healthy and Homemade Recipes for the Pickiest, Most Deserving Eaters on the Planet by Brenda Bradshaw and Lauren Bramley (Random House, 2004)

Better Baby Food: Your Essential Guide to Nutrition, Feeding, and Cooking for All Babies and Toddlers by Daina Kalnins and Joanne Saab (Robert Rose, 2008)

Better Food for Kids: Your Essential Guide to Nutrition for All Children from Age 2 to 6 by Diana Kalnins and Joanne Saab (Robert Rose, 2002)

Child of Mine: Feeding with Love and Good Sense by Ellyn Satter (Bull Publishing, 2000)

Food to Grow On: Give Your Kids a Healthy Lifestyle for Keeps by Susan and Rena Mendelson (HarperCollins, 2005)

Dietitians of Canada
www.dietitians.ca
For ideas and tools to build a good meal plan for children, go to the "Let's Make a Meal" page under "Eat Well, Live Well."

Health Canada
www.hc-sc.gc.ca
For Canada's Food Guide, select "Food & Nutrition," then "Canada's Food Guide" and "Choosing Food."

Product Safety

Canada Food Inspection Agency
www.inspection.gc.ca
For up-to-date information on food recalls and safety advisories.

Canadian Consumer Information Gateway
www.consumerinformation.ca
Information on purchasing safe products for children.

Canadian Toy Testing Council
www.toy-testing.org
The *Toy Report* is available at bookstores, from your local library, or online at the CTTC's website. This buying guide rates toys by age group for play value and includes precautions for safe use.

Health Canada
www.hc-sc.gc.ca
To check that your baby's furniture and toys meet current safety standards, select "Consumer Product Safety," and then select "Children's Products."

For product advisories and recalls, select "Consumer Product Safety" and then select "Advisories, Warnings and Recalls."

Sexuality

Books on sexuality:

Mommy Laid an Egg, Or Where Do Babies Come From? by Babette Cole (Chronicle Books, 1996)

What's the Big Secret? Talking about Sex with Girls and Boys by Marc Brown and Laurie Krasny Brown (Little, Brown & Co., 2000)

Where Did I Come From? by Peter Mayle (Citadel Press, 1999)

Special Needs

Ability Online Support Network
www.ablelink.org
An Internet community for children with disabilities and illnesses.

**Canadian Association of Speech-Language Pathologists
and Audiologists**
www.caslpa.ca
Information about speech therapy, or to find out about resources in
your community.

Canadian Association of the Deaf
www.cad.ca
Information on various issues to do with hearing problems.

Canadian National Institute for the Blind
www.cnib.ca
Links to local CNIB offices, where you can find support and
resources.

**CanChild Centre for Childhood Disability Research
at McMaster University**
www.canchild.ca
Information about disability research, and resources for families
learning about disabilities.

Learning Disabilities Association of Canada
www.ldac-taac.ca
Information and support for people with learning disabilities.

Travel

Canadian Air Transport Security Authority
www.catsa-acsta.gc.ca
For up-to-date information on travelling with breast milk and
formula in Canada, select "For Travellers" and "Permitted and
Non-Permitted Items."

Foreign Affairs and International Trade Canada
www.voyage.gc.ca
Travel advisories and addresses of Canadian embassies and consulates
around the world.

Public Health Agency of Canada
www.phac-aspc.gc.ca
For international travel health advisories, a list of travel medicine
clinics, and health tips for travel, select "Travel Health."

Transport Canada
www.tc.gc.ca
For information on how your child can travel safely in each stage of
his life, and to check current product advisories, select "Main Page"
and then select "Child Safety."

Index

D

dairy products. *See* milk and alternatives

daycare
  aggressive behaviour, 154, 230
  anxiety, 452
  appropriate time to adjust, 232
  common illnesses contracted, 298–303
  dealing with separation anxiety, 138–139
  ear infections and, 350
  infection risks, 101
  nightmares and, 214
  part-time, 157–158
  sexual abuse concerns, 282–283
  signs of problem, 137
  using breast milk at, 113

daycare facilities
  choosing, 158–160
  environment, 156–157
  features of good settings, 156
  safety issues, 266

daydreaming, 455

daytime incontinence, 285

deafness, causes of, 75, 97, 98

death, causes of, 24, 98, 401

decongestants, 249

DEET, 270

defiance, 292–294

dehydration
  with fever, 333
  in illnesses, 297
  signs of, 165, 337, 339–340, 342
  treatment for, 339, 340–341

dental health
  brushing teeth, 140
  decay, 93
  guidelines for dental care, 93–94
  juice and, 120
  natal teeth, 107
  pacifier use, 58, 59
  primary teeth, 90–92
  teaching brushing teeth, 254–256
  teething, 92, 249

dental injuries, 390

dentist visits, 94, 255

depression
  with new baby, 33–35
  when weaning, 175

dessert, 263

developmental milestones
  birth to 12 months old, 45–48
  slow development, 49–51, 135–136
  12 to 24 months old, 133–134

dexterity, 239

diabetes, 101, 103

diabetic mothers, 75

diaper bags, first-aid kits for, 22–24

diaper change tables, 384

diaper pins, 55

diaper rash
  causes of, 13, 81, 82, 84
  prevention of, 41
  treatment for, 55, 82

diapers
  change tables, 384
  changing procedure, 55
  choices in, 12–13
  hygiene, 364–365
  indications of enough to eat, 112
  number and appearance in first month, 53–54
  number and appearance in first week, 40, 53
  number of wet, 339
  washing, 56

diarrhea
  causes of, 329, 337–339
  crying and, 61
  diaper rash and, 81
  with fever, 342
  following taking medication, 370
  in food allergies, 171
  for longer than a week, 342
  for more than a few days, 164
  signs of, 54
  in stomach flu, 334
  with stool withholding, 285–286

sudden onset, 163
treatment for, 337, 339–342
vaccine for rotovirus, 106
when teething, 92
when travelling, 196

diastasis rectii, 107

diction, 279

digestive system. *See* gastrointestinal problems

digital ear thermometers, 247

digits, extra, 108

dining room, babyproofing, 24–25

diphtheria, 96, 98

dirt, eating, 116, 309–310

discharge
  after circumcision, 14
  from eye, 344, 352–353
  from nose, 348
  from orange-red scratch, 302
  from umbilical cord, 79

discipline
  birth to 12 months old, 442
  effective, 440–441
  four to five years old, 292–294
  three to five years old, 444
  12 to 24 months old, 144–148, 442–443
  two to three years old, 220–225, 443

dishwashers, 25

dishwashing liquid, 25

disobedience, 289

disorganization, 455

disposable diapers, advantages and disadvantages, 12–13

distractible, 455

divorce, 431

dizziness, 171, 269, 323

doctors
  choosing, 7–10
  questions when choosing, 7–8
  well-child visits, 8

dolls, 243

doorknob covers, 29

doors, 29, 265, 385

doorstops, 29

DPTP-Hib. *See* 5-in-1 vaccine

drapes, 25, 27–28